Study Guide and Examination Review for

ADVANCED EMERGENCY CARE
FOR
PARAMEDIC PRACTICE

Shirley A. Jones, M.S.Ed., M.H.A., EMT-P

Allied Health Education, Program Director - EMS
Methodist Hospital of Indiana, Indianapolis, Indiana

6 5 4 3 2 1
ISBN 0-397-54931-8

Any procedure or practice described in this book should be applied by the health care practitioner under appropriate supervision in accordance with professional standards of care used with regard to the unique circumstances that apply in each practice situation. Care has been taken to confirm the accuracy of information presented and to describe generally accepted practices. However, the authors, editors, and publisher cannot accept any responsibility for errors or omissions or for any consequences from application of the information in this book and make no warranty, express or implied, with respect to the contents of the book.

Every effort has been made to ensure drug selections and dosages are in accordance with current recommendations and practice. Because of ongoing research, changes in government regulations and the constant flow of information on drug therapy, reactions, and interactions, the reader is cautioned to check the package insert for each drug for indications, dosages, warnings, and precautions, particularly if the drug is new or infrequently used.

To my best friend, Sue, for her support and help
in putting this project together

CONTRIBUTORS

Daniel Finley, M.Ed., NREMT-P
Instructor
Austin Community College, Austin, Texas

Alice "Twink" Gorgen, R.N., B.S.N., N.R.P.M., C.E.N., NREMT-P
Paramedic Nurse Coordinator, Omaha Fire Division
Prehospital Education Program, Creighton University, Omaha, Nebraska

Karen Hill Less, M.Ed., NREMT-P
Instructor - Clinical Coordinator
Austin Community College, Austin, Texas

Douglas D. Key, B.S., EMT-P
Chief Operating Officer
MedStar Ambulance, Fort Worth, Texas

Kay L. Strombeck, B.A., EMT-P
Training Coordinator
State Emergency Management Agency, Indianapolis, Indiana

vi

CONTENTS

PREFACE

This Study Guide and Examination Review workbook has been designed to accompany the textbook, *Advanced Emergency Care for Paramedic Practice*. In order to assist students in learning the enormous amount of material in the text, the workbook has been designed to reinforce the most important concepts and techniques described in the text. After thoroughly studying each text chapter, the student should be able to successfully complete the corresponding chapters and assignments in the workbook. How to study and test-taking tips are discussed in the beginning of this workbook and should be used as a guide for the student.

If students carefully complete this workbook as they progress through their Emergency Medical Technician-Intermediate (EMT-I) or Emergency Medical Technician-Paramedic (EMT-P) course, their learning and comprehension will be enhanced considerably. After answering each workbook assignment, students should check their answers at the end of the workbook and consult the textbook carefully to be sure they understand each of the important points.

While many of the workbook problems require only recall of specific information, others are designed to make students think about problem situations they will encounter as practicing EMT-Is or EMT-Ps. Flash cards on EKGs, drugs, and Advanced Cardiac Life Support Treatment Protocols (© American Heart Association: *Textbook of Advanced Cardiac Life Support*, 2nd ed. Dallas, Texas: American Heart Association, 1987)) are included at the end of the chapter assignments.

The primary purpose of this Study Guide and Examination Review is to offer tools that allow the student to evaluate fundamental knowledge and skills that are considered important in the practice of emergency medical services. Although it is ideally suited for use with the textbook, *Advanced Emergency Care for Paramedic Practice*, the workbook can also be used with other texts, or by anyone interested in examining their knowledge in emergency medical services without reference to a specific text.

TO THE STUDENT

During your course of study as an Emergency Medical Technician-Intermediate (EMT-I) or Emergency Medical Technician-Paramedic (EMT-P), you will be constantly preparing for and taking examinations. This beginning portion of the Study Guide and Examination Review workbook reviews study skills and test-taking techniques. The study tips give you information on how to use your time more efficiently and effectively for studying. The discussion on how to take a test reviews different types of test questions and gives you hints on how to master each.

The workbook is perforated so that assignments can be torn out and turned in to your instructor or kept in a separate notebook as you complete each assignment or group of assignments. Flash cards are included for EKGs, drugs, and Advanced Cardiac Life Support Treatment Protocols. The flash cards are perforated and can be torn out of the workbook and assembled to help you with your memorization and recognition skills.

The author welcomes the comments, criticisms, and ideas of the student for the improvement of future editions.

HOW TO STUDY

One key to your success in the classroom is based on how well you study. Your progress will be determined by tests that cover both clinical and classroom material. If you have been out of school for a number of years, you are encouraged to talk with your instructor about study methods that might work best for you. Remember too that spelling, punctuation, and math skills are extremely important in the field of emergency medical services. If you are weak in these areas, pick up a review text in your local bookstore and spend some time refamiliarizing yourself with this material. You will not regret it when you get to the sections in your EMT-I or EMT-P course covering documentation or pharmacology.

EFFECTIVE CLASSROOM SKILLS

* Practice good classroom manners: Arrive in class on time. Be courteous to other students and do not interrupt or cause disruptions by talking or making jokes.
* Listen: Pay attention and avoid day dreaming even if the material is not very interesting. Develop the ability to concentrate. If the instructor has distracting gestures, focus on his or her face and not on the gestures.
* Participate: Be involved in the classroom and ask questions. Remember, there is no such thing as a dumb question.
* Keep up-to-date with course work: Turn in assignments on time. Keep up with your reading assignments.
* Know the instructor's requirements: Each instructor has different requirements. Make sure you have a copy of the course rules and regulations.
* Take good class notes: Effective note-taking is essential in keeping up with course material and helps you remember what you have learned in class. Record both facts and ideas. Circle, star, or underline material when your instructor emphasizes certain points. These are sure to be on the exam.
* Attend classes regularly: Missing classes even if you know the material will only hurt you in the long run. What if you miss that 100-point quiz or are not informed about the time change for the emergency department clinical? Or what if your medical director shows up to discuss some new drug being considered for use in prehospital care?

ORGANIZE YOUR STUDY TIME

* Use the right study equipment: Stay away from that favorite couch where you take naps. A sturdy chair, desk or table, and good lighting are all important in keeping you awake and alert.
* Select a specific place to study: Let others in your household know where you are studying so that they will respect your space.
* Avoid distractions: Make sure the television and radio are turned off. Noise distractions do not allow for proper concentration.
* Recite and review: Your class notes should be reviewed within twenty-four hours of taking them. This kind of review will serve to fix the lecture firmly in your mind.
* Be a good reader: Concentrate on what you are reading, remember as much as possible, and apply or associate what you read to your own experience.
* Reward yourself for studying: Normal attention span is about 45 minutes. After about 45 minutes, take a 15-minute break; take the dog for a walk, walk around the house, or have a light snack.
* Know how to use your textbook: Read the Preface; this will tell you how the text is organized. Skim through the assignment to see how much you need to learn. As you read, highlight key points or write them down in your notebook.

* Evaluate yourself: Use your workbook to see how much you have learned.
* Learn to use the library: Know the parts of a book and journal, as well as its title, author, publisher, date of publication, and edition.

HOW TO TAKE TESTS

Grades for a particular course or portion of a course are arrived at by the instructor's evaluation of a student's performance. Instructors use tests to aid them in this evaluation process. A test indicates the progress of both student and instructor.

TEST-TAKING SKILLS

Test-taking skills involve learning the strategy and techniques to understand what is being asked in a question and to respond accordingly. "Test" is a word that evokes many responses. Each student has a different approach to taking a test or preparing for one. Students often do poorly on tests because they develop a negative attitude, i.e., "I'll never understand this!", or because they do not know how to use what they have learned to answer questions. The following are some points to remember when you are getting ready to take a test.

Preparing for the Test

* Attend class regularly.
* Develop a positive attitude.
* Take good class notes and review then daily.
* Read your assignments.
* Predict questions by reviewing notes and objectives.
* To measure how effectively you have learned the material, quiz yourself by using the workbook and checking your answers.
* Determine the type of test to be given (practical or written).
* Know the date, room, and time when the test is being given.

Types of Test Questions

Multiple-Choice Items

A multiple-choice question is a problem in the form of a statement or question with a suggested series of answers. The statement or question may ask you to identify the INCORRECT choice, so be sure to read each question carefully. You may also be asked, in the directions, to give the BEST answer. In this case you will be forced to choose among several alternatives, all of which appear to be correct.

You first want to eliminate the answers that are obviously wrong. Then look for clues such as a statement with a word or phrase missing. Words in the statement or question such as *a*, *an*, *is*, or *are* will indicate whether the answer is singular or plural. Also remember the length of the question does not always indicate the length of the answer.

There are three types of multiple-choice items: simple, completion, and compound. The *simple* format asks you to complete a sentence or answer a question. The following are examples of the simple multiple-choice item.

1. The upper airway and lower airway are separated by the:
   a. epiglottis.
   b. tongue.
   c. vocal cords.
   d. cricoid cartilage.

The correct answer is *d*. By definition, the upper airway ends at the cricoid cartilage.

2. Organophosphate and carbamate insecticide exposures can occur from which route(s)?
   a. Inhalation
   b. Ingestion
   c. Skin contact
   d. All of the above

The correct answer is *d*. The complications of aspiration and additional injuries are possible with these exposures.

The *completion* format presents you with a reading passage with words or data deleted and blanks inserted in their place. These items usually test your recognition, recall, and problem-solving abilities.

1. If a red blood cell is placed into a(an) _____ solution, it will lose water to the surrounding solution and shrink.
   a. hypertonic
   b. hypotonic
   c. isotonic
   d. ultratonic

The correct answer is *a*. Examples of hypertonic solutions include: $D_5 0.9\%$ NaCl, $D_5 0.45\%$ NaCl, $D_{10}W$, and D_5LR.

2. Arteries, by definition, are blood vessels that carry blood _____ the heart.
   a. away from
   b. through
   c. to
   d. both b and c

The correct answer is *a*. Arteries carry blood to the body, while veins carry blood to the heart.

The *compound* format asks you to select from a number of possible combinations of answers. You must pick the right combination. These involve a good deal of critical thinking, and you must be careful to look at each alternative or you may miss something.

1. In patients with smoke inhalation the signs include:
   I. hoarseness.
   II. cough.
   III. singed nasal hair.
   IV. labored breathing.
   V. blisters around the mouth.
      a. I, II, and IV.
      b. I, II, III, and V.
      c. I, II, III, and IV.
      d. I, II, III, IV, and V.

The correct answer is *b*. Labored breathing is a symptom; hoarseness, cough, singed nasal hair, and blisters around the mouth are signs.

2. Abnormal respiratory patterns that result from neurologic impediments include which of the following?
   I. Cheyne-Stokes respiration
   II. Shallow tachypnea
   III. Central neurogenic hyperventilation
   IV. Ataxic breathing
      a. I, II, and III.
      b. II, III, and IV.
      c. I, II, and IV.
      d. I, III, and IV.

The correct answer is *d*. The respiratory system is often affected by neurologic impediments. Respiratory patterns may be normal or may fall under one of several variations, such as Cheyne-Stokes respiration, central neurogenic hyperventilation, ataxic breathing, or apneustic breathing. Shallow tachypnea is a result of compensatory mechanisms rather than a result of neurologic impediments.

Essay Items

This is generally the hardest type of test question. It relies on your ability to remember the information and to organize it in a different manner. Read through all the essay questions before you start to write and allot time to each question. Divide the time available for the test according to the importance of the questions. A question that is worth 25 percent of the test should get 25 percent of the available time. Read each question, carefully underlining the key words. An essay item usually begins with a specific command or action word that tells you how the question is to be answered. (Examples include *Name*, *Define*, *Explain*, *Discuss*, *Compare*, *List*, *Outline*, *Describe*, and *Contrast*.)

When you begin writing the answer, start with an opening sentence that describes the major points. Then list the specific information in paragraph form. The conclusion should summarize and pull points together. You may want to begin by writing an outline on the back of a piece of paper.

Matching Items

These are usually two columns of words or phrases. Answer the ones you know first. If the instructor is test-wise, you will not be given the same number of items in each column; there will always be an extra word or phrase left over.

True and False Items

A partially true statement is false. Look for words like *never*, *always*, *none*, and *all*; these are usually part of false statements. Look for words like *many*, *seldom*, *frequently*, and *often*; these leave room for exceptions and are often true.

DAY OF THE TEST

Make sure you get a good nights sleep and:

* Be on time.
* If the test is given after a meal (i.e., lunch), eat lightly. A full stomach will make you drowsy and not very attentive.
* Bring extra pencils or pens, and calipers, calculator, and watch if needed.
* Know how much time is allotted for the test.
* Follow the directions; ask for clarification if needed.
* Make a quick survey of the whole test before writing any answer. This overview will help you determine how quickly you will need to work.
* Do some easy questions first to gain confidence.
* Answer all the questions; partial credit is better than none.
* Do not change answers too quickly as you check your test before turning it in. If there is any doubt, leave the first answer. The first impression, as psychological tests have shown, is usually more reliable.

CHAPTER 1

Roles and Responsibilities

STUDY GUIDE ASSIGNMENT 1-1

- Professionalism
- Ethics
- Responsibilities of the Paramedic

Reading Assignment: pages 4-7

Matching Items

Match each of the terms in the left column with the BEST definition in the right column by placing the letter of that definition in the space next to the term. Each definition may be used once or not at all.

_____ 1. profession
_____ 2. professionalism
_____ 3. ethics
_____ 4. code of ethics
_____ 5. run report

A. An example that serves to promote uniformity and indicates what is expected of members of a profession

B. System of principles that identify conduct deemed morally desirable

C. Specialized body of knowledge or expertise

D. A governmental agency grants permission for regulation

E. Medical and legal document

F. A position in which integrity and diligence are assumed

Multiple-Choice Items

Read each question carefully. For each item, select the answer that BEST completes the statement or answers the question, and place the letter of that answer in the space provided.

_____ 1. You are called on the scene of a car/bicycle accident where a drunk driver has hit a little girl on a bicycle. Another paramedic is taking care of the little girl, and your patient, the drunk driver, has several minor lacerations on his face. You would:
   a. refuse to care for the driver.
   b. assist the other paramedic with the little girl.
   c. bandage the driver's injuries and transport him to the hospital.
   d. summon another person to help the driver.

_____ 2. For the paramedic, the term _____ refers to the ideal conduct in the relationship of the paramedic to the patient, as well as to other paramedics and to the public.
   a. a profession
   b. professionalism
   c. medical ethics
   d. ethics

_____ 3. You request orders for 4 mg of morphine for your patient, who is in extreme pain. The physician okays this order and says to give another 4 mg in 5 minutes. You accidently give the patient the full 8 mg. Upon arrival at the emergency department you would:
   a. tell the physician that you gave the medication according to her orders.
   b. tell the physician about the medication error.
   c. document on the run report that 4 mg of morphine was administered in 5 minute intervals.
   d. both a and c.

_____ 4. The paramedic is responsible for:
   I. the safety and well-being of the patient.
   II. emergency management of the patient.
   III. record keeping.
   IV. equipment maintenance.
       a. I and III
       b. I, II, and III
       c. I, II, and IV
       d. I, II, III, and IV

_____ 5. The patient run report should include:
   a. basic identification of the patient.
   b. the times at which events occurred.
   c. management techniques rendered.
   d. all of the above.

STUDY GUIDE ASSIGNMENT 1-2

- Certification
- Licensure
- Reciprocity
- Continuing Education
- National Organizations

Reading Assignment: pages 7-8

Matching Items

Match each of the terms in the left column with the BEST definition in the right column by placing the letter of that definition in the space next to the term. **Each definition may be used once or not at all.**

_____ 1. certification

_____ 2. licensure

_____ 3. reciprocity

_____ 4. continuing education

A. Must be regulated by a governmental agency

B. Regulated by governmental or nongovernmental agencies

C. Not regulated by any agency

D. A state recognizes another state's certification or licensure

E. Training that may be mandatory for certification or licensure

CHAPTER 2

The Emergency Medical Services System

STUDY GUIDE ASSIGNMENT 2-1

- Medical Control
- Emergency Medical Services System Components
- Vehicles and Equipment

Reading Assignment: pages 10-14

Matching Items

Match each of the terms in the left column with the BEST definition in the right column by placing the letter of that definition in the space next to the term. Each definition may be used once or not at all.

_____ 1. medical control (medical direction)

_____ 2. protocols

_____ 3. standing orders

_____ 4. off-line medical control

_____ 5. on-line medical control

_____ 6. KKK standards

A. Voice communication between the paramedic and emergency physician

B. Treatment performed in life-threatening situations without direct voice contact with the physician

C. Voice communication between the paramedic and communications operator

D. Monitoring by the physician of all medical aspects of the EMS system

E. Administrative components of medical control

F. Guidelines for the management of many types of medical conditions

G. Federal design specifications for ambulances

Multiple-Choice Items

Read each question carefully. For each item, select the answer that BEST completes the statement or answers the question, and place the letter of that answer in the space provided.

_____ 1. A term that has the same meaning as medical control is:

    a. medical direction.

    b. medical supervision.

c. medical administration.

d. medical sponsorship.

_____ 2. You are on the scene of an accident and need to administer an antiarrhythmic drug to your patient, but you cannot contact the hospital because your radio was just broken. If you give the medication without speaking with the physician, you are operating under:

a. administration.

b. guidelines.

c. protocols.

d. standing orders.

_____ 3. The administration of protocols and standing orders falls under:

a. on-line medical control.

b. off-line medical control.

c. in-line medical control.

d. affiliation.

_____ 4. The physician supervises patient care given by the paramedic at the scene and en route to the hospital via communication called:

a. on-line medical control.

b. off-line medical control.

c. in-line medical control.

d. affiliation.

_____ 5. The day-to-day operations of the EMS system and personnel are monitored by the _____ physician.

a. on-line medical control

b. off-line medical control

c. in-line medical control

d. affiliation

_____ 6. The following areas fall under the operational units of the EMS delivery system:

  I. support services

 II. system operations

III. system management

IV. initial operations

 V. system evaluation

   a. I, II, III, and V

   b. II, III, and V

   c. I, III, IV, and V

   d. I, II, III, IV, and V

_____ 7. Federal design specifications by which ambulances are manufactured are known as:

a. design standards.

b. EMS standards.

c. KKK standards.

d. ambulance standards.

STUDY GUIDE ASSIGNMENT 2-2

- Aeromedical Transport
- Personnel
- Citizen Access
- Communications
- Medical Standards
- Hospital Care
- The Emergency Medical Services System in Operation
- The Emergency Medical Services System in Retrospect

Reading Assignment: pages 14-18

Matching Items

Match each of the terms in the left column with the BEST definition in the right column by placing the letter of that definition in the space next to the term. Each definition may be used once or not at all.

_____ 1. aeromedical transport
_____ 2. 911
_____ 3. simplex system
_____ 4. duplex system
_____ 5. run reviews

A. Ability to transmit or receive, but not both simultaneously

B. Emergency code for lights and siren

C. Nationally recognized emergency telephone number by which an EMS system can quickly respond to a call

D. Air transportation of ill or injured people

E. Can be used to expose gaps or identify needed additions to operational and treatment protocols

F. Ability to receive and transmit at the same time

Multiple-Choice Items

Read each question carefully. For each item, select the answer that BEST completes the statement or answers the question, and place the letter of that answer in the space provided.

_____ 1. The need for air transport is based on several factors. Included among these are the:
  I. smoothness of transport required for the patient.
  II. specific location of the patient.
  III. time involved in transport.
  IV. time of day.
  V. severity of the patient's condition.
    a. I, III, and IV
    b. II, III, and V
    c. I, II, III, and V
    d. I, II, III, IV, and V

_____ 2. The most specific danger encountered by emergency personnel who are working around helicopters is:
   a. the tail area.
   b. the rotors.
   c. loose objects.
   d. noise.

_____ 3. An EMS professional who performs most of the skills of an emergency physician is an:
   a. EMT.
   b. EMT-A.
   c. EMT-I.
   d. EMT-P.

_____ 4. The initial element of any EMS system is:
   a. patient care.
   b. citizen access.
   c. medical standards.
   d. patient assessment.

_____ 5. The professional who enables a network of assistance to be activated as needed is known as a(n):
   a. communication operator.
   b. EMT.
   c. EMT-P.
   d. on-line operator.

_____ 6. If your radio communication did not allow you to be linked to the telephone system of your base hospital, and if it had only a single channel, it would be called a _____ system.
   a. simplex
   b. multiplex
   c. duplex
   d. monoplex

CHAPTER 3

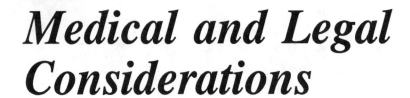

Medical and Legal Considerations

STUDY GUIDE ASSIGNMENT 3-1

- Classifications of Law
- Medical Practices Act
- State Emergency Medical Services Legislation
- Motor Vehicle Laws
- Additional Laws That Affect the Paramedic
- Good Samaritan Law
- Governmental Immunity

Reading Assignment: pages 20-24

Matching Items

Match each of the terms in the left column with the BEST definition in the right column by placing the letter of that definition in the space next to the term. Each definition may be used once or not at all.

C   1. criminal law

A   2. civil law

F   3. tort

H   4. administrative law

B   5. medical practices act

G   6. living will

J   7. Do Not Resuscitate

E   8. Good Samaritan Law

I   9. sovereign immunity

A. Private law between two persons or parties

B. Legislation that governs the practice of medicine

C. Conduct or offenses that legally have been classified as "public wrongs" or crimes "against the state"

D. Lack of provision for continued care

E. Statutes of immunity for emergency medical providers; they vary from state to state

F. Any wrongful act that does not involve a breach of contract and from which a civil suit can be brought

G. Document in which patients express their desire not to be kept alive through "extraordinary" treatment

H. The government's authority to enforce rules, regulations, and pertinent statutes of governmental agencies

I. If allowed, it relieves governmental employees from liability for certain types of negligent acts

J. A physician's order not to give cardiopulmonary resuscitation to patients who have cardiopulmonary or respiratory arrests

Multiple-Choice Items

Read each question carefully. For each item, select the answer that BEST completes the statement or answers the question, and place the letter of that answer in the space provided.

a 1. The law that may allow a patient to seek recovery of money from an ambulance service because he or she received poor care by the paramedic is called a(n) _____ law.
   a. civil
   b. administrative
   c. state
   d. criminal

b 2. The KKK standards required of ambulance manufacturers fall under _____ law.
   a. civil
   b. administrative
   c. state
   d. criminal

d 3. If your patient had been caught breaking into someone's home, he or she would have been violating a(n) _____ law.
   a. civil
   b. administrative
   c. state
   d. criminal

? b 4. The medical practices act:
   a. is the same in all states.
   b. has been repealed.
   c. is a federal law.
   d. may vary from state to state.

d 5. Violation of the medical practices act is one source of _____ liability.
   a. state
   b. criminal
   c. administrative
   d. civil

? b 6. The motor vehicle code:
   a. is the same in all states.
   b. is not legally enforceable.
   c. is a federal law.
   d. may vary from state to state.

d 7. The use of lights and sirens in accordance to any state's motor vehicle code is:
   a. not a defense to liability.
   b. a defense to liability.
   c. only one factor in determination of fault.
   d. both a and c.

STUDY GUIDE ASSIGNMENT 3-2

- Privilege
- Malpractice Actions
- Consent

Reading Assignment: pages 24-26

Matching Items

Match each of the terms in the left column with the BEST definition in the right column by placing the letter of that definition in the space next to the term. Each definition may be used once or not at all.

A	1.	privilege
D	2.	confidentiality
G	3.	malpractice
C	4.	causation
H	5.	consent
L	6.	informed consent
K	7.	competent
M	8.	incompetent
B	9.	expressed consent
I	10.	implied consent
E	11.	involuntary consent
J	12.	parens patriae

A. Legal principle that refers to a statutory restriction on testimony

B. Written or verbal statement by a patient that expresses a desire and willingness to receive medical treatment

C. The link between a breach of duty and the element of injury in a malpractice claim

D. Patient's right to expect that the communications made in a relationship of trust will not be disclosed

E. Permission to treat a patient granted by the authority of law, regardless of the patient's desire

F. Verbal or written denial of medical treatment

G. Negligent conduct of a professional person; its claim is a common basis for civil liability

H. Verbal or written acceptance of medical treatment

I. Situation in which a patient is unable to communicate consent to treatment and a life-threatening injury or illness requires prompt medical attention

J. Legal doctrine that gives authority to the State, for various reasons, to acts in lieu of the parents to protect the welfare and health of a minor

K. Reflects a health care provider's judgment that a patient is capable of giving consent to treatment

L. Patient's agreement to medical treatment after adequate information about the treatment, its risks and consequences, and any alternative methods of treatment have been explained

M. Reflects a health care provider's judgment that a patient is not capable of giving consent to treatment

STUDY GUIDE ASSIGNMENT 3-3

- Patient Refusal
- Bases of Liability
- Problem Areas for the Paramedic
- Insurance and Liability Protection

Reading Assignment: pages 26-28

Matching Items

Match each of the terms in the left column with the BEST definition in the right column by placing the letter of that definition in the space next to the term. Each definition may be used once or not at all.

B 1. signature of release
D 2. abandonment
H 3. battery
G 4. assault
I 5. false imprisonment
E 6. libel
C 7. slander
A 8. invasion of privacy

A. Claim based on unauthorized release of confidential or private information that causes the plaintiff damages

B. Witnessed statement in writing from a patient who refuses treatment or transport

C. Pertains to verbal defamatory statements about one person to another

D. Lack of provision for continued care

E. Tort action based on a written defamatory statement, falsely or inaccurately made, that damages a person's character, name, or reputation

F. Touching a person with consent

G. Situation in which a patient has a reasonable apprehension of immediate bodily harm without giving consent, such as with a threat of restraints or a hypodermic injection

H. Touching a patient without consent

I. Claim based on an intentional and unjustifiable detention of an unwilling, conscious person

CHAPTER **4**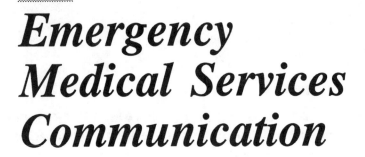

Emergency Medical Services Communication

STUDY GUIDE ASSIGNMENT 4-1

- Radio Communications
- Emergency Medical Services Communications System Capabilities

Reading Assignment: pages 30-32

Matching Items

Match each of the terms in the left column with the BEST definition in the right column by placing the letter of that definition in the space next to the term. Each definition may be used once or not at all.

_____ 1. base station
_____ 2. simplex
_____ 3. mobile repeater
_____ 4. satellite receiver system
_____ 5. telemetry
_____ 6. frequency
_____ 7. 911
_____ 8. enhanced 911

A. Strategically placed remote receivers that receive signals from a mobile radio

B. Vehicle unit that receives radio communications and rebroadcasts the communications

C. Unit of measurement for the number of cycles per unit of time

D. System that offers such capabilities as immediate display of the caller's telephone number and identification of the caller's location

E. A fixed location that contains a transmitter and a receiver

F. Ability to transmit and receive at the same time

G. Nationally recognized emergency telephone number by which an EMS system can quickly respond to a call

H. In EMS communications systems, the use of the communications system to transmit patient data, typically an EKG

I. Ability to transmit or receive, but not both simultaneously

STUDY GUIDE ASSIGNMENT 4-2

- Technological Components
- Emergency Medical Services Communications Operator
- The Emergency Medical Services Incident Sequence
- Radio Technique
- Equipment Maintenance

Reading Assignment: pages 33-39

Matching Items

Match each of the terms in the left column with the BEST definition in the right column by placing the letter of that definition in the space next to the term. Each definition may be used once or not at all.

_____ 1. Federal Communications Commission (FCC)

_____ 2. very-high frequency (VHF)

_____ 3. ultra-high frequency (UHF)

_____ 4. EMS communications operator

_____ 5. squelch

A. Frequency band that extends from about 300 MHz to 3000 MHz

B. Frequency band that extends from about 3000 MHz to 6000 MHz

C. Regulatory agency for radio communications that licenses communications systems and assigns radio frequencies, among other things

D. The person responsible for knowing the capabilities of the various components of the EMS system so that the proper units can be dispatched

E. Frequency band that extends from about 30 MHz to 300 MHz

F. Special receiver circuit that suppresses the unwanted radio noise that would otherwise be heard between transmissions

CHAPTER 5

Rescue Management

STUDY GUIDE ASSIGNMENT 5-1

- Principles of Safety
- Assessment of the Scene
- Gaining Access
- Disentanglement
- Removal
- Emergency Care and Transportation

Reading Assignment: pages 42-50

Matching Items

Match each of the terms in the left column with the BEST definition in the right column by placing the letter of that definition in the space next to the term. Each definition may be used once or not at all.

_____ 1. turnout gear
_____ 2. bunker coat
_____ 3. self-contained breathing apparatus (SCBA)
_____ 4. self-contained underwater breathing apparatus (SCUBA)
_____ 5. hazards
_____ 6. disentanglement
_____ 7. extrication

A. The coat worn to protect the paramedic from blood and body fluids

B. Protective clothing designed for structural fire fighting

C. The many dangers present in the line of duty

D. The freeing from entanglement; a label for tools used for this purpose

E. Respiratory protection device that provides a totally enclosed system of air; used by divers

F. The coat worn for structural fire fighting

G. Removal of the patient from the scene of accident or injury

H. Respiratory protection device that provides a totally enclosed system of air; used by the fire service

CHAPTER 6

Disaster Management

STUDY GUIDE ASSIGNMENT 6-1

- Defining Levels of Intensity
- The Disaster Plan

Reading Assignment: pages 52-62

Matching Items

Match each of the terms in the left column with the BEST definition in the right column by placing the letter of that definition in the space next to the term. Each definition may be used once or not at all.

D   1. disaster
E   2. emergency
B   3. major incident
F   4. triage
H   5. critical incident
C   6. Critical Incident Stress Debriefing (CISD)
A   7. Incident Command System (ISC)

A. System in which the highest-ranking officers from each agency share responsibility for scene management

B. Event that causes injury or death and damage to property or environment to a degree greater than that which occurs on a routine basis

C. Group support that is provided for extremely distressing events

D. Any event that overwhelms the existing manpower, facilities, equipment, and capabilities of a responding agency or institution

E. Situation that could not have been reasonably foreseen, threatens public health, welfare, or safety, and requires immediate action

F. Process of prioritization of medical care, treatment, and transportation

G. System in which the mayor takes responsibility for command of a disaster

H. Event that has a powerful emotional impact and results in an acute stress reaction

CHAPTER 7

Stress Management

STUDY GUIDE ASSIGNMENT 7-1

- The Stress Process
- Types of Stress Reactions

Reading Assignment: pages 64-69

Matching Items

Match each of the terms in the left column with the BEST definition in the right column by placing the letter of that definition in the space next to the term. Each definition may be used once or not at all.

_____ 1. stress
_____ 2. stressor
_____ 3. fight or flight
_____ 4. acute stress reaction
_____ 5. delayed stress reaction
_____ 6. cumulative stress reactions

A. State of physical and psychological arousal that appears as a response to some external stimulus

B. Universal reaction to a stressor that is regulated by the sympathetic nervous system

C. Occurs after exposure to any situation that has a powerful emotional impact

D. Destructive process that occurs over many years and is not associated with a recognized critical incident

E. Destructive process that occurs over many years and is associated with a recognized critical incident

F. External stimulus that results in stress

G. Acute stress reaction that occurs days or weeks after the critical event

STUDY GUIDE ASSIGNMENT 7-2

- Specific Paramedic Stressors
- Coping with Stress
- The Grieving Process in Death and Dying
- Dealing with Death and Dying

Reading Assignment: pages 69-73

Matching Items

Match each of the terms in the left column with the BEST definition in the right column by placing the letter of that definition in the space next to the term. Each definition may be used once or not at all.

_____ 1. acceptance
_____ 2. anger
_____ 3. bargaining
_____ 4. coping
_____ 5. defense mechanism
_____ 6. denial
_____ 7. depression
_____ 8. humor
_____ 9. isolation
_____ 10. rationalization
_____ 11. repression

A. The second stage of the grieving process, which can be projected toward anything or anyone

B. Any behavior that protects an individual from both internal and external stressors

C. Psychological defense mechanism by which an individual blocks out or refuses to acknowledge stressful circumstances

D. Stage one of the grieving process, which helps bring about the partial acceptance of the death

E. The fourth stage of the grieving process, wherein a great sense of loss becomes evident

F. Psychological defense mechanism by which individuals attempt to suppress distressing thoughts or ideas

G. Coping effort that may be internal, unnoticed, and sometimes unconscious; automatic effort to adjust to stressful situations

H. The seventh stage of the grieving process

I. Disassociates and accepts the inevitable without fear or despair

J. Third stage of the grieving process, in which the patient enters into some type of "agreement" in an attempt to postpone the inevitable

K. Defense mechanism that can reduce tension by providing an outlet for the person faced with a distressing situation

L. Justification of one's actions or inaction

CHAPTER 8

Medical Terminology and Human Systems

STUDY GUIDE ASSIGNMENT 8-1

■ Medical Terminology
Reading Assignment: pages 78-80

Matching Items

Match each of the terms in the left column with the BEST definition in the right column by placing the letter of that definition in the space next to the term. Each definition may be used once or not at all.

_____ 1. word root
_____ 2. prefix
_____ 3. suffix
_____ 4. combining vowel
_____ 5. combining form

A. Last part of a word

B. Labels the term

C. Part of a medical term that usually indicates the tissue, organ, or body system that is involved

D. First part of a word or the beginning of a word

E. Word root followed by a vowel that facilitates pronunciation; combines a word root with a suffix or other root

F. Links the root to the suffix or to another root to ease pronunciation

Multiple-Choice Items

Read each question carefully. For each item, select the answer that BEST completes the statement or answers the question, and place the letter of that answer in the space provided.

_____ 1. The word root brachi- means:
    a. wrist.
    b. arm.
    c. chest.
    d. muscle.

_____ 2. The word root somat- means:
    a. body.
    b. limb.
    c. fibers.
    d. brain.

_____ 3. The word root gloss- means:
    a. viscera.
    b. kidney.
    c. mouth.
    d. tongue.

_____ 4. The prefix ab- means:
    a. outer.
    b. away from.
    c. on or upon.
    d. to or toward.

_____ 5. The prefix hypo- means:
    a. down or from.
    b. backward.
    c. under.
    d. beside.

_____ 6. The prefix ana- means:
    a. up or toward.
    b. beside.
    c. excessive.
    d. above.

_____ 7. The prefix dis- means:
    a. opposed or against.
    b. around.
    c. outer.
    d. apart.

_____ 8. The suffix -emesis means:
    a. inflammation.
    b. pain.
    c. abnormal fear.
    d. vomit.

_____ 9. The suffix -algia means:
    a. inflammation.
    b. abnormal fear.
    c. pain.
    d. vomit.

_____ 10. The suffix -pnea means:
    a. cell.
    b. breathing.
    c. flow or discharge.
    d. blood condition.

_____ 11. The suffix -emia means:
    a. abnormal fear.
    b. blood condition.
    c. pain.
    d. small.

_____ 12. The common abbreviation for history is:
   a. Hx.
   b. PI.
   c. PO.
   d. HI.

_____ 13. The common abbreviation PRN means:
   a. every day.
   b. every hour.
   c. when necessary.
   d. four times a day.

STUDY GUIDE ASSIGNMENT 8-2

▪ Human Systems
Reading Assignment: pages 80-87

Matching Items

Match each of the terms in the left column with the BEST definition in the right column by placing the letter of that definition in the space next to the term. Each definition may be used once or not at all.

_____ 1. abduction
_____ 2. adduction
_____ 3. anterior
_____ 4. circumduction
_____ 5. distal
_____ 6. erect
_____ 7. extension
_____ 8. flexion
_____ 9. frontal
_____ 10. inferior
_____ 11. lateral
_____ 12. laterally recumbent
_____ 13. medial
_____ 14. posterior
_____ 15. prone
_____ 16. proximal
_____ 17. rotation
_____ 18. sagittal
_____ 19. superior
_____ 20. supine
_____ 21. transverse

A. Dorsal or back surface
B. Movement away from the midline of the body
C. An imaginary line that divides the body into right and left halves
D. Front surface of the body
E. Plane that passes vertically through the body and divides the body into anterior and posterior portions
F. Side lying position of the body
G. Lying on the back face upward; also the position of the hand or foot facing upward
H. Away from the point of origin or attachment
I. Movement toward the midline of the body
J. Side surface of the body
K. The swinging of a part in a circle; it involves displacement of the axis
L. Plane that divides the body or any of its parts horizontally into superior and inferior positions; sometimes referred to as a cross section
M. Nearest point of origin or attachment
N. In a straight position, or the movement of the limbs into a straight position
O. The turning of a part on its own axis
P. On top or toward the head

20

Q. Lying on the stomach with the face down; also the position of the hand or foot when facing down

R. Toward the midline

S. Away from the midline

T. On the bottom or toward the feet

U. Standing upright

V. The act of bending or the condition of being bent

Labeling Items

Read each question carefully and place your answer in the space provided.

1. Label the four planes of the body identified in the drawing by filling in the blank next to each letter, which corresponds with the same letter in the drawing. The four planes are to be selected from the answers that follow the drawing.

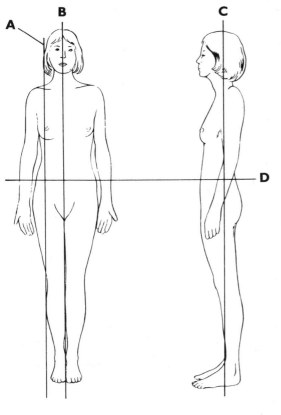

A. _____

B. _____

C. _____

D. _____

midsaggital   superior   transverse
frontal   saggital

2. Label the eight cavities of the body identified in the drawing by filling in the blank next to each letter, which corresponds with the same letter in the drawing. The eight cavities are to be selected from the answers that follow the blanks.

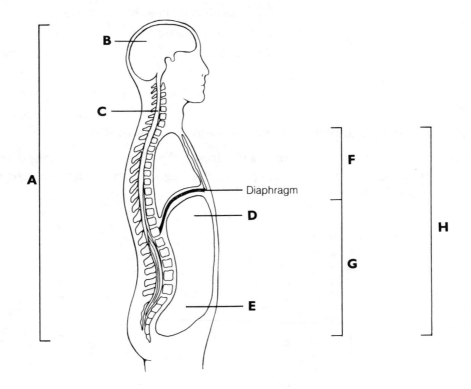

A. _____   E. _____

B. _____   F. _____

C. _____   G. _____

D. _____   H. _____

thoracic	ventral	pelvic
dorsal	superior	spinal
cranial	abdominal	abdominopelvic

CHAPTER 9

Patient Assessment

STUDY GUIDE ASSIGNMENT 9-1

- Scene Survey
- Scene Control
- Primary Survey

Skill 9-1: Patient Assessment

Reading Assignment: pages 90-103

Matching Items

Match each of the terms in the left column with the BEST definition in the right column by placing the letter of that definition in the space next to the term. Each definition may be used once or not at all.

_____ 1. scene survey
_____ 2. mechanism of injury
_____ 3. scene control
_____ 4. primary survey
_____ 5. rapport
_____ 6. surname
_____ 7. open-ended questions
_____ 8. direct questions

A. Questions that allow patients to tell the story in their own words

B. Questions with "yes" or "no" answers

C. A person's last name

D. Complete head-to-toe evaluation of the patient

E. Paramedic's control of the scene to insure personal safety and to be able to properly assess and manage the patient

F. Quick, yet observant, evaluation of potential hazards, mechanism of injury, and clues to medical illness that are provided by the patient's environment

G. Harmonious or sympathetic relationship

H. First step once the paramedic is at the patient's side; a rapid evaluation, lasting less than 45 seconds, to determine the patient's status in terms of responsiveness, airway, breathing, and circulation

I. Helps the paramedic determine patient injuries in a trauma call

STUDY GUIDE ASSIGNMENT 9-2

- Secondary Survey
Reading Assignment: pages 103-120

Matching Items

Match each of the terms in the left column with the BEST definition in the right column by placing the letter of that definition in the space next to the term. Each definition may be used once or not at all.

_____ 1. AVPU system
_____ 2. arousability
_____ 3. auscultation
_____ 4. capillary refill test
_____ 5. chief complaint
_____ 6. cyanosis
_____ 7. diastolic pressure
_____ 8. head-to-toe survey
_____ 9. hypertension
_____ 10. hypotension
_____ 11. Korotkoff's sounds
_____ 12. level of consciousness
_____ 13. medical history
_____ 14. palpation
_____ 15. percussion
_____ 16. present illness
_____ 17. pulse
_____ 18. respiration
_____ 19. systolic pressure
_____ 20. vital signs

A. Process of listening, especially with a stethoscope, to the lungs and abdomen to assess respiratory and gastrointestinal status

B. Determination of the chronology, nature, and severity of the patient's current illness or injury

C. Breathing

D. Maximum pressure against the arteries when the heart contracts

E. Slightly bluish or purplish discoloration of the skin and mucous membranes as a result of hypoxia

F. Survey of a patient that begins with the head and neck and proceeds to the chest and back, abdomen, and extremities

G. Series of sounds sometimes used to record blood pressure

H. Abnormally high blood pressure

I. Constant force of blood on the arteries when the heart is resting

J. A noninvasive test to judge the rate of blood flow through peripheral capillary beds

K. Normal blood pressure

L. Assessment of a patient by touch or feel

M. Survey taken to identify a patient's past health problems that may affect the current illness or injury

N. Important to the secondary survey; includes respiration, pulse, and blood pressure

O. Condition described according to the patient's response to various types of verbal or painful stimuli

P. An acronym for responsiveness

Q. The patient's answer to the question "Why did you call us today?"

R. Evaluation of the patient's ability to respond to simple commands, mental ability, and general orientation

S. Abnormally low blood pressure

T. Evaluation tool that involves striking or tapping the patient's skin to determine the size, location, and density of an underlying structure

U. The effect on an artery caused by the movement of blood from the heart as it contracts

Multiple-Choice Items

Read each question carefully. For each item, select the answer that BEST completes the statement or answers the question, and place the letter of that answer in the space provided.

____ 1. The _____ includes a patient interview, is a more thorough physical evaluation, and proposes to find less obvious and less acute problems.
   a. patient history
   b. primary assessment
   c. secondary assessment
   d. surveillance assessment

____ 2. During a patient interview, the paramedic should use the _____ question technique for a patient with an altered level of consciousness or when limited time makes it impossible to use other methods.
   a. direct
   b. non-verbal
   c. open-ended
   d. suggestive

____ 3. The primary component(s) of a patient history is(are):
   a. the patient's chief complaint.
   b. the history of the present illness.
   c. a medical history.
   d. all of the above.

____ 4. Determining _____ is NOT a purpose of taking the history of the present illness.
   a. chronology of illnesses
   b. nature of the illness
   c. severity of the illness
   d. types of medications

____ 5. During your patient assessment, you ask the following questions: Has this ever happened before? Have you ever had surgery? Are you under a physician's care for any reason? These questions are part of the:
   a. chief complaint.
   b. history of present illness.
   c. medical history.
   d. diagnostic signs.

____ 6. During the secondary survey, the sense of hearing is used directly or is aided by the stethoscope. This skill is known as:
   a. inspection.
   b. auscultation.
   c. palpation.
   d. auditation.

____ 7. During your evaluation of the level of consciousness, which of the following is(are) included in the neurologic exam?
   a. Pupil size
   b. Pattern of breathing
   c. Motor status
   d. All of the above

____ 8. When assessing the arousability of a patient, which of the following should you NOT do?
   a. Use descriptive terms such as lethargic and stuporous to describe your patient.
   b. Describe exactly how the patient responded to the stimuli.
   c. Utilize the AVPU system.
   d. Utilize the Glasgow Coma Scale.

____ 9. The normal adult respiratory rate is _____ breaths per minute.
   a. 10 to 15
   b. 12 to 15
   c. 12 to 20
   d. 15 to 24

____ 10. When assessing a pulse, the paramedic should evaluate:
   a. its rate.
   b. its rhythm.
   c. its strength.
   d. all of the above.

____ 11. A slow pulse rate, bradycardia, can occur under which of the following circumstances?
   a. In a fit athlete
   b. As a result of the use of digitalis
   c. With increasing intracranial pressure
   d. All of the above

____ 12. The _____ pressure represents the constant force of blood on the arteries when the heart is resting.
   a. deficit
   b. wedge
   c. systolic
   d. diastolic

____ 13. Which of the following statements is NOT true about blood pressure?
   a. The width of the bladder should be at least 20% greater than the extremity.
   b. A standing blood pressure is acceptable.
   c. A wide cuff can be used on the thigh.
   d. All of the above.

___ 14. Korotkoff's sounds are a series of sounds sometimes used to record blood pressure. The first diastolic figure should be identified during:
   a. phase II.
   b. phase III.
   c. phase IV.
   d. phase V.

___ 15. Which of the following statements is(are) true about a child's blood pressure?
   a. Crying and anxiety usually increase the blood pressure.
   b. A normal diastolic pressure is typically estimated to be two-thirds of the systolic pressure.
   c. The normal systolic pressure is estimated as age times 2 plus 80.
   d. All of the above.

___ 16. A pulse pressure of 20 mm Hg in an adult could be caused by:
   a. fever.
   b. increased intracranial pressure.
   c. cardiac tamponade.
   d. all of the above.

___ 17. During the tilt test, if the patient's pulse and blood pressure when the patient is sitting are no different from when she or he is standing, the paramedic should suspect:
   a. early stages of hypovolemic shock.
   b. normal hemodynamic compensation.
   c. cardiogenic shock.
   d. anaphylactic shock.

___ 18. Using the _____ route is the most appropriate method of evaluating a child's temperature.
   a. rectal
   b. oral
   c. axillary
   d. any of the above

___ 19. Bilateral dilated and fixed pupils can result from:
   a. narcotic poisoning.
   b. glaucoma medicine.
   c. subdural hematoma.
   d. atropine sulfate.

___ 20. What should be suspected, if during the chest assessment, the paramedic feels a crackling sensation as his or her finger pads move over the patient's skin?
   a. Subcutaneous emphysema
   b. Crepitus
   c. Rales
   d. Wheezes

___ 21. _____ is(are) heard during inspiration and is(are) caused by fluid in the alveoli.
   a. Wheezes
   b. Rales
   c. Rhonchi
   d. Stridor

_____ 22. The primary purpose of prehospital auscultation of heart sounds is to:
   a. document heart murmurs.
   b. establish a presence of mitral valve prolapse.
   c. establish a presence and regularity of heart activity.
   d. document a presence of pericardial rubs.

_____ 23. In _____ posturing, all four extremities are rigid and fully extended.
   a. decorticate
   b. decerebrate
   c. abducted
   d. flexion

STUDY GUIDE ASSIGNMENT 9-3

- Trauma Scoring Systems
- Re-evaluation of the Patient
- Communication of Patient Data

Reading Assignment: pages 120-124, Appendix C

Multiple-Choice Items

Read each question carefully. For each item, select the answer that BEST completes the statement or answers the question, and place the letter of that answer in the space provided.

_____ 1. The Adult Trauma Score places a numerical value on the assessment of which of the following?
   a. Respiratory rate and expansion
   b. Systolic blood pressure
   c. Capillary refill
   d. All of the above

_____ 2. During your assessment of a 25-year-old male patient, you find that your patient's eyes open to painful stimuli, he babbles incomprehensibly, and he withdraws from pain. His Glasgow Coma Scale is:
   a. 5.
   b. 7.
   c. 8.
   d. 10.

STUDY GUIDE ASSIGNMENT 9-4

Performance Checklist: Patient Assessment

The following skill should be practiced until you reach competency. Practice can be done in classroom settings using other students as patients, or in clinical rotations in the hospital or out on the ambulance or rescue unit. You may evaluate yourself, work with another student, or have a preceptor or instructor evaluate you using this form.

Instructions

1. Place a check mark in the "C" ("competent") column if you used the recommended technique the first time you performed each activity.
2. Place a check mark in the "A" ("acceptable") column if you used the recommended technique but it took you several times to perform each activity.
3. Place a check mark in the "U" ("unsatisfactory") column if you used some but not all of each recommended technique.
4. Place a check mark in the "NP" ("not performed") column if you forgot to perform that particular technique.
5. The section for comments provides space to make notes about what further practice you need, what errors you made, how you can improve your skill, and so on.

Performance Checklist: Patient Assessment

C	A	U	NP	C = competent; A = acceptable; U = unsatisfactory; NP = not performed
☐	☐	☐	☐	Visually observe the patient and the surrounding area
☐	☐	☐	☐	Assemble and check:

Primary equipment	*Accessory equipment and supplies*
▪ Blood pressure cuff	▪ Gloves
▪ Stethoscope	▪ Watch
▪ Penlight	▪ Scissors

C	A	U	NP	
☐	☐	☐	☐	Check responsiveness
☐	☐	☐	☐	Check airway
☐	☐	☐	☐	Check breathing
☐	☐	☐	☐	Check circulation
☐	☐	☐	☐	Check for obvious external hemorrhage
☐	☐	☐	☐	Evaluate and document vital signs. (May be performed by partner during exam or after patient assessment)
☐	☐	☐	☐	Inspect and palpate scalp
☐	☐	☐	☐	Inspect eyes
☐	☐	☐	☐	Inspect and palpate face, nose, and mouth
☐	☐	☐	☐	Inspect and palpate ears
☐	☐	☐	☐	Inspect and palpate neck
☐	☐	☐	☐	Inspect and palpate the chest
☐	☐	☐	☐	Evaluate breath sounds
☐	☐	☐	☐	Inspect and palpate abdomen
☐	☐	☐	☐	Inspect and palpate pelvic region
☐	☐	☐	☐	Inspect and palpate extremities
☐	☐	☐	☐	Inspect and palpate back

OUTCOME: ☐ Pass ☐ Fail ☐ Retest

Comments:

Student's Signature _____ Date _____

Instructor's Signature _____ Date _____

31

CHAPTER 10

Airway Management and Ventilation

STUDY GUIDE ASSIGNMENT 10-1

- Anatomy and Physiology
- Upper Airway Obstructions

Reading Assignment: pages 126-129

Matching Items

Match each of the terms in the left column with the BEST definition in the right column by placing the letter of that definition in the space next to the term. Each definition may be used once or not at all.

_____ 1. epiglottis
_____ 2. glottis
_____ 3. coughing
_____ 4. pharynx
_____ 5. nasopharynx
_____ 6. oropharynx
_____ 7. laryngopharynx
_____ 8. larynx
_____ 9. vocal cord
_____ 10. dyspnea
_____ 11. laryngeal spasm
_____ 12. laryngeal edema

A. Thin, leaf-shaped structure that is located within the larynx at the juncture of the larynx and esophagus and that protects the lower airways from foreign bodies

B. Upper end of the trachea that lies below the root of the tongue and contains the vocal cords

C. Subdivision of the pharynx that leads to the larynx and esophagus

D. Final generation of the airways before the alveoli are reached

E. Acute, involuntary, transitory contraction of the larynx and esophagus

F. Throat; that portion of the airway between the nasal cavity and the larynx

G. Subdivision of the pharynx, located posterior to the nose

H. Shortness of breath

I. Opening between the vocal cords

J. Swelling in and around the larynx

K. Modified form of respiration that serves to remove foreign bodies that inadvertently enter the larynx

33

L. One of two thin, reedlike folds of tissue within the larynx that vibrate as air passes between them

M. Portion of the pharynx that lies between the soft palate and the upper portion of the epiglottis

Labeling Items

Read each question carefully and place your answer in the space provided.

1. Label the eight structures of the upper airway identified in the drawing by filling in the blank next to each letter, which corresponds with the same letter in the drawing. The eight structures are to be selected from the answers that follow the blanks.

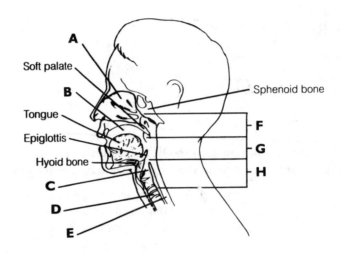

A. _____   E. _____

B. _____   F. _____

C. _____   G. _____

D. _____   H. _____

larynx	nasopharynx	laryngopharynx
oral cavity	trachea	esophagus
glottis	nasal cavity	oropharynx

2. Label the five structures of the larynx identified in the drawing by filling in the blank next to each letter, which corresponds with the same letter in the drawing. The five structures are to be selected from the answers that follow the blanks.

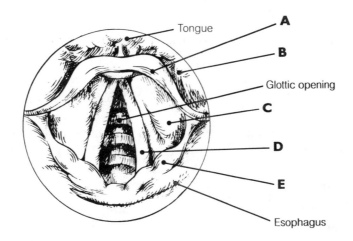

Tongue

A

B

Glottic opening

C

D

E

Esophagus

A. _____   D. _____

B. _____   E. _____

C. _____

vocal folds   epiglottis   cricoid cartilage
vallecula   arytenoid cartilage   vestibular fold

Multiple-Choice Items

Read each question carefully. For each item, select the answer that BEST completes the statement or answers the question, and place the letter of that answer in the space provided.

____ 1. The upper airway and lower airway are separated by the:
  a. epiglottis.
  b. tongue.
  c. vocal cords.
  d. cricoid cartilage.

____ 2. The act of simple hyperventilation can result in:
  a. decreased oxygen.
  b. increased carbon dioxide.
  c. dehydration.
  d. overhydration.

____ 3. The mucous layer in the nose is important because its **major functions are** to:
  I. keep the area moist.
  II. prevent infection.
  III. help humidify air.
  IV. reduce friction of air flow.

a. I and II
b. II and III
c. I, II, and III
d. I, II, III, and IV

_____ 4. When transporting patients who have had tracheostomies, airway care includes:
a. antibiotics.
b. frequent suctioning.
c. high-flow oxygen.
d. humidified, warmed air.

_____ 5. The _____ is(are) very important for the functioning of the tympanic membrane.
a. eustachian tube
b. adenoids
c. oropharynx
d. lymphatic glands

_____ 6. The larynx protects the lower airway by using the epiglottis and the:
a. vocal cords.
b. gag reflex.
c. cricoid cartilage.
d. cough reflex.

_____ 7. In the patient who has had a tracheostomy, the _____ reflex is diminished.
a. gag
b. sneeze
c. cough
d. sigh

_____ 8. The narrowest part of the adult airway, and the most frequent site of foreign body obstruction, is the:
a. epiglottis.
b. larynx at the cricoid cartilage.
c. larynx at the vocal cords.
d. carina.

_____ 9. Laryngeal spasm can have a variety of causes. Which of the following causes can be controlled by paramedics?
a. Near drowning
b. Exposure to chlorine gas
c. Deep suctioning
d. Prolonged vomiting

_____ 10. Common causes of airway obstruction due to laryngeal edema include:
I. tracheal intubation.
II. anaphylaxis.
III. a blow to the anterior neck.
IV. epiglottitis.
a. I, II, and III
b. II, III, and IV
c. I, II, and IV
d. I, II, III, and IV

STUDY GUIDE ASSIGNMENT 10-2

▪ Assessment of the Airway
Reading Assignment: pages 129-131

Matching Items

Match each of the terms in the left column with the BEST definition in the right column by placing the letter of that definition in the space next to the term. Each definition may be used once or not at all.

_____ 1. head-tilt/chin-lift
_____ 2. jaw-thrust
_____ 3. finger sweep
_____ 4. hypoxemia
_____ 5. hypercarbia
_____ 6. retractions
_____ 7. subcutaneous emphysema
_____ 8. auscultation
_____ 9. stridor

A. Harsh-sounding respirations due to airway obstruction

B. The presence of an abnormally high concentration of carbon dioxide in the blood

C. The presence of an abnormally low concentration of carbon dioxide in the blood

D. Method of opening the airway that requires forward displacement of the jaw without any tilting of the head

E. Method of opening the airway that involves tilting back the patient's head by placing one hand on the forehead and applying firm backward pressure

F. Shortening or drawing in of the intercostal and clavicle muscles; an indication of respiratory distress

G. Dilation of the subcutaneous space as a result of the presence of air

H. Process of listening, especially with a stethoscope, to the lungs and abdomen to assess respiratory and gastrointestinal status

I. Decreased partial pressure of oxygen in arterial blood

J. Removal of a foreign body from a patient's mouth with gloved fingers

Multiple-Choice Items

Read each question carefully. For each item, select the answer that BEST completes the statement or answers the question, and place the letter of that answer in the space provided.

_____ 1. A mechanism of injury such as striking a fence should increase the suspicion of:
   a. lung puncture.
   b. laryngeal trauma.
   c. lung contusion.
   d. carina separation.

_____ 2. Opening the airway in the trauma patient requires the use of which one of the following airway maneuvers?
   a. Head-tilt/chin-lift
   b. Head-tilt/jaw-thrust

    c.   Jaw-thrust

    d.   Head to the side

_____ 3. The best way to differentiate between the patient with a chronic condition from the patient with an acute onset is by:

    a.   a good physical assessment.

    b.   history of the episode.

    c.   lung sounds.

    d.   medications.

_____ 4. During the assessment, observations of which of the following often indicate hypoxemia or hypercarbia?

    I.   Restlessness

    II.   Slurred speech

    III.   Combativeness

    IV.   Drowsiness

        a.   I, II, and III

        b.   II, III, and IV

        c.   I, II, and IV

        d.   I, III, and IV

_____ 5. Of the following, which sign is MOST indicative of hypoxemia?

    a.   Central cyanosis

    b.   Tachycardia

    c.   Peripheral cyanosis

    d.   Hyperventilation

_____ 6. An asthma patient's pulse fading in and out according to inhalation and exhalation is MOST likely to indicate which of the following?

    a.   Significant lower airway obstruction is present.

    b.   Subcutaneous emphysema is developing.

    c.   Severe hypoxemia and hypercarbia are present.

    d.   If the patient is an adolescent, this is a normal variation of pulse.

STUDY GUIDE ASSIGNMENT 10-3

▪ Management of Airway Disorders
Reading Assignment: pages 131-174

Matching Items

Match each of the terms in the left column with the BEST definition in the right column by placing the letter of that definition in the space next to the term. Each definition may be used once or not at all.

_____ 1. oxygen

_____ 2. FiO$_2$

_____ 3. pin-indexing system

_____ 4. flowmeter

_____ 5. simple mask

A. Device that essentially serves as a tongue hook, holding the tongue at its base to prevent it from falling back against the posterior pharyngeal wall

B. Safety mechanism on an oxygen cylinder that allows only the attachment of an oxygen pressure regulator

_____ 6. nasal cannula

_____ 7. nonrebreathing mask

_____ 8. Venturi mask

_____ 9. oropharyngeal airway

_____ 10. nasopharyngeal airway

_____ 11. bag-valve-mask device

C. An odorless, tasteless gas necessary for all cellular life and proper metabolism

D. Hand-held external device used to assist or control ventilation; it can deliver 100% oxygen

E. Permanent attachment to oxygen pressure regulator to permit the regulated release of oxygen in liters per minute

F. This device, placed through the nose, is used to maintain an open upper airway by preventing the tongue from obstructing the posterior pharynx

G. The flow of oxygen is directed into a bag that is attached to the mask

H. Fraction of inspired oxygen

I. Suctions blood or mucous from endotracheal tubes

J. Specialized mask that enables delivery of precise concentrations of oxygen between 24% and 50%

K. Contains an inlet for oxygen delivery and small vents on either side of the mask to allow for escape of exhaled gas

L. An apparatus capable of delivering up to 44% oxygen when operated at a maximum of 6 L/min

Multiple-Choice Items

Read each question carefully. For each item, select the answer that BEST completes the statement or answers the question, and place the letter of that answer in the space provided.

_____ 1. Which of the following airway devices BEST protects the lower airway?
   a. Oropharyngeal airway
   b. Endotracheal tube
   c. Pharyngeo-tracheal lumen
   d. Esophageal obturator

_____ 2. Simply increasing the amount of oxygen in the inspired air usually increases the amount of oxygen in the alveoli unless the patient is suffering from:
   a. air hunger.
   b. a diffusion disorder.
   c. shortness of breath.
   d. upper respiratory infection .

_____ 3. An oxygen cannula is an acceptable oxygen delivery device even for those who breathe through the mouth, because:
   a. the concentration of oxygen delivered is not high.
   b. sooner or later everyone breathes through the nose.
   c. dead air space in the nasopharynx acts as a reservoir.
   d. none of these; the nasal cannula is NOT an acceptable device for mouth breathers.

_____ 4. An airway best used for the patient whose airway requires maintenance for only a short period of time is the:
a. oropharyngeal airway.
b. endotracheal tube.
c. pharyngeo-tracheal lumen.
d. esophageal obturator.

_____ 5. An endotracheal tube should be considered for the patient who:
a. gags on an oropharyngeal airway.
b. tolerates suctioning.
c. accepts an oropharyngeal airway without gagging.
d. has suffered a head injury.

_____ 6. Correct measurement of the nasopharyngeal airway is done by measuring the:
a. nostril size.
b. distance between the nose and the earlobe.
c. distance between the nose and the chin.
d. distance between the corner of the mouth and the earlobe.

_____ 7. Suctioning should NOT be done for more than _____ seconds.
a. 5
b. 10
c. 20
d. 30

_____ 8. Oxygen-powered demand valves should NOT be used in children for which of the following reasons?
a. Face pieces do not adequately cover a child's face.
b. It is difficult to regulate the rate of respirations.
c. These devices can be used only on intubated patients.
d. It is too easy to cause a pneumothorax or gastric rupture.

_____ 9. The primary limiting factor of positive-pressure ventilation devices is the:
a. percent of oxygen delivered.
b. seal of the mask.
c. amount of pressure delivered.
d. requirement for manual operation.

_____ 10. The main functions of the laryngoscope blade are to provide direct visualization of the larynx and vocal cords and to:
a. align the structures of the upper and lower airways.
b. lift the tongue and enlarge the pharynx.
c. open the passage between the vocal cords.
d. lift the epiglottis and enlarge the larynx.

_____ 11. A first-line airway technique is use of a(an):
a. endotracheal tube.
b. EGTA.
c. oropharyngeal airway.
d. esophageal obturator airway.

STUDY GUIDE ASSIGNMENT 10-4

Performance Checklist: Endotracheal Intubation, Oral
Performance Checklist: Endotracheal Intubation, Nasal
Performance Checklist: Pharyngeo-Tracheal Lumen Airway
Performance Checklist: Esophageal Obturator Airway and Esophageal
Gastric Tube Airway

The following skills should be practiced until you reach competency. Practice can be done in classroom settings using manikins, or in clinical rotations in the hospital or out on the ambulance or rescue unit. You may evaluate yourself, work with another student, or have a preceptor or instructor evaluate you using these forms.

Instructions

1. Place a check mark in the "C" ("competent") column if you used the recommended technique the first time you performed each activity.
2. Place a check mark in the "A" ("acceptable") column if you used the recommended technique but it took you several times to perform each activity.
3. Place a check mark in the "U" ("unsatisfactory") column if you used some but not all of each recommended technique.
4. Place a check mark in the "NP" ("not performed") column if you forgot to perform that particular technique.
5. The section for comments provides space to make notes about what further practice you need, what errors you made, how you can improve your skill, and so on.

Performance Checklist: Endotracheal Intubation, Oral

C	A	U	NP	C = competent; A = acceptable; U = unsatisfactory; NP = not performed
☐	☐	☐	☐	Check responsiveness
☐	☐	☐	☐	Check airway
☐	☐	☐	☐	Check breathing
☐	☐	☐	☐	Check circulation
☐	☐	☐	☐	Assemble and check:

Primary equipment
- Laryngoscope handle
- Laryngoscope blade
- Endotracheal (ET) tube
- Stylet
- 10-mL syringe

Accessory equipment and supplies
- Suction unit
- Suction catheter
- Bag-valve-mask device
- Oxygen
- Stethoscope
- Magill forceps
- Tape- or tube-securing device
- Protective eye wear
- Mask
- Gloves

C	A	U	NP	
☐	☐	☐	☐	Remove potential airway obstructions
☐	☐	☐	☐	Position patient's head
☐	☐	☐	☐	Hyperventilate patient
☐	☐	☐	☐	Insert blade
☐	☐	☐	☐	Lift blade
☐	☐	☐	☐	Expose and visualize:

- Epiglottis
- Vocal cords

C	A	U	NP	
☐	☐	☐	☐	Insert ET tube
☐	☐	☐	☐	Inflate cuff
☐	☐	☐	☐	Assess breath sounds
☐	☐	☐	☐	Correct improperly placed ET tube
☐	☐	☐	☐	Stabilize ET tube
☐	☐	☐	☐	Reassess breath sounds
☐	☐	☐	☐	Correct ET tube placement as indicated

OUTCOME: ☐ Pass   ☐ Fail   ☐ Retest

Comments:

Student's Signature _____ Date _____

Instructor's Signature _____ Date _____

Performance Checklist: Endotracheal Intubation, Nasal

C	A	U	NP	
				C = competent; A = acceptable; U = unsatisfactory; NP = not performed
☐	☐	☐	☐	Check responsiveness
☐	☐	☐	☐	Check airway
☐	☐	☐	☐	Check breathing
☐	☐	☐	☐	Check circulation
☐	☐	☐	☐	Assemble and check:

Primary equipment
- Endotracheal (ET) tube
- 10-mL syringe

Accessory equipment and supplies
- Water soluble lubricant
- Suction unit
- Suction catheter
- Bag-valve-mask device
- Oxygen
- Stethoscope
- Tape- or tube-securing device
- Protective eye wear
- Mask
- Gloves

C	A	U	NP	
☐	☐	☐	☐	Remove potential airway obstruction
☐	☐	☐	☐	Position patient's head
☐	☐	☐	☐	Hyperventilate patient
☐	☐	☐	☐	Choose a naris
☐	☐	☐	☐	Insert ET tube
☐	☐	☐	☐	Inflate cuff
☐	☐	☐	☐	Assess breath sounds
☐	☐	☐	☐	Correct improperly placed ET tube
☐	☐	☐	☐	Stabilize ET tube
☐	☐	☐	☐	Reassess breath sounds
☐	☐	☐	☐	Correct ET tube placement as indicated

OUTCOME:　　☐ Pass　　　☐ Fail　　　☐ Retest

Comments:

Student's Signature _____ Date _____

Instructor's Signature _____ Date _____

Performance Checklist: Pharyngeo-Tracheal Lumen Airway

C	A	U	NP	C = competent; A = acceptable; U = unsatisfactory; NP = not performed
☐	☐	☐	☐	Check responsiveness
☐	☐	☐	☐	Check airway
☐	☐	☐	☐	Check breathing
☐	☐	☐	☐	Check circulation
☐	☐	☐	☐	Assemble and check:

Primary equipment
- Pharyngo-tracheal lumen (PtL) airway

Accessory equipment and supplies
- Suction unit
- Suction catheter
- Bag-valve-mask device
- Oxygen
- Stethoscope
- Protective eye wear
- Mask
- Gloves

C	A	U	NP	
☐	☐	☐	☐	Remove potential airway obstructions
☐	☐	☐	☐	Position patient's head
☐	☐	☐	☐	Hyperventilate patient
☐	☐	☐	☐	Insert PtL airway
☐	☐	☐	☐	Stabilize the tube
☐	☐	☐	☐	Close white port cap
☐	☐	☐	☐	Ventilate into the #1 inflation valve
☐	☐	☐	☐	Determine location of the #3 long clear tube
☐	☐	☐	☐	Ventilate through proper tube
☐	☐	☐	☐	Assess breath sounds
☐	☐	☐	☐	Correct tube placement as indicated
☐	☐	☐	☐	Reassess breath sounds periodically

OUTCOME: ☐ Pass   ☐ Fail   ☐ Retest

Comments:

Student's Signature _____ Date _____

Instructor's Signature _____ Date _____

Performance Checklist: Esophageal Obturator Airway and Esophageal Gastric Tube Airway

C	A	U	NP	C = competent; A = acceptable; U = unsatisfactory; NP = not performed
☐	☐	☐	☐	Check responsiveness
☐	☐	☐	☐	Check airway
☐	☐	☐	☐	Check breathing
☐	☐	☐	☐	Check circulation
☐	☐	☐	☐	Assemble and check:

Primary equipment
- Esophageal obturator airway (EOA) or esophageal gastric tube airway (EGTA)
- 35-mL syringe

Accessory equipment and supplies
- Water-soluble lubricant
- Suction unit
- Bag-valve-mask device
- Oxygen
- Stethoscope
- Protective eye wear
- Mask
- Gloves

C	A	U	NP	
☐	☐	☐	☐	Remove potential airway obstructions
☐	☐	☐	☐	Position patient's head
☐	☐	☐	☐	Hyperventilate patient
☐	☐	☐	☐	Insert EOA or EGTA
☐	☐	☐	☐	Assess breath sounds to determine tube position
☐	☐	☐	☐	Correct tube placement as indicated
☐	☐	☐	☐	Inflate tube cuff
☐	☐	☐	☐	Reassess breath sounds periodically

OUTCOME: ☐ Pass ☐ Fail ☐ Retest

Comments:

Student's Signature _____ Date _____

Instructor's Signature _____ Date _____

STUDY GUIDE ASSIGNMENT 10-5

Performance Checklist: Surgical Cricothyroidotomy
Performance Checklist: Translaryngeal Jet Ventilation

The following skills should be practiced until you reach competency. Practice can be done in classroom settings using manikins, or in clinical rotations in the hospital or out on the ambulance or rescue unit. You may evaluate yourself, work with another student, or have a preceptor or instructor evaluate you using these forms.

Instructions

1. Place a check mark in the "C" ("competent") column if you used the recommended technique the first time you performed each activity.
2. Place a check mark in the "A" ("acceptable") column if you used the recommended technique but it took you several times to perform each activity.
3. Place a check mark in the "U" ("unsatisfactory") column if you used some but not all of each recommended technique.
4. Place a check mark in the "NP" ("not performed") column if you forgot to perform that particular technique.
5. The section for comments provides space to make notes about what further practice you need, what errors you made, how you can improve your skill, and so on.

Performance Checklist: Surgical Cricothyroidotomy

C	A	U	NP	C = competent; A = acceptable; U = unsatisfactory; NP = not performed
☐	☐	☐	☐	Check responsiveness
☐	☐	☐	☐	Check airway
☐	☐	☐	☐	Check breathing
☐	☐	☐	☐	Check circulation
☐	☐	☐	☐	Assemble and check:

Primary equipment
- #10 Scalpel blade and handle
- 5.0-mm or 6.0-mm endotracheal (ET) tube
- 10-mL syringe
- Hemostat

Accessory equipment and supplies
- Sterile gauze pads
- Antiseptic swabs
- Suction unit
- Suction catheter
- Bag-valve-mask device
- Oxygen
- Stethoscope
- Tape
- Protective eye wear
- Mask
- Sterile gloves

C	A	U	NP	
☐	☐	☐	☐	Position patient
☐	☐	☐	☐	Hyperventilate patient
☐	☐	☐	☐	Prepare the area
☐	☐	☐	☐	Locate the cricothyroid membrane
☐	☐	☐	☐	Perform incision
☐	☐	☐	☐	Insert hemostat
☐	☐	☐	☐	Insert ET tube
☐	☐	☐	☐	Inflate tube cuff
☐	☐	☐	☐	Assess breath sounds
☐	☐	☐	☐	Correct placement of ET tube as indicated
☐	☐	☐	☐	Stabilize ET tube
☐	☐	☐	☐	Dispose of scalpel blade

OUTCOME: ☐ Pass   ☐ Fail   ☐ Retest

Comments:

Student's Signature _____ Date _____

Instructor's Signature _____ Date _____

54

Performance Checklist: Translaryngeal Jet Ventilation

C	A	U	NP	C = competent; A = acceptable; U = unsatisfactory; NP = not performed
☐	☐	☐	☐	Check responsiveness
☐	☐	☐	☐	Check airway
☐	☐	☐	☐	Check breathing
☐	☐	☐	☐	Check circulation
☐	☐	☐	☐	Assemble and check:

Primary equipment
- 12- or 14-gauge over-the-needle catheter

Accessory equipment and supplies
- Antiseptic swabs
- Suction unit
- Suction catheter
- Jet ventilator
- Oxygen
- Stethoscope
- Tape
- Protective eye wear
- Mask
- Sterile gloves

C	A	U	NP	
☐	☐	☐	☐	Position patient
☐	☐	☐	☐	Hyperventilate patient
☐	☐	☐	☐	Prepare the area
☐	☐	☐	☐	Locate the cricothyroid membrane
☐	☐	☐	☐	Insert the needle
☐	☐	☐	☐	Advance catheter
☐	☐	☐	☐	Withdraw the needle
☐	☐	☐	☐	Correct placement of catheter as indicated
☐	☐	☐	☐	Assess breath sounds
☐	☐	☐	☐	Stabilize the catheter
☐	☐	☐	☐	Dispose of needle

OUTCOME: ☐ Pass   ☐ Fail   ☐ Retest

Comments:

Student's Signature _____ Date _____

Instructor's Signature _____ Date _____

CHAPTER 11

Pathophysiology of Shock and Fluid Management

STUDY GUIDE ASSIGNMENT 11-1

■ Pathophysiology of Shock
Reading Assignment: pages 176-191

Matching Items

Match each of the terms in the left column with the BEST definition in the right column by placing the letter of that definition in the space next to the term. Each definition may be used once or not at all.

_____ 1. aerobic
_____ 2. anaerobic
_____ 3. stroke volume
_____ 4. cardiac output
_____ 5. diffusion
_____ 6. osmosis
_____ 7. active transport
_____ 8. isotonic
_____ 9. hypertonic
_____ 10. hypotonic

A. In the absence of oxygen

B. In the presence of oxygen

C. The amount of blood pumped by the heart each minute

D. Constant movement of molecules from an area of higher concentration to an area of lower concentration

E. A fluid with a lower osmotic pressure than another fluid

F. A fluid with the same osmotic pressure as another fluid

G. A fluid with a higher osmotic pressure than another fluid

H. Blood is shunted from an inactive capillary bed to one that is more active

I. The passage of water through a semipermeable membrane that separates solutions of different concentrations

J. Amount of blood ejected by the left ventricle with each contraction of the heart

K. The crossing of electrolytes against the diffusion gradient or osmotic gradient

Matching Items

Match each of the terms in the left column with the BEST definition in the right column by placing the letter of that definition in the space next to the term. Each definition may be used once or not at all.

_____ 11. extracellular
_____ 12. intracellular
_____ 13. electrolyte
_____ 14. cation
_____ 15. anion
_____ 16. sodium
_____ 17. potassium

A. Substance composed of charged particles or ions when placed in water
B. Negatively charged ion
C. Neutral ion
D. Positively charged ion
E. Chief intracellular ion in blood plasma
F. Fluid outside of the cells
G. Fluid within cell membranes
H. Chief extracellular ion in blood plasma

Matching Items

Match each of the terms in the left column with the BEST definition in the right column by placing the letter of that definition in the space next to the term. Each definition may be used once or not at all.

_____ 18. blood
_____ 19. erythrocyte
_____ 20. hemoglobin
_____ 21. hematocrit
_____ 22. leukocyte
_____ 23. lymphocyte
_____ 24. platelet
_____ 25. antigen
_____ 26. antibody

A. Red blood cell
B. Volume percentage of red blood cells in whole blood
C. Protein that contains iron
D. Protective protein substance formed in the body as a result of contact with an antigen
E. Foreign substance that induces the formation of antibodies
F. Buffer that regulates the pH in the body
G. White blood cell
H. Lymph cell
I. Thick fluid that lies within the intravascular space
J. Fragment of a cell

Matching Items

Match each of the terms in the left column with the BEST definition in the right column by placing the letter of that definition in the space next to the term. Each definition may be used once or not at all.

_____ 27. acid
_____ 28. base
_____ 29. pH
_____ 30. buffer
_____ 31. respiratory acidosis
_____ 32. respiratory alkalosis

A. Excess amount of alkaline in the body
B. Excess amount of protein in the blood
C. Excess amount of acids in the body
D. A chemical compound that gives up or donates a hydrogen ion
E. Inverse logarithm of the hydrogen ion concentration

_____	33.	metabolic acidosis
_____	34.	metabolic alkalosis

F. A chemical compound that accepts or receives a hydrogen ion

G. Acidosis as a result of impaired respiration

H. A chemical system set up in the body to respond to changes in the hydrogen ion concentration to maintain a normal pH

I. Alkalosis as a result of excessive ventilation

STUDY GUIDE ASSIGNMENT 11-2

▪ Pathophysiology of Shock
Reading Assignment: Pages 176-191

Multiple-Choice Items

Read each question carefully. For each item, select the answer that BEST completes the statement or answers the question, and place the letter of that answer in the space provided.

a 1. All of the following are components of the Fick principle EXCEPT:
    a. active transport of oxygen into the cellular mitochondria.
    b. delivery of oxygenated red blood cells to the tissue cells.
    c. off-loading of oxygen by the red blood cells at the cellular level.
    d. on-loading of oxygen by the red blood cells in the lungs.

b 2. _____ is the process in which there is constant movement of molecules from an area of higher concentration to an area of lower concentration.
    a. Active transport
    b. Diffusion
    c. Menhidrosis
    d. Osmosis

d 3. _____ is the process in which water moves toward a more concentrated solution (water movement from area of lower concentration to an area of higher concentration).
    a. Active transport
    b. Diffusion
    c. Menhidrosis
    d. Osmosis

a 4. _____ is the process in which non-water molecules move in a direction opposite to that in which they would normally flow (that is, from an area of lower concentration to an area of higher concentration) through the utilization of energy.
    a. Active transport
    b. Diffusion
    c. Menhidrosis
    d. Osmosis

_a_ 5. When a red blood cell is placed into a(an) _____ solution, it loses water to the surrounding solution and shrinks.
   a. hypertonic
   b. hypotonic
   c. isotonic
   d. ultratonic

_b_ 6. When a red blood cell is placed into a(an) _____ solution, it absorbs water from the surrounding solution, swells, and may burst (if sufficiently swollen).
   a. hypertonic
   b. hypotonic
   c. isotonic
   d. ultratonic

_c_ 7. Total body water accounts for _____ % of total body weight.
   a. 15
   b. 45
   c. 60
   d. 80

_c_ 8. _____ are substances whose molecules dissociate into electrically charged particles called ions when placed in water.
   a. Acids
   b. Bases
   c. Electrolytes
   d. Substates

_d_ 9. The chief extracellular ion in the blood plasma is:
   a. calcium.
   b. chloride.
   c. potassium.
   d. sodium.

_c_ 10. The chief intracellular ion is:
   a. calcium.
   b. chloride.
   c. potassium.
   d. sodium.

_c_ 11. The force or weight of a fluid pushing against the capillary wall, resulting in forcing of water from the capillary, is called:
   a. active transport.
   b. barometric pressure.
   c. hydrostatic pressure.
   d. osmotic pressure.

_b_ 12. The average adult male who weighs 70 kg (154 lbs) has about _____ liters of blood in his cardiovascular system.
 a. 4
 b. 5
 c. 6
 d. 7

_b_ 13. Plasma is the fluid portion of the blood and represents _____% of blood volume.
 a. 25
 b. 55
 c. 65
 d. 80

_a_ 14. The blood cell responsible for carrying oxygen and carbon dioxide is the:
 a. erythrocyte.
 b. leukocyte.
 c. lymphocyte.
 d. thrombocyte.

_b_ 15. Hematocrit is the term used to identify the volume percentage of red blood cells in whole blood. The average adult male has a hematocrit of:
 a. 33.
 b. 45.
 c. 55.
 d. 60.

_b_ 16. The blood cell responsible for destroying foreign organisms and fighting infection is the:
 a. erythrocyte.
 b. leukocyte.
 c. platelet.
 d. thrombocyte.

_d_ 17. The blood cell responsible for blood coagulation (clotting) is the:
 a. erythrocyte.
 b. leukocyte.
 c. lymphocyte.
 d. platelet.

_d_ 18. An acid is a chemical compound that:
 a. accepts bicarbonate ions.
 b. donates bicarbonate ions.
 c. accepts hydrogen ions.
 d. donates hydrogen ions.

_c_ 19. A base is a chemical compound that:
 a. accepts bicarbonate ions.
 b. donates bicarbonate ions.
 c. accepts hydrogen ions.
 d. donates hydrogen ions.

_C_ 20. The normal pH range for human blood is:
   a. 6.90-7.10.
   b. 7.15-7.25.
   c. 7.35-7.45.
   d. 7.50-7.60.

_a_ 21. Death can occur if the blood pH drops below _____ for more than a few hours.
   a. 6.8
   b. 6.9
   c. 7.1
   d. 7.3

_a_ 22. Several body mechanisms work to regulate acid-base balance. The most important and most rapidly acting is the _____ system.
   a. buffer
   b. protein
   c. renal
   d. respiratory

_C_ 23. The respiratory system contributes to acid-base balance by regulating the retention and elimination of:
   a. bicarbonate.
   b. carbonic acid.
   c. carbon dioxide.
   d. oxygen.

_C_ 24. Your patient is a 34-year-old man in coma from a heroin overdose. He is breathing 6 times per minute, shallowly. At the hospital, you learn that his PCO_2 is very high and his PO_2 is low. The blood pH is 7.15. These readings and patient presentation are consistent with:
   a. metabolic acidosis.
   b. metabolic alkalosis.
   c. respiratory acidosis.
   d. respiratory alkalosis.

_d_ 25. Your patient is a 16-year-old cheerleader who has become overly excited at a football game. She complains of dizziness, tightness in her chest, and "pins and needles" tingling in her arms and legs. Her breathing rate is deep and rapid. At the hospital, you learn that her PCO_2 is very low and her PO_2 is only slightly high. The pH is 7.6. These readings and patient presentation are consistent with:
   a. metabolic acidosis.
   b. metabolic alkalosis.
   c. respiratory acidosis.
   d. respiratory alkalosis.

_a_ 26. Your patient is a 54-year-old diabetic male who is stuporous. His wife says he has not taken his insulin in several days. His skin is flushed; his breathing is deep and rapid with a fruity odor. He appears dehydrated. The PCO_2 and PO_2 are within normal limits, but his pH is 7.1. These readings and patient presentation are consistent with:

   a.   metabolic acidosis.

   b.   metabolic alkalosis.

   c.   respiratory acidosis.

   d.   respiratory alkalosis.

_b_ 27. Your patient is 42-year-old female who has a history of peptic ulcer disease. She seems nervous and complains of muscle twitching. Her husband states that because her ulcer has been acting up, she has eaten several rolls of antacid tablets and has consumed most of a box of baking soda mixed into water. Her PCO_2 and PO_2 are within normal limits, but her pH is 7.7. These readings and patient presentation are consistent with:

   a.   metabolic acidosis.

   b.   metabolic alkalosis.

   c.   respiratory acidosis.

   d.   respiratory alkalosis.

STUDY GUIDE ASSIGNMENT 11-3

- Stages of Shock
- Assessment of the Patient in Shock
- Management

Skill 11-1. Pneumatic Anti-shock Garment

Reading Assignment: pages 191-203

Multiple-Choice Items

Read each question carefully. For each item, select the answer that BEST completes the statement or answers the question, and place the letter of that answer in the space provided.

_d_ 1. In compensated shock, the body adjusts for shock in each of the following ways EXCEPT increased:

   a.   heart contractions.

   b.   heart rate.

   c.   peripheral vascular resistance.

   d.   vagal activity.

_d_ 2. Oxygen therapy is an important component of management of the shock patient. Resuscitation of the shock patient should include _____ % or greater oxygen, with assisted or controlled ventilation to ensure adequate volume of air movement.

   a.   40

   b.   50

   c.   65

   d.   85

C 3. When the pneumatic anti-shock garment is applied to a shock patient in a cold environment, and then the patient is moved to a warmer area, the garment may:
   a. become looser.
   b. come apart due to inactivation of the Velcro fasteners.
   c. get tighter.
   d. spontaneously deflate.

C 4. Which of the following conditions are indications for the use of the pneumatic anti-shock garment?
   I. Fractured femur
   II. Fractured pelvis
   III. Hypovolemic shock
   IV. Intra-abdominal hemorrhage
   V. Severe blood loss
   VI. Thoracic trauma with associated hemorrhage
      a. I, II, III, V, and VI
      a. I, II, III, V, and VI
      b. I, II, III, IV, and VI
      c. I, II, III, IV, and V
      d. II, III, IV, V, and VI

d 5. The intravenous solution of choice for hypovolemic shock is:
   a. D_5W.
   b. lactated Ringer's.
   c. normal saline.
   d. b or c.

STUDY GUIDE ASSIGNMENT 11-4

Performance Checklist: Pneumatic Anti-Shock Garment

The following skill should be practiced until you reach competency. Practice can be done in classroom settings using other students as patients, or in clinical rotations in the hospital or out on the ambulance or rescue unit. You may evaluate yourself, work with another student, or have a preceptor or instructor evaluate you using this form.

Instructions

1. Place a check mark in the "C" ("competent") column if you used the recommended technique the first time you performed each activity.
2. Place a check mark in the "A" ("acceptable") column if you used the recommended technique but it took you several times to perform each activity.
3. Place a check mark in the "U" ("unsatisfactory") column if you used some but not all of each recommended technique.
4. Place a check mark in the "NP" ("not performed") column if you forgot to perform that particular technique.
5. The section for comments provides space to make notes about what further practice you need, what errors you made, how you can improve your skill, and so on.

Performance Checklist: Pneumatic Anti-Shock Garment

C	A	U	NP	
				C = competent; A = acceptable; U = unsatisfactory; NP = not performed
☐	☐	☐	☐	Check responsiveness
☐	☐	☐	☐	Check airway
☐	☐	☐	☐	Check breathing
☐	☐	☐	☐	Check circulation
☐	☐	☐	☐	Assemble and check:

Primary equipment
- Pneumatic anti-shock garment (PASG)
- Inflation device

Accessory equipment and supplies
- Long backboard
- Cervical collar
- Gloves
- Stethoscope
- Blood pressure cuff

C	A	U	NP	
☐	☐	☐	☐	Apply cervical immobilization as indicated
☐	☐	☐	☐	Log-roll patient onto long backboard and PASG
☐	☐	☐	☐	Secure abdominal section
☐	☐	☐	☐	Secure leg sections
☐	☐	☐	☐	Reassess patient
☐	☐	☐	☐	Connect pump tubing
☐	☐	☐	☐	Inflate the PASG
☐	☐	☐	☐	Reassess patient

OUTCOME: ☐ Pass   ☐ Fail   ☐ Retest

Comments:

Student's Signature _____ Date _____

Instructor's Signature _____ Date _____

CHAPTER 12

General Pharmacology

STUDY GUIDE ASSIGNMENT 12-1

- General Drug Information
- Drug Sources and Legislation
- Drug Names
- Drug References and Resources

Reading Assignment: pages 206-209

Matching Items

Match each of the terms in the left column with the BEST definition in the right column by placing the letter of that definition in the space next to the term. **Each definition may be used once or not at all.**

_A_ 1. Pure Food and Drug Act of 1906

_E_ 2. Harrison Narcotic Act of 1914

_J_ 3. Controlled Substance Act

_I_ 4. Schedule I drugs

_H_ 5. Schedule II drugs

_G_ 6. Schedule III drugs

_N_ 7. Schedule V drugs

_C_ 8. Drug Enforcement Agency

_K_ 9. Food and Drug Administration

_B_ 10. Public Health Service

_F_ 11. United States Pharmacopeia

_M_ 12. Hospital Formulary

_D_ 13. Physicians' Desk Reference

A. Mandates the labeling of preparations that contain certain habit-forming drugs and prohibits making false claims about a drug's actions

B. Federal agency that inspects and licenses establishments that manufacture drugs

C. Federal agency responsible for the enforcement of drug legislation

D. Common resource for drug information

E. Regulates the manufacture, import, sale, and use of opium and cocaine and their derivatives

F. Government publication that lists the official name of a drug

G. Drugs that are used in medical care but do not have a high potential for abuse

H. Drugs that are used in medical care but have a high potential for abuse

I. Drugs that do not have a medical use

J. Classifies drugs according to their usefulness and abuse potential

K. Agency that regulates the manufacturing, research, and testing of drugs and monitors any adverse effects of drugs new to the market

L. Lists names of physicians by specialty

M. Published by the American Society of Hospital Pharmacists; provides information on drugs and is continuously updated as new information is published

N. Drugs that are used in medical care and may be dispensed without a prescription

Multiple-Choice Items

Read each question carefully. For each item, select the answer that BEST completes the statement or answers the question, and place the letter of that answer in the space provided.

_b_ 1. Drugs such as epinephrine and insulin are derived from _____ sources.
   a. plant
   b. animal
   c. mineral
   d. synthetic

_a_ 2. The _____ was the first major federal law that mandated labeling of preparations that contain certain habit-forming drugs and prohibited making false claims about a drug's action.
   a. Pure Food and Drug Act
   b. Harrison Narcotic Act
   c. Controlled Substance Act
   d. Narcotic Control Act

_d_ 3. The agency responsible for the enforcement of drug legislation is the:
   a. Federal Trade Commission.
   b. Food and Drug Administration.
   c. Public Health Service.
   d. Drug Enforcement Agency.

STUDY GUIDE ASSIGNMENT 12-2

- Forms of Drugs
- Drug Pharmacokinetics
- Drug Pharmacodynamics
Reading Assignment: pages 209-219

Matching Items

Match each of the terms in the left column with the BEST definition in the right column by placing the letter of that definition in the space next to the term. Each definition may be used once or not at all.

_c_ 1. parenteral drugs
_a_ 2. pharmacokinetics
_d_ 3. intradermal
_f_ 4. intramuscular
_g_ 5. subcutaneous

A. Study of the movement of drugs in the body as they are absorbed, distributed, metabolized, and excreted

B. Administration route that injects the drug directly into the bloodstream

_b_ 6. intravenous

_h_ 7. topical

C. Liquid drugs administered into the body by a subcutaneous, intramuscular, or intravenous route

D. Route of administration of a drug that involves injecting it directly into the skin

E. Administration of a drug that melts at body temperature

F. Route of administration of a drug that involves the injection of small quantities into a muscle

G. Administration of a drug by injection into the fatty tissue beneath the skin

H. Administration of a drug through a surface membrane, such as the skin or a mucous membrane

Matching Items

Match each of the terms in the left column with the BEST definition in the right column by placing the letter of that definition in the space next to the term. Each definition may be used once or not at all.

_g_ 8. syrup

_L_ 9. emulsion

_o_ 10. aqueous solution

_J_ 11. magma

_M_ 12. spirit

_P_ 13. elixir

_N_ 14. tincture

_D_ 15. extract

_H_ 16. liniment

_K_ 17. lotion

_E_ 18. ointment

_I_ 19. capsule

_F_ 20. tablet

_B_ 21. pill

_Q_ 22. suppository

_A_ 23. powder

A. Finely divided or ground drug mixture that is solid and dry

B. Mixture of a drug with some cohesive material, which is then molded into a form convenient for swallowing

C. Alcoholic extracts of vegetable drugs and contain 1 gram of drug per milliliter of solution

D. Active ingredient of animal or vegetable drug; may be liquid or powder

E. Semisolid medication in a petroleum or lanolin base for prolonged contact with the skin

F. Powdered drug formed into small disk

G. Aqueous solution of 85% sucrose

H. Suspension that contains oil, soap, water, or alcohol designed for external application to the skin by rubbing

I. Made from a gelatin container designed to dissolve quickly in the stomach

J. Bulky suspension of insoluble preparation in water

K. Liquid preparation designed for external application

L. Suspension of fats or oils in water with an emulsifying agent that keeps it in solution

M. Concentrated alcoholic solution of volatile substance; also called essence

N. Chemical and plant substances dissolved in an alcoholic solution

O. Drug or combination of drugs dissolved in water

P. Alcoholic preparation that has been sweetened and is used to act as a vehicle for other medications

Q. Mixture of a drug in a firm base that melts at body temperature

STUDY GUIDE ASSIGNMENT 12-3

- Forms of Drugs
- Drug Pharmacokinetics
- Drug Pharmacodynamics

Reading Assignment: pages 209-219

Multiple-Choice Items

Read each question carefully. For each item, select the answer that BEST completes the statement or answers the question, and place the letter of that answer in the space provided.

___d___ 1. A drug that is dissolved in water is known as a(an):
  a. emulsion.
  b. fluid extract.
  c. aqueous suspension.
  d. aqueous solution.

___d___ 2. Which of the following statements is NOT true about oral administration of a drug?
  a. It is generally the most popular method.
  b. Most drugs are efficiently absorbed from the gastrointestinal tract.
  c. Dosages often must be lower than if they were administered by another route.
  d. Plasma drug levels peak rapidly and then fall off.

___b___ 3. The primary parenteral administration route for drug administration by paramedics is generally:
  a. intradermal.
  b. intravenous.
  c. intramuscular.
  d. subcutaneous.

___d___ 4. If peripheral IV access is impossible, which of the following drugs can be given via the tracheal route?
  a. Epinephrine
  b. Lidocaine
  c. Narcan
  d. All of the above

_b_ 5. If two drugs given to a patient have an affinity for the same proteins, a large displacement of drug may occur, causing more drug to be free and to act on receptors. This action is known as:
   a. antagonism.
   b. synergism.
   c. adrenergic.
   d. potentiation.

_a_ 6. The _____ is highly selective and not all drugs are allowed to cross it. It prevents many drugs from leaving the blood and crossing the cerebrospinal fluid into the brain.
   a. blood-brain barrier
   b. corpus callosum
   c. cerebral cortex
   d. hypothalamus

_a_ 7. Which of the following statements is NOT true about drug metabolism?
   a. The primary organ used in metabolism is the kidney.
   b. Microsomes begin to react by metabolizing the drug into components capable of being excreted.
   c. Increased production of the microsomes occurs to manage the increased drug exposure.
   d. When exposure to the drug ceases, the number of microsomal structures declines.

_d_ 8. Receptors may be occupied or blocked by substances called:
   a. adrenergics.
   b. synaptic bridges.
   c. agonists.
   d. antagonists.

_b_ 9. Which of the following is NOT an effect of sympathetic stimulation?
   a. Increased heart rate
   b. Bronchiole constriction
   c. Increased metabolism
   d. All of the above; that is, all ARE effects of sympathetic stimulation

_d_ 10. When β_1 adrenergic receptors are stimulated, they cause an increase in the heart's:
   a. inotropic effect.
   b. chronotropic effect.
   c. dromotropic effect.
   d. all of the above.

_a_ 11. _____ is an almost pure β agent and causes vasodilation, bronchodilation, and increased heart inotropic and chronotropic effects. It is a drug used in the prehospital setting as a chemical pacemaker.
   a. Isoproterenol
   b. Dobutamine
   c. Propranolol
   d. Norepinephrine

_d_ 12. Acetylcholine breakdown can be inhibited by which of the following?
   a. Organophosphate poisoning
   b. Physostigmine
   c. Endrophonium
   d. All of the above

STUDY GUIDE ASSIGNMENT 12-4

- Calculating Drug Dosages
- Drug Administration

Reading Assignment: pages 219-260

Multiple-Choice Items

Read each question carefully. For each item, select the answer that BEST completes the statement or answers the question, and place the letter of that answer in the space provided.

_____ 1. A tablespoon is equal to _____ mL.
   a. 5
   b. 15
   c. 30
   d. 60

_____ 2. A patient weighs 215 pounds, which equals _____ kilograms.
   a. 86
   b. 96
   c. 98
   d. 103

_____ 3. Addition: 5.1 + 8.25 + 3.006
   a. 4.341
   b. 11.766
   c. 16.032
   d. 16.356

_____ 4. Subtraction: 52.7 - 23.81
   a. 18.54
   b. 28.26
   c. 28.89
   d. 28.90

_____ 5. Multiplication: 7.5 X 125
   a. 166
   b. 937.5
   c. 950
   d. 9375

_____ 6.   Division: 7.8 divided by 0.25
   a.   .32
   b.   3.125
   c.   31.2
   d.   312.0

_____ 7.   You receive an order to administer Valium 2.5 mg from a syringe that contains 10 mg in 2 mL. The delivered dose will be:
   a.   0.50 mL.
   b.   1.0l mL.
   c.   1.5l mg.
   d.   2.0l mg.

_____ 8.   You receive an order to give a 50-mg bolus of lidocaine from a syringe that contains 100 mg in 10 mL. The delivered dose will be:
   a.   0.50 mL.
   b.   2.5l mg.
   c.   5.00 mL.
   d.   7.5l mg.

_____ 9.   ou receive an order to administer lidocaine at 4 mg/minute; the premixed bag contains 2 g in 500 mL D$_5$W. How many drops per microgtt/minute do you give?
   a.   15
   b.   30
   c.   60
   d.   120

_____ 10.   Because of the decreased absorption from muscle in low-perfusion states, the preferred method of administering medication is through the _____ route.
   a.   intradermal
   b.   intramuscular
   c.   subcutaneous
   d.   intravenous

_____ 11.   During a subcutaneous injection, the needle penetrates the skin at a ____ degree angle.
   a.   30
   b.   45
   c.   55
   d.   90

_____ 12.   Indications for intraosseous infusion may include which of the following?
   a.   Cardiac arrest
   b.   Shock
   c.   Extensive burns
   d.   All of the above

STUDY GUIDE ASSIGNMENT 12-5

Performance Checklist: Intradermal Injection
Performance Checklist: Subcutaneous Injection
Performance Checklist: Intramuscular Injection
Performance Checklist: Peripheral Venipuncture
Performance Checklist: Central Line Placement (Femoral)
Performance Checklist: Central Line Placement (Internal Jugular, Anterior Approach)
Performance Checklist: Central Line Placement (Internal Jugular, Middle Approach)
Performance Checklist: Central Line Placement (Internal Jugular, Posterior Approach)
Performance Checklist: Central Line Placement (Subclavian Approach)
Performance Checklist: Intraosseous Infusion

The following skills should be practiced until you reach competency. Practice can be done in classroom settings using manikins, or in clinical rotations in the hospital or out on the ambulance or rescue unit. You may evaluate yourself, work with another student, or have a preceptor or instructor evaluate you using these forms.

Instructions

1. Place a check mark in the "C" ("competent") column if you used the recommended technique the first time you performed each activity.
2. Place a check mark in the "A" ("acceptable") column if you used the recommended technique but it took you several times to perform each activity.
3. Place a check mark in the "U" ("unsatisfactory") column if you used some but not all of each recommended technique.
4. Place a check mark in the "NP" ("not performed") column if you forgot to perform that particular technique.
5. The section for comments provides space to make notes about what further practice you need, what errors you made, how you can improve your skill, and so on.

Performance Checklist: Intradermal Injection

C	A	U	NP	C = competent; A = acceptable; U = unsatisfactory; NP = not performed
☐	☐	☐	☐	Check responsiveness
☐	☐	☐	☐	Check airway
☐	☐	☐	☐	Check breathing
☐	☐	☐	☐	Check circulation
☐	☐	☐	☐	Confirm and review the medication order
☐	☐	☐	☐	Explain procedure to patient
☐	☐	☐	☐	Check for patient allergies
☐	☐	☐	☐	Assemble and check:

Primary equipment
- Medication
- 3-mL syringe
- 25-gauge needle

Accessory equipment and supplies
- Antiseptic swabs
- Gloves

C	A	U	NP	
☐	☐	☐	☐	Select the injection site
☐	☐	☐	☐	Prepare the injection site
☐	☐	☐	☐	Insert the needle
☐	☐	☐	☐	Perform the injection
☐	☐	☐	☐	Dispose of the needle

OUTCOME:　　☐ Pass　　　☐ Fail　　　☐ Retest

Comments:

Student's Signature _____ Date _____

Instructor's Signature _____ Date _____

Performance Checklist: Subcutaneous Injection

C	A	U	NP	C = competent; A = acceptable; U = unsatisfactory; NP = not performed
☐	☐	☐	☐	Check responsiveness
☐	☐	☐	☐	Check airway
☐	☐	☐	☐	Check breathing
☐	☐	☐	☐	Check circulation
☐	☐	☐	☐	Confirm and review the medication order
☐	☐	☐	☐	Explain procedure to patient
☐	☐	☐	☐	Check for patient allergies
☐	☐	☐	☐	Assemble and check:

Primary equipment
- Medication
- 3-mL syringe
- 25-gauge needle

Accessory equipment and supplies
- Antiseptic swabs
- Gloves

C	A	U	NP	
☐	☐	☐	☐	Select the injection site
☐	☐	☐	☐	Prepare the injection site
☐	☐	☐	☐	Insert the needle
☐	☐	☐	☐	Pull back on the plunger
☐	☐	☐	☐	Withdraw needle if blood vessel was entered
☐	☐	☐	☐	Perform the injection
☐	☐	☐	☐	Gently massage area
☐	☐	☐	☐	Dispose of the needle

OUTCOME: ☐ Pass   ☐ Fail   ☐ Retest

Comments:

Student's Signature _____ Date _____

Instructor's Signature _____ Date _____

Performance Checklist: Intramuscular Injection

C	A	U	NP	C = competent; A = acceptable; U = unsatisfactory; NP = not performed
☐	☐	☐	☐	Check responsiveness
☐	☐	☐	☐	Check airway
☐	☐	☐	☐	Check breathing
☐	☐	☐	☐	Check circulation
☐	☐	☐	☐	Confirm and review the medication order
☐	☐	☐	☐	Explain procedure to patient
☐	☐	☐	☐	Check for patient allergies
☐	☐	☐	☐	Assemble and check:

Primary equipment	*Accessory equipment and supplies*
▪ Medication	▪ Antiseptic swabs
▪ Syringe	▪ Gloves
▪ Needle	

C	A	U	NP	
☐	☐	☐	☐	Select the injection site
☐	☐	☐	☐	Prepare the injection site
☐	☐	☐	☐	Insert the needle
☐	☐	☐	☐	Pull back on the plunger
☐	☐	☐	☐	Withdraw needle if blood vessel was entered
☐	☐	☐	☐	Perform the injection
☐	☐	☐	☐	Gently massage area
☐	☐	☐	☐	Dispose of the needle

OUTCOME: ☐ Pass   ☐ Fail   ☐ Retest

Comments:

Student's Signature _____ Date _____

Instructor's Signature _____ Date _____

Performance Checklist: Peripheral Venipuncture

C	A	U	NP	C = competent; A = acceptable; U = unsatisfactory; NP = not performed
☐	☐	☐	☐	Check responsiveness
☐	☐	☐	☐	Check airway
☐	☐	☐	☐	Check breathing
☐	☐	☐	☐	Check circulation
☐	☐	☐	☐	Explain procedure to patient
☐	☐	☐	☐	Assemble and check:

Primary equipment	*Accessory equipment and supplies*
■ Intravenous (IV) solution	■ Antiseptic swabs
■ IV tubing and administration set	■ Tape
■ IV catheter	■ Sterile gauze squares
■ Tourniquet	■ Syringe
	■ Gloves

C	A	U	NP	
☐	☐	☐	☐	Apply tourniquet
☐	☐	☐	☐	Select the injection site
☐	☐	☐	☐	Prepare the injection site
☐	☐	☐	☐	Insert the needle
☐	☐	☐	☐	Thread catheter into the vein
☐	☐	☐	☐	Withdraw the needle
☐	☐	☐	☐	Release tourniquet
☐	☐	☐	☐	Start fluid flow
☐	☐	☐	☐	Reattempt venipuncture as appropriate
☐	☐	☐	☐	Secure the catheter
☐	☐	☐	☐	Adjust flow rate
☐	☐	☐	☐	Dispose of the needle

OUTCOME: ☐ Pass   ☐ Fail   ☐ Retest

Comments:

Student's Signature _____ Date _____

Instructor's Signature _____ Date _____

Performance Checklist: Central Line Placement (Femoral)

C	A	U	NP	C = competent; A = acceptable; U = unsatisfactory; NP = not performed
☐	☐	☐	☐	Check responsiveness
☐	☐	☐	☐	Check airway
☐	☐	☐	☐	Check breathing
☐	☐	☐	☐	Check circulation
☐	☐	☐	☐	Assess need for central line
☐	☐	☐	☐	Assemble and check:

Primary equipment	*Accessory equipment and supplies*
▪ Intravenous (IV) solution	▪ Antiseptic swabs
▪ IV tubing and administration set	▪ Sterile gauze squares
▪ 16-gauge catheter	▪ Tape
▪ 10-mL syringe	▪ Protective eye wear
	▪ Mask
	▪ Gloves

C	A	U	NP	
☐	☐	☐	☐	Position the patient
☐	☐	☐	☐	Locate the femoral artery
☐	☐	☐	☐	Prepare the selected site
☐	☐	☐	☐	Insert the needle
☐	☐	☐	☐	Aspirate the syringe
☐	☐	☐	☐	Withdraw needle if femoral artery has been entered
☐	☐	☐	☐	Start fluid flow
☐	☐	☐	☐	Adjust flow rate
☐	☐	☐	☐	Secure the catheter
☐	☐	☐	☐	Dispose of the needle

OUTCOME: ☐ Pass   ☐ Fail   ☐ Retest

Comments:

Student's Signature _____ Date _____

Instructor's Signature _____ Date _____

Performance Checklist: Central Line Placement
(Internal Jugular, Anterior Approach)

C	A	U	NP	C = competent; A = acceptable; U = unsatisfactory; NP = not performed
☐	☐	☐	☐	Check responsiveness
☐	☐	☐	☐	Check airway
☐	☐	☐	☐	Check breathing
☐	☐	☐	☐	Check circulation
☐	☐	☐	☐	Assess need for central line
☐	☐	☐	☐	Assemble and check:

Primary equipment
- Intravenous (IV) solution
- IV tubing and administration set
- 16-gauge catheter
- 10-mL syringe

Accessory equipment and supplies
- Antiseptic swabs
- Sterile gauze squares
- Tape
- Protective eye wear
- Mask
- Gloves

C	A	U	NP	
☐	☐	☐	☐	Position the patient
☐	☐	☐	☐	Find landmarks for venipuncture
☐	☐	☐	☐	Prepare the selected site
☐	☐	☐	☐	Insert the needle
☐	☐	☐	☐	Aspirate the syringe
☐	☐	☐	☐	Start fluid flow
☐	☐	☐	☐	Adjust flow rate
☐	☐	☐	☐	Secure the catheter
☐	☐	☐	☐	Dispose of the needle

OUTCOME: ☐ Pass ☐ Fail ☐ Retest

Comments:

Student's Signature _____ Date _____

Instructor's Signature _____ Date _____

86

Performance Checklist: Central Line Placement
(Internal Jugular, Middle Approach)

C	A	U	NP	C = competent; A = acceptable; U = unsatisfactory; NP = not performed
☐	☐	☐	☐	Check responsiveness
☐	☐	☐	☐	Check airway
☐	☐	☐	☐	Check breathing
☐	☐	☐	☐	Check circulation
☐	☐	☐	☐	Assess need for central line
☐	☐	☐	☐	Assemble and check:

Primary equipment
- Intravenous (IV) solution
- IV tubing and administration set
- 16-gauge catheter
- 10-mL syringe

Accessory equipment and supplies
- Antiseptic swabs
- Sterile gauze squares
- Tape
- Protective eye wear
- Mask
- Gloves

C	A	U	NP	
☐	☐	☐	☐	Position the patient
☐	☐	☐	☐	Find landmarks for venipuncture
☐	☐	☐	☐	Prepare the selected site
☐	☐	☐	☐	Insert the needle
☐	☐	☐	☐	Aspirate the syringe
☐	☐	☐	☐	Start fluid flow
☐	☐	☐	☐	Adjust flow rate
☐	☐	☐	☐	Secure the catheter
☐	☐	☐	☐	Dispose of the needle

OUTCOME:　　☐ Pass　　　　☐ Fail　　　　☐ Retest

Comments:

Student's Signature _____ Date _____

Instructor's Signature _____ Date _____

Performance Checklist: Central Line Placement
(Internal Jugular, Posterior Approach)

C	A	U	NP	C = competent; A = acceptable; U = unsatisfactory; NP = not performed
☐	☐	☐	☐	Check responsiveness
☐	☐	☐	☐	Check airway
☐	☐	☐	☐	Check breathing
☐	☐	☐	☐	Check circulation
☐	☐	☐	☐	Assess need for central line
☐	☐	☐	☐	Assemble and check:

Primary equipment
- Intravenous (IV) solution
- IV tubing and administration set
- 16-gauge catheter
- 10-mL syringe

Accessory equipment and supplies
- Antiseptic swabs
- Sterile gauze squares
- Tape
- Protective eye wear
- Mask
- Gloves

C	A	U	NP	
☐	☐	☐	☐	Position the patient
☐	☐	☐	☐	Find landmarks for venipuncture
☐	☐	☐	☐	Prepare the selected site
☐	☐	☐	☐	Insert the needle
☐	☐	☐	☐	Aspirate the syringe
☐	☐	☐	☐	Start fluid flow
☐	☐	☐	☐	Adjust flow rate
☐	☐	☐	☐	Secure the catheter
☐	☐	☐	☐	Dispose of the needle

OUTCOME: ☐ Pass ☐ Fail ☐ Retest

Comments:

Student's Signature _____ Date _____

Instructor's Signature _____ Date _____

90

Performance Checklist: Central Line Placement
(Subclavian Approach)

C	A	U	NP	C = competent; A = acceptable; U = unsatisfactory; NP = not performed
☐	☐	☐	☐	Check responsiveness
☐	☐	☐	☐	Check airway
☐	☐	☐	☐	Check breathing
☐	☐	☐	☐	Check circulation
☐	☐	☐	☐	Assess need for central line
☐	☐	☐	☐	Assemble and check:

Primary equipment
- Intravenous (IV) solution
- IV tubing and administration set
- 16-gauge catheter
- 10-mL syringe

Accessory equipment and supplies
- Antiseptic swabs
- Sterile gauze squares
- Tape
- Protective eye wear
- Mask
- Gloves

C	A	U	NP	
☐	☐	☐	☐	Position the patient
☐	☐	☐	☐	Find landmarks for venipuncture
☐	☐	☐	☐	Prepare the selected site
☐	☐	☐	☐	Insert the needle
☐	☐	☐	☐	Aspirate the syringe
☐	☐	☐	☐	Start fluid flow
☐	☐	☐	☐	Adjust flow rate
☐	☐	☐	☐	Secure the catheter
☐	☐	☐	☐	Dispose of the needle

OUTCOME: ☐ Pass   ☐ Fail   ☐ Retest

Comments:

Student's Signature _____ Date _____

Instructor's Signature _____ Date _____

Performance Checklist: Intraosseous Infusion

C	A	U	NP	C = competent; A = acceptable; U = unsatisfactory; NP = not performed
☐	☐	☐	☐	Check responsiveness
☐	☐	☐	☐	Check airway
☐	☐	☐	☐	Check breathing
☐	☐	☐	☐	Check circulation
☐	☐	☐	☐	Assess need for intraosseous infusion
☐	☐	☐	☐	Assemble and check:

Primary equipment
- Intravenous (IV) solution
- IV tubing and administration set
- Rigid spinal needle with stylet or intraosseous needle
- 10-mL syringe filled with sterile saline

Accessory equipment and supplies
- Antiseptic swabs
- Tape
- Sterile gauze squares
- Protective eye wear
- Mask
- Gloves

C	A	U	NP	
☐	☐	☐	☐	Position the patient
☐	☐	☐	☐	Find landmarks for needle insertion
☐	☐	☐	☐	Prepare the site
☐	☐	☐	☐	Insert the needle
☐	☐	☐	☐	Aspirate the syringe
☐	☐	☐	☐	Start fluid flow
☐	☐	☐	☐	Adjust flow rate
☐	☐	☐	☐	Secure the needle
☐	☐	☐	☐	Dispose of the needle

OUTCOME: ☐ Pass   ☐ Fail   ☐ Retest

Comments:

Student's Signature _____ Date _____

Instructor's Signature _____ Date _____

CHAPTER 13

Kinematics of Trauma

STUDY GUIDE ASSIGNMENT 13-1

■ Physics
Reading Assignment: pages 264-268

Matching Items

Match each of the terms in the left column with the BEST definition in the right column by placing the letter of that definition in the space next to the term. Each definition may be used once or not at all.

C	1.	kinematics
F	2.	Conservation of Energy law
G	3.	Newton's first law of motion
A	4.	Newton's second law of motion
D	5.	force
K	6.	mass
H	7.	acceleration
J	8.	deceleration
E	9.	kinetic energy
B	10.	velocity

A. The force of an object is equal to its mass multiplied by its acceleration

B. Speed

C. The science of motion that involves the transfer of energy from an external source to a victim's body

D. Equal to an object's mass multiplied by its acceleration

E. The energy of motion

F. Energy can be neither created nor destroyed, but its form can be changed

G. A body, whether in motion or at rest, remains in that state until acted on by an outside force

H. Change in velocity

I. Energy can be both created and destroyed

J. Force applied to a moving body to stop or reduce its motion

K. Weight

Matching Items

Match each of the terms in the left column with the BEST definition in the right column by placing the letter of that definition in the space next to the term. Each definition may be used once or not at all.

D	11.	energy exchange
G	12.	density
C	13.	blunt trauma
A	14.	penetrating trauma

A. Type of impact to tissue that causes it to move in a lateral direction away from the penetrating instrument, creating a cavity in the tissue

B. Number of particles in one square meter

F ___ 15. permanent cavity
E ___ 16. temporary cavity

C. Type of impact to tissue that causes it to move in an anterior-posterior direction consistent with the angle of impact

D. The loss of velocity or energy by one body to another

E. Shortly after impact, tissues move back to their original position

F. A permanent hole; its size depends on the elasticity of the damaged tissue

G. Number of particles per unit of volume

STUDY GUIDE ASSIGNMENT 13-2

- Penetrating Trauma
- Blunt Trauma

Reading Assignment: pages 268-283

Matching Items

Match each of the terms in the left column with the BEST definition in the right column by placing the letter of that definition in the space next to the term. Each definition may be used once or not at all.

F ___ 1. blast
B ___ 2. cavitation
G ___ 3. fragmentation
H ___ 4. malleability
D ___ 5. momentum
I ___ 6. pressure waves
C ___ 7. profile
A ___ 8. whiplash

A. Severe cervical strain

B. Created by the acceleration of tissue particles away from the pathway of the missile

C. Frontal area

D. Motion

E. Severe lumbar pain

F. An explosive force

G. When a bullet breaks into several parts

H. The ability of a projectile to change shape

I. Waves that radiate outward from a blast

Multiple-Choice Items

Read each question carefully. For each item, select the answer that BEST completes the statement or answers the question, and place the letter of that answer in the space provided.

_b_ 1. In penetrating trauma, all of the following are factors that affect the frontal area of the penetrating object:
    I. size of the penetrating object.
    II. tumble or rotation of the missile.
    III. direction of travel.
    IV. fragmentation of the missile.
        a. I and II
        b. I, II, and IV
        c. I, III, and IV
        d. I, II, III, and IV

_b_ 2. Penetrating trauma fragmentation:
    a. decreases the frontal area.
    b. increases the frontal area.
    c. does not change the frontal area.
    d. changes the speed of the missile.

_a_ 3. Examples of low-energy weapons in penetrating trauma include all of the following:
    I. ice pick.
    II. knife.
    III. needle.
    IV. handgun.
        a. I, II, and III
        b. I, II and IV
        c. I and IV
        d. I, II, III, and IV

_d_ 4. Mechanism of injury is an important consideration because:
    a. this information helps the paramedic focus on the initial assessment.
    b. it will provide valuable information to subsequent caregivers.
    c. it can help the paramedic reconstruct the incident.
    d. all of the above.

_c_ 5. The crashes involved in an automotive accident include the:
    I. car.
    II. rebound.
    III. occupants.
    IV. internal organs.
        a. I and III
        b. I and IV
        c. I, III, and IV
        d. I, II, III, and IV

_a_ 6. The most common site of injury in automotive accidents involving unrestrained occupants is the:
   a. head.
   b. thorax.
   c. abdomen.
   d. long bones.

_c_ 7. The five patterns of collisions are:
   a. frontal, rear-end, torsional, flexion, and passive.
   b. frontal, rear-end, lateral, torsional, and suspended.
   c. frontal, rear-end, lateral, rotational, and rollover.
   d. frontal, rear-end, rotational, passive and torsional.

_a_ 8. In frontal collisions, the unrestrained occupant's body can follow one of two pathways. These are:
   a. down-and-under, and up-and-over.
   b. up-and-over, and flexion.
   c. flexion and extension.
   d. forward and rearward.

_c_ 9. In rear-end collisions the most common injury is to the:
   a. chest.
   b. abdomen.
   c. cervical spine.
   d. lower extremities.

_c_ 10. The stages of the pedestrian-car collision include the:
   I. car-body impact.
   II. body-to-car hood thrust.
   III. body-to-ground fall.
   IV. body-tire impact.
      a. I, II, and IV
      b. I and IV
      c. I, II, and III
      d. I, II, III, and IV

_c_ 11. In a child involved in a pedestrian-car collision, the injury is:
   a. likely to be posterior.
   b. likely to be lateral.
   c. likely to be frontal.
   d. unlikely to involve one portion of the body over another.

_b_ 12. In motorcycle accidents the four types of collisions are:
   a. head-on, angular, frontal, and ejection.
   b. head-on, angular, ejection, and laying the bike down.
   c. head-on, angular, rear-end, and laying the bike down.
   d. head-on, angular, rear-end, and ejection.

_a_ 13. In sports injuries, cervical compression and vertebral fractures may be due to all of the following EXCEPT:
- a. rotation.
- b. hyperextension.
- c. hyperflexion.
- d. lateral flexion.

_c_ 14. In rapid-deceleration injuries, the organ(s) in the thorax most likely to be injured is(are) the:
- a. lungs.
- b. heart.
- c. aorta.
- d. trachea.

_d_ 15. In rapid-deceleration injuries of the liver, the cause of a resulting laceration is the:
- a. ligamentum arteriosum.
- b. ligamentum diverticulum.
- c. ligamentum porticum.
- d. ligamentum teres.

_a_ 16. In explosions the energy is converted into:
- a. light, heat, and pressure.
- b. light, heat, and sound.
- c. heat, sound, and force.
- d. heat, velocity, and force.

_c_ 17. The extent of damage from a blast depends on the:
- a. force and direction of travel.
- b. force and velocity.
- c. force and distance between the blast and the individual.
- d. force and the time.

CHAPTER 14

Soft-Tissue and Burn Injuries

STUDY GUIDE ASSIGNMENT 14-1

- Anatomy and Physiology of the Skin
- Soft-Tissue Injuries

Reading Assignment: pages 286-292

Matching Items

Match each of the terms in the left column with the BEST definition in the right column by placing the letter of that definition in the space next to the term. Each definition may be used once or not at all.

D 1. epidermis
A 2. melanin
F 3. dermis
J 4. ecchymosis
B 5. hematoma
H 6. abrasion
I 7. laceration
G 8. avulsion
C 9. amputation

A. Agent responsible for skin pigmentation

B. Blood clot that forms at the site of an injury

C. Removal of a limb or any appendage of the body

D. Outer, thinner layer of skin; the body's first line of defense against the external environment

E. Subcutaneous layer of the skin

F. Thick layer of dense, fibrous connective tissue that lies beneath the epidermis

G. The tearing loose of a flap of skin, which may either remain hanging or tear off altogether

H. A scratching of the skin surface without penetration of all layers of the skin

I. Jagged wound that bleeds freely and is the result of snagging or tearing of tissues

J. Characteristic black and blue mark

Multiple-Choice Items

Read each question carefully. For each item, select the answer that BEST completes the statement or answers the question, and place the letter of that answer in the space provided.

a 1. A wound is defined as:
   a. a traumatically induced injury that disrupts normal continuity of the tissue, organ, or bone affected.
   b. an injury to the tissues.
   c. a disruption in function.
   d. an alteration in the integrity of a body part.

_d_ 2. Types of closed wounds include:
   a. contusions.
   b. hematomas.
   c. crush injuries.
   d. all of the above.

_b_ 3. Ecchymosis is caused by:
   a. edema.
   b. blood accumulation resulting in a black and blue mark.
   c. migration of white blood cells into the affected area.
   d. cell destruction due to trauma.

_d_ 4. Open wounds that should result in the transport of the patient include wounds:
   a. that have spurted blood.
   b. with embedded or impaled objects.
   c. inflicted by a human or animal bite.
   d. all of the above.

_c_ 5. An abrasion is defined as a:
   a. tearing of the tissue that leaves a jagged wound.
   b. wound that penetrates through all layers of the skin.
   c. scratching of the skin surface without penetration of all layers of the skin.
   d. tearing loose of a flap of skin.

_a_ 6. Tetanus may be a serious complication of any open soft-tissue injury and is caused by a:
   a. soil bacterium.
   b. virus.
   c. parasite.
   d. none of the above.

_c_ 7. When dealing with an avulsion in which the flap is still attached, the paramedic should:
   a. remove the flap and dress it with a sterile dressing.
   b. remove the flap and place it in a moist gauze pad.
   c. align the flap in its normal position and dress the wound.
   d. disregard the flap and treat the avulsion just like any other injury.

_c_ 8. The three general types of amputations are:
   a. complete, partial, and near-complete.
   b. complete, degloving, and avulsed.
   c. complete, partial, and degloving.
   d. complete, near-complete, and degloving.

_d_ 9. A _____ amputation results in less bleeding than the other types.
   a. partial
   b. near-complete
   c. degloving
   d. complete

_c_ 10. When dealing with an amputated body part, the paramedic should:
   I. rinse the part with a saline solution and then dry it.
   II. wrap the part in dry sterile gauze.
   III. cover the open end with a saline-soaked sponge.

IV. place the part in dry ice.
V. place the part in a plastic bag.
  a. I, II, and III
  b. I, II, and IV
  c. I, II, III, and V
  d. I, II, III, IV, and V

_a_ 11. The only time an impaled object should be removed is when:
  a. it causes an airway compromise.
  b. it is difficult to deal with.
  c. the patient is uncomfortable.
  d. none of these; impaled objects should NEVER be removed.

STUDY GUIDE ASSIGNMENT 14-2

■1 Burn Injuries
Reading Assignment: pages 292-302

Matching Items

Match each of the terms in the left column with the BEST definition in the right column by placing the letter of that definition in the space next to the term. Each definition may be used once or not at all.

_C_ 1. thermal burn
_B_ 2. electrical burn
_G_ 3. chemical burn
_F_ 4. radiation burn
_D_ 5. superficial burn
_E_ 6. partial-thickness burn
_A_ 7. full-thickness burn

A. Characterized by destruction of both epidermis and dermis

B. Caused by contact with low- or high-voltage electricity

C. Results from heat conducted by hot liquids, solids, and super-heated gases, as well as a flame burn that results from fire

D. Confined to the epidermal layers of the skin

E. Involves the deep epidermal layers of the skin and always causes injury to the upper layers of the dermis

F. Occurs from overexposure to ultraviolet light or from the heat of an atomic explosion

G. Results from wet or dry corrosive substances coming in contact with the skin

H. Determines what percent of the body is burned

Multiple-Choice Items

Read each question carefully. For each item, select the answer that BEST completes the statement or answers the question, and place the letter of that answer in the space provided.

_b_ 1. The four major sources of burn injuries are:
  a. thermal, electrical, chemical, and liquid.
  b. thermal, electrical, chemical, and radiation.

c. thermal, electrical, liquid, and radiation.

d. thermal, electrical, liquid, and flash.

_d_ 2. The three classifications of injuries in burns are:

a. full-thickness, dermal, and partial-thickness.

b. dermal, partial-thickness, and superficial.

c. superficial, dermal, and full-thickness.

d. superficial, partial-thickness, and full-thickness.

_a_ 3. The rule of palms, used in determining the extent of body surface area burned, assumes that the palm of the patient represents _____ percent.

a. 1

b. 2

c. 3

d. 4

_d_ 4. The severity of injury is determined by the depth and extent of the burn as well as by the:

a. location of the burn.

b. age of the patient.

c. general health of the patient.

d. all of the above.

_c_ 5. The age of the patient is an important factor in determining outcome. Those patients whose age is of greatest concern are:

a. the very young, under 5 years.

b. the very old, over 60 years.

c. both the very young and the very old.

d. those patients between the ages of 5 and 34 years.

_c_ 6. Carbon monoxide's affinity for hemoglobin is _____ times greater than that of oxygen:

a. 2

b. 20

c. 200

d. 2000

_b_ 7. Early signs and symptoms of carbon monoxide poisoning include:

a. headache, coma, and seizures.

b. headache, nausea, and loss of manual dexterity.

c. headache, paralysis, and arrhythmias.

d. headache, seizures, and cardiac arrest.

_b_ 8. In patients with smoke inhalation the signs include:

I. hoarseness.

II. cough.

III. singed nasal hair.

IV. labored breathing.

V. blisters around the mouth.

a. I, II, and IV

b. I, II, III, and V

c. I, II, III, and IV

d. I, II, III, IV, and V

a 9. The MOST important aspect of the scene survey is:
   a. to assess potential hazards to the paramedic.
   b. to ascertain the number of patients involved.
   c. to ascertain the location of all patients and family members.
   d. to determine which hospital patients will be transported to.

d 10. The primary survey includes:
   a. airway, breathing, circulation, and secondary exam.
   b. airway, breathing, circulation, and treatment.
   c. airway, breathing, circulation, and hemorrhage control.
   d. responsiveness, airway, breathing, and circulation.

c 11. In the secondary survey, a medical history includes:
   a. allergies, medications, recent surgeries, and family history.
   b. allergies, hospital preference, and physician's name.
   c. allergies, medications, and past medical history, with events leading up to this incident.
   d. allergies, medications, physician's name, and medical history.

d 12. In the management of thermal burns, the first priority is to:
   a. establish an airway.
   b. administer 100% oxygen.
   c. ensure adequate ventilation.
   d. stop the burning process.

a 13. In treating electrical burns, fluid becomes necessary to:
   a. flush the kidneys of myoglobin.
   b. restore circulating volume because of hypovolemia.
   c. maintain blood pressure.
   d. none of these; fluid is NOT necessary in electrical burns.

c 14. When flushing chemical burns with irrigating solutions, you should:
   a. flush for at least 10 minutes.
   b. flush for at least 15 minutes.
   c. flush for at least 20-30 minutes.
   d. none of these; flushing time is NOT a critical factor.

d 15. The greatest amount of intravascular fluid loss occurs within the first _____ after the burn.
   a. hour
   b. 2 hours
   c. 4 hours
   d. 8 to 12 hours

c 16. The primary goal of fluid resuscitation is to keep the heart rate under:
   a. 80.
   b. 90.
   c. 110.
   d. 130.

CHAPTER 15

Injuries to the Head, Neck, and Spine

STUDY GUIDE ASSIGNMENT 15-1

▪ Injuries to the Head
Reading Assignment: pages 304-318

Matching Items

Match each of the terms in the left column with the **BEST** definition in the right column by placing the letter of that definition in the space next to the term. **Each definition may be used once or not at all.**

D   1.   auricle
L   2.   tympanic membrane
K   3.   eustachian tube
G   4.   cerebrospinal fluid
H   5.   conjunctiva
I   6.   iris
F   7.   lens
A   8.   retina
C   9.   lacrimal gland
E   10.   sebaceous gland
B   11.   cribriform plate

A.   Innermost layer of the eye that has specialized nerve cells sensitive to light and color

B.   Portion of the ethmoid bone that separates the roof of the nose from the cranial cavity

C.   Tear gland

D.   Skin-covered cartilaginous framework that projects from the head and is part of the outer ear

E.   Oil-secreting gland of the skin

F.   Structure behind the iris that changes shape to focus light rays on the back of the eye

G.   Thin, watery liquid found in the subarachnoid space and spinal column

H.   Paper-thin covering that lines the exposed portion of the white part of the eye

I.   Colored portion of the eye

J.   White part of the eye

K.   Allows air to pass into or out of the middle ear and leads to the upper part of the throat

L.   Eardrum

Matching Items

Match each of the terms in the left column with the BEST definition in the right column by placing the letter of that definition in the space next to the term. **Each definition may be used once or not at all.**

E 12. reticular activating system
J 13. Cushing's triad
R 14. cerebral herniation
D 15. transtentorial herniation
I 16. decorticate
P 17. decerebrate
C 18. cerebral concussion
Q 19. amnesia
N 20. cerebral contusion
B 21. depressed skull fracture
G 22. basilar skull fracture
K 23. raccoon's eyes
A 24. Battle's sign
L 25. epidural hematoma
O 26. subdural hematoma
F 27. subarachnoid hemorrhage
H 28. intracerebral hemorrhage

A. Discoloration behind the ears

B. Fracture in which bone fragments are driven into the brain

C. Transient episode of neuronal dysfunction after a violent jar or shock to the brain, with a rapid return to normal neurologic activity

D. Occurs when the falx cerebri is displaced

E. Functions in general wakefulness and causes awakening from deep sleep

F. Bleeding that occurs between the arachnoid membrane and the pia mater

G. Results from the extension of linear fractures onto the floor of the skull

H. Occurs from bleeding within the brain itself

I. Flexion of the upper extremities with the lower extremities rigid and extended

J. Threefold phenomenon associated with increasing intracranial pressure

K. Typical appearance when blood travels into the periorbital subcutaneous tissue

L. Bleeding that occurs because the meningeal arteries are torn

M. Extension of the upper extremities and flexion of the lower extremities

N. Bruising and bleeding of the brain

O. Bleeding that occurs between the dura mater and arachnoid membrane, usually as a result of injury

P. Type of posture in which the upper extremities extend and rotate inward with palms facing lateral, and the lower extremities extend and are rigid

Q. Memory deficit

R. Protrusion of a portion of the brain through an opening in the wall of the cranial cavity

Labeling Items

Read each question carefully and place your answer in the space provided.

1. Label the six structures of the ear identified in the drawing by filling in the blank next to each letter, which corresponds with the same letter in the drawing. The six structures are to be selected from the answers that follow the blanks.

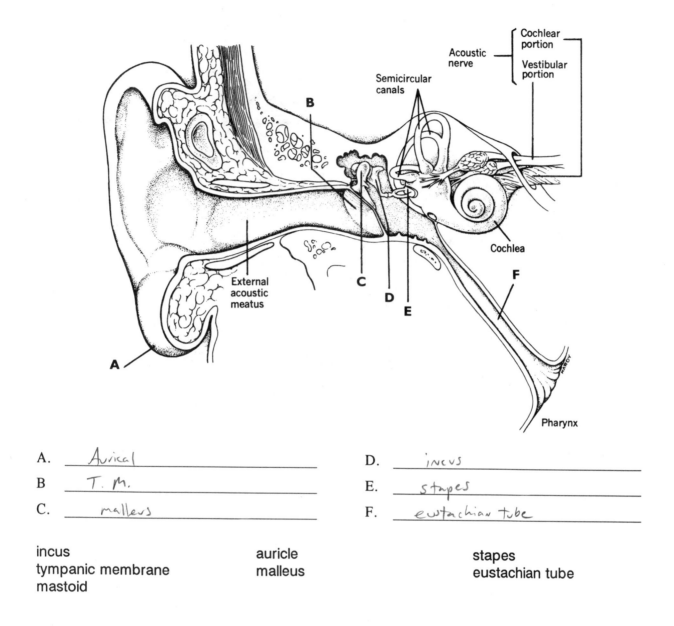

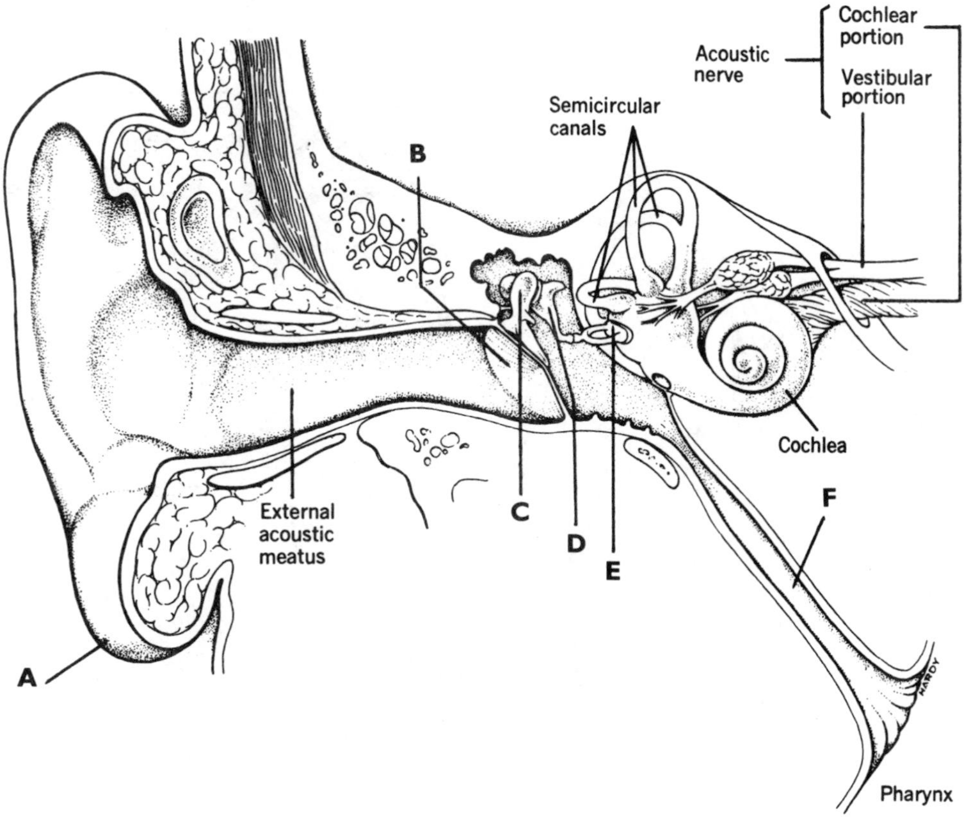
Acoustic nerve
Cochlear portion
Vestibular portion
Semicircular canals
B
External acoustic meatus
C
D
E
Cochlea
F
A
HARDY
Pharynx

A. Aurical

B T. M.

C. malleus

D. incus

E. stapes

F. eustachian tube

incus
tympanic membrane
mastoid
auricle
malleus
stapes
eustachian tube

2. Label the nine structures of the eye identified in the drawing by filling in the blank next to each letter, which corresponds with the same letter in the drawing. The nine structures are to be selected from the answers that follow the blanks.

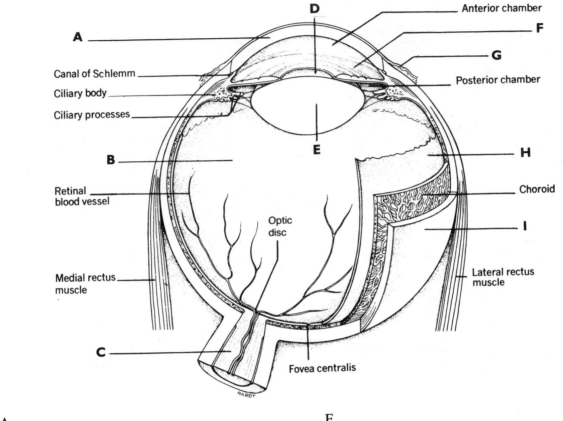

Labels on diagram: A, D, Anterior chamber, F, G, Posterior chamber, Canal of Schlemm, Ciliary body, Ciliary processes, B, E, H, Retinal blood vessel, Optic disc, Choroid, I, Medial rectus muscle, Lateral rectus muscle, C, Fovea centralis, HARDY

A. _____   F. _____

B. _____   G. _____

C. _____   H. _____

D. _____   I. _____

E. _____

pupil   iris   optic nerve
lens   retinal nerve   retina
sclera   cornea   conjunctiva
vitreous body

STUDY GUIDE ASSIGNMENT 15-2

▪ Injuries to the Head
Reading Assignment: pages 304-318

Multiple-Choice Items

Read each question carefully. For each item, select the answer that BEST completes the statement or answers the question, and place the letter of that answer in the space provided.

_d_ 1. Loss of fluid from the ear may indicate:
a. infection.
b. basilar skull fracture.
c. cribriform plate fracture.
d. b and c.

_c_ 2. If cerebrospinal fluid is noted to be leaking from the ear, the paramedic should:
a. note the finding but do nothing further.
b. apply direct pressure to stop the fluid leak.
c. gently pack the ear with sterile dressings.
d. realize that this is an ominous sign and nothing can be done for the patient.

_d_ 3. The paramedic may be able to remove a foreign object by:
a. flushing the eye with saline.
b. drawing the upper lid down over the lower lid.
c. everting the upper lid over a cotton swab and removing the object with the corner of a sterile gauze pad.
d. all of the above.

_b_ 4. An avulsed eye should be treated in the same manner as:
a. any other eye injury.
b. an eye impaled by an object.
c. a lacerated orbit.
d. none of the above.

_c_ 5. Bleeding from the nose can occur as a result of:
I. a fracture of the skull.
II. facial injuries.
III. intracerebral hemorrhage.
IV. infections within the nose.
a. I, II, and III
b. I and II
c. I, II and IV
d. I, II, III, and IV

_d_ 6. Bleeding from the nose that is due to causes other than skull fracture may be controlled by:
a. pinching the nostrils closed.
b. applying a rolled bandage between the upper lip and gum.
c. packing the nostrils with gauze and applying pressure.
d. all of the above.

_a_ 7. Cerebral perfusion pressure is dependent on:
a. mean arterial pressure minus intracranial pressure.
b. mean arterial pressure plus intracranial pressure.
c. mean arterial pressure minus diastolic pressure.
d. mean arterial pressure plus diastolic pressure.

_C_ 8. Cushing's triad is related to:
   a. increasing blood pressure, increasing pulse, and changes in mentation.
   b. increasing blood pressure, decreasing pulse, and changes in mentation.
   c. increasing blood pressure, decreasing pulse, and changes in respiratory pattern.
   d. decreasing blood pressure, decreasing pulse, and changes in respiratory pattern.

_a_ 9. The three levels of herniation measure or involve:
   a. vital signs, pupil reaction, and response to stimuli.
   b. vital signs, pupil reaction, and blood pressure.
   c. vital signs, blood pressure, and pulse rate.
   d. vital signs, blood pressure, and respirations.

_d_ 10. Decorticate posturing involves:
   a. extension of the upper and lower extremities.
   b. extension of the upper extremities and flexion of the lower extremities.
   c. flexion of the upper and lower extremities.
   d. flexion of the upper extremities and extension of the lower extremities.

_b_ 11. In cerebral herniation, decerebrate posturing is associated with the signs and symptoms in level:
   a. one.
   b. two.
   c. three.
   d. four.

_C_ 12. Cerebral concussion is defined as:
   a. a traumatic loss of consciousness.
   b. a traumatic loss of consciousness with brain injury.
   c. a traumatic temporary loss of consciousness without brain injury.
   d. a loss of consciousness without associated mental deficit.

_d_ 13. Antegrade and retrograde amnesia are associated with:
   a. epidural hematoma.
   b. subdural hematoma.
   c. basilar skull fracture.
   d. cerebral concussion.

_a_ 14. Cerebral contusion is defined as:
   a. bruising or bleeding of the brain.
   b. laceration of brain tissue.
   c. cerebral edema.
   d. a temporary loss of consciousness.

_d_ 15. Raccoon's eyes are indicative of:
   a. basilar skull fracture.
   b. direct trauma to the orbit.
   c. later findings, developing over 6-12 hours after the injury.
   d. all of the above.

_b_ 16. In epidural hematomas the most common cause is:
   a. a tear of a vessel from a venous source.
   b. a tear of the middle meningeal artery.
   c. venous bleeding.
   d. infection.

_c_ 17. The signs and symptoms of a subarachnoid hemorrhage include:
  a. symptoms that develop over days to weeks.
  b. blood leaking from the ears and nose.
  c. abrupt onset of headache, nausea, and vomiting.
  d. none of the above.

_d_ 18. The parameters of the Glasgow Coma Scale include:
  a. vital signs, motor response, and verbal response.
  b. vital signs, motor response, and eye opening.
  c. vital signs, verbal response, and eye opening.
  d. motor response, verbal response, and eye opening.

_a_ 19. Unilateral dilated pupils in the presence of head trauma indicate compression of cranial nerve number:
  a. 3.
  b. 4.
  c. 6.
  d. 10.

_d_ 20. Cervical spinal immobilization should be carried out on patients who demonstrate:
  a. a mechanism that suggests violent action to the spine.
  b. a severe head injury.
  c. a loss of consciousness or altered mentation following head injury.
  d. all of the above.

_b_ 21. When hyperventilating patients with head trauma, the paramedic should ventilate at a rate:
  a. of 12-20 ventilations per minute.
  b. of 24-30 ventilations per minute.
  c. greater than 36 ventilations per minute.
  d. equivalent to the patient's respirations.

_b_ 22. In a patient suffering from an isolated head injury, the flow rate of the IV should be _____ ml/hr.
  a. 10
  b. 50
  c. 200
  d. 500

_c_ 23. The two conditions that aggravate cerebral edema are:
  a. hypotension and bradycardia.
  b. hypotension and hypoxia.
  c. hypoxia and hypercarbia.
  d. hypotension and hypercarbia.

STUDY GUIDE ASSIGNMENT 15-3

▪ Soft Tissue Injuries to the Neck
▪ Injuries to the Spine
Reading Assignment: pages 318-323

Multiple-Choice Items

Read each question carefully. For each item, select the answer that BEST completes the statement or answers the question, and place the letter of that answer in the space provided.

_d_ 1. The principal signs of injury to the soft tissues of the neck include:
   a. loss of voice.
   b. hoarseness.
   c. palpable fracture over the anterior neck.
   d. all of the above.

_a_ 2. When a large vessel in the neck has been severed, it is important to realize that air can be introduced. Therefore, the paramedic should:
   a. place an occlusive dressing over the wound and apply direct pressure.
   b. apply a gauze dressing over the wound and apply direct pressure.
   c. transport the patient immediately to a medical facility, because nothing can be done in the field.
   d. not put direct pressure on the wound, because doing so would limit blood flow to vital organs.

_d_ 3. The term axial loading refers to:
   a. hyperextension of the spine.
   b. hyperflexion of the spine.
   c. rotation of the spine.
   d. compression of the spine.

_c_ 4. Shock secondary to spinal cord injury is due to the following two mechanisms:
   a. dilation of vessels and tachycardia.
   b. constriction of vessels and bradycardia.
   c. dilation of vessels and normal pulse rate or slight bradycardia due to unchecked vagal tone.
   d. hypovolemia and hypercarbia.

_d_ 5. Indicators of spinal trauma include:
   a. the mechanism of injury.
   b. guarding of the neck or back.
   c. pain on palpation of the posterior neck.
   d. all of the above.

_b_ 6. Log-rolling methods that call for elevating an arm over the head or that do not include keeping the ankles elevated while rolling the patient should:
   a. be discussed with your medical director.
   b. not be used.
   c. be considered safe and appropriate techniques.
   d. be used only if the patient has a lumbar injury.

_c_ 7. When immobilizing children, it is often necessary to:
   a. use a smaller board because body size is smaller.
   b. improvise because nothing fits.
   c. pad under the torso because of the size of the head relative to the body.
   d. pad under the head because of the size of the torso relative to the head.

CHAPTER 16

Thoracic Injuries

STUDY GUIDE ASSIGNMENT 16-1

- Assessment of Thoracic Injuries
- Pathophysiology of Thoracic Injuries
- Injuries That Cause Inadequate Ventilation
- Injuries That Cause Inadequate Cardiac Output
- Injuries That Cause Inadequate Circulating Blood Volume

Skill 16-1: Thoracentesis
Skill 16-2: Pericardiocentesis
Reading Assignment: pages 326-340

Matching Items

Match each of the terms in the left column with the BEST definition in the right column by placing the letter of that definition in the space next to the term. Each definition may be used once or not at all.

I __ 1. cardiac contusion
B __ 2. cardiac tamponade
C __ 3. flail chest
H __ 4. hemothorax
J __ 5. paradoxical motion
G __ 6. tension pneumothorax
K __ 7. open pneumothorax
F __ 8. pulmonary contusion
D __ 9. pericardiocentesis
E __ 10. thoracentesis

A. Accumulation of blood in the cerebellum

B. Condition that occurs when extensive pericardial fluid restricts diastolic filling of the heart

C. Two or more adjacent ribs each fractured in at least two places

D. Effective emergency treatment for life-threatening cardiac tamponade

E. Fastest and easiest treatment for a tension pneumothorax

F. Bruise on the lung that frequently accompanies rib fractures and flail chest

G. May result from a fractured rib that punctures the lung tissue; leakage of air into the pleural space continues to occur with no avenue of escape from the pleural space for the accumulating air and pressure

H. Condition in which blood accumulates in the pleural space

I. A bruise to the heart

J. Condition that occurs when the flail segment of the chest moves in a direction opposite to that of the rest of the chest wall during respiration

K. An open wound connects the pleural space to the outside environment

Multiple-Choice Items

Read each question carefully. For each item, select the answer that BEST completes the statement or answers the question, and place the letter of that answer in the space provided.

_b_ 1. Initial assessment in the primary survey includes all of the following:
   I. responsiveness.
   II. breathing.
   III. circulation.
   IV. vital signs.
     a. II and III
     b. I, II, and III
     c. II, III, and IV
     d. I, II, III, and IV

_a_ 2. Initial auscultation of the chest wall should be done over the:
   a. anterior lung fields and the epigastrium.
   b. anterior and posterior lung fields.
   c. posterior lung fields and the epigastrium.
   d. anterior lung fields only.

_b_ 3. Unilateral absent or diminished breath sounds indicate:
   a. pericardial tamponade.
   b. pneumothorax.
   c. mediastinal air.
   d. transection of the aorta.

_c_ 4. Thoracic injuries are classified by the effects that they have on the function of _____ systems:
   a. neurologic and respiratory
   b. neurologic and cardiovascular
   c. respiratory and cardiovascular
   d. respiratory and neurologic

_a_ 5. The most important consideration in treating a rib fracture is to:
   a. recognize the potential for associated injuries.
   b. provide pain relief.
   c. immobilize the fracture by taping or binding.
   d. realize that rib fractures represent a minor injury.

_c_ 6. The definition of a flail chest is:
   a. two ribs fractured.
   b. three or more ribs fractured.
   c. two or more adjacent ribs fractured in two or more places.
   d. multiple rib fractures.

_d_ 7. The major pathologic process of a flail chest is:
   a. pneumothorax.
   b. hemothorax.
   c. tension pneumothorax.
   d. pulmonary contusion.

_b_ 8. Paradoxical motion is defined as:
   a. a flail segment that moves in the same direction as the remainder of the chest wall.
   b. a flail segment that moves in the opposite direction from the remainder of the chest wall.
   c. a flail segment that does not move with the remainder of the chest wall.
   d. a flail segment that moves with each beat of the heart.

_d_ 9. Treatment of the patient with a large flail chest may include:
   a. endotracheal intubation.
   b. supplemental oxygen.
   c. positive-pressure ventilation.
   d. all of the above.

_c_ 10. The detrimental effect of a pulmonary contusion is directly related:
   a. only to the size of the contused area.
   b. only to the amount of lung tissue that is unable to function.
   c. to the size of the contused area and the amount of lung tissue unable to function.
   d. to the number of rib fractures involved.

_a_ 11. A treatment that may actually worsen the respiratory compromise of diaphragmatic rupture is:
   a. inflation of the abdominal section of the pneumatic anti-shock garment.
   b. massive infusion of intravenous fluids.
   c. endotracheal intubation with positive-pressure ventilation.
   d. splinting of rib fractures.

_d_ 12. A simple pneumothorax may occur from a:
   a. fractured rib.
   b. blunt force to the chest.
   c. spontaneous cause in an otherwise normal patient.
   d. all of the above.

_c_ 13. The mediastinal shift associated with tension pneumothorax results in:
   a. ventilatory compromise.
   b. cardiovascular compromise.
   c. a and b.
   d. worsening of thoracic bleeding.

_c_ 14. A specific field treatment of a severely compromised patient secondary to tension pneumothorax may be:
   a. supplemental oxygen.
   b. positive-pressure ventilation.
   c. thoracentesis.
   d. intravenous fluid administration.

_c_ 15. Complications of thoracentesis include:
   a. puncture or laceration of the lung tissue.
   b. puncture or laceration of intercostal vessels.
   c. a and b.
   d. puncture of the large intestine.

_b_ 16. The difference between an open pneumothorax and a simple pneumothorax is:
  a. that a simple pneumothorax is more severe.
  b. that in an open pneumothorax a wound connects the pleural space to the outside.
  c. in the mechanism of injury.
  d. that a simple pneumothorax builds up intense pressure.

_d_ 17. The treatment of an open pneumothorax includes:
  a. thoracentesis.
  b. rapid infusion of intravenous fluids.
  c. inflation of the pneumatic anti-shock garment.
  d. an airtight dressing and supplemental oxygen.

_c_ 18. A hemothorax produces signs and symptoms similar to those of a(n):
  a. cardiac tamponade.
  b. diaphragmatic rupture.
  c. pneumothorax.
  d. aortic tear.

_c_ 19. When cardiac contusion affects the electrical system of the myocardium, it may cause:
  I. ST depression.
  II. tachycardia.
  III. bradycardia.
  IV. atrial fibrillation.
  V. premature ventricular contractions.
    a. I, II, and IV
    b. I, III, and V
    c. II, IV, and V
    d. III and V

_a_ 20. The cause of patient decline in cardiac tamponade is due to:
  a. decreasing cardiac output due to restriction of blood flow.
  b. increasing cardiac output due to restriction of blood flow.
  c. compromise of the respiratory system due to increased myocardial pressure.
  d. neurological compromise secondary to decreased cerebral perfusion.

_c_ 21. Aggressive treatment of life-threatening cardiac tamponade may include:
  a. atropine sulfate.
  b. thoracentesis.
  c. pericardiocentesis.
  d. sodium bicarbonate.

_d_ 22. Whether intrathoracic bleeding should be suspected depends on the mechanism of injury and on:
  a. whether the patient's speech pattern has changed.
  b. whether there are changes in vital signs.
  c. the pattern of other injuries.
  d. b and c.

_b_ 23. The most important component of the management of thoracic trauma is the prevention of:
   a. hypoxia only.
   b. hypoxia and anaerobic metabolism.
   c. coma.
   d. anaerobic metabolism only.

_d_ 24. Steps taken to ensure adequate oxygenation of red blood cells include:
   a. supplemental oxygen.
   b. adequate ventilation.
   c. treatment of the specific pathophysiologic processes.
   d. all of the above.

_b_ 25. It is the responsibility of the paramedic, upon initial approach to the patient with suspected thoracic trauma, to do all of the following EXCEPT:
   a. rapidly examine the patient.
   b. diagnose all injuries.
   c. assess the scene.
   d. evaluate the history and mechanism of injury.

STUDY GUIDE ASSIGNMENT 16-2

Performance Checklist: Thoracentesis
Performance Checklist: Pericardiocentesis

The following skills should be practiced until you reach competency. Practice can be done in classroom settings using manikins, or in clinical rotations in the hospital or out on the ambulance or rescue unit. You may evaluate yourself, work with another student, or have a preceptor or instructor evaluate you using these forms.

Instructions

1. Place a check mark in the "C" ("competent") column if you used the recommended technique the first time you performed each activity.
2. Place a check mark in the "A" ("acceptable") column if you used the recommended technique but it took you several times to perform each activity.
3. Place a check mark in the "U" ("unsatisfactory") column if you used some but not all of each recommended technique.
4. Place a check mark in the "NP" ("not performed") column if you forgot to perform that particular technique.
5. The section for comments provides space to make notes about what further practice you need, what errors you made, how you can improve your skill, and so on.

Performance Checklist: Thoracentesis

C	A	U	NP	C = competent; A = acceptable; U = unsatisfactory; NP = not performed
☐	☐	☐	☐	Check responsiveness
☐	☐	☐	☐	Check airway
☐	☐	☐	☐	Check breathing
☐	☐	☐	☐	Check circulation
☐	☐	☐	☐	Assess the need for thoracentesis
☐	☐	☐	☐	Assemble equipment:

Primary equipment
- 14-gauge over-the-needle catheter

Accessory equipment and supplies
- Flutter valve (if available)
- Antiseptic swabs
- Protective eye wear
- Mask
- Gloves

C	A	U	NP	
☐	☐	☐	☐	Position the patient
☐	☐	☐	☐	Find landmarks for thoracentesis
☐	☐	☐	☐	Prepare the site
☐	☐	☐	☐	Insert the needle
☐	☐	☐	☐	Advance the catheter
☐	☐	☐	☐	Withdraw the needle
☐	☐	☐	☐	Dispose of the needle

OUTCOME: ☐ Pass   ☐ Fail   ☐ Retest

Comments:

Student's Signature _____ Date _____

Instructor's Signature _____ Date _____

Performance Checklist: Pericardiocentesis

C	A	U	NP	C = competent; A = acceptable; U = unsatisfactory; NP = not performed
☐	☐	☐	☐	Check responsiveness
☐	☐	☐	☐	Check airway
☐	☐	☐	☐	Check breathing
☐	☐	☐	☐	Check circulation
☐	☐	☐	☐	Assess the need for pericardiocentesis
☐	☐	☐	☐	Assemble equipment:

Primary equipment
- 18-gauge spinal or cardiac needle
- Syringe

Accessory equipment and supplies
- Antiseptic swabs
- Protective eye wear
- Mask
- Gloves

C	A	U	NP	
☐	☐	☐	☐	Position the patient
☐	☐	☐	☐	Find landmarks for pericardiocentesis
☐	☐	☐	☐	Prepare the site
☐	☐	☐	☐	Insert the needle
☐	☐	☐	☐	Aspirate the syringe
☐	☐	☐	☐	Withdraw the needle
☐	☐	☐	☐	Dispose of the needle

OUTCOME: ☐ Pass ☐ Fail ☐ Retest

Comments:

Student's Signature _____ Date _____

Instructor's Signature _____ Date _____

Abdominal Trauma

STUDY GUIDE ASSIGNMENT 17-1

- Mechanisms of Abdominal Trauma
- Complications of Abdominal Trauma
- Specific Intra-abdominal Injuries

Reading Assignment: pages 342-347

Matching Items

Match each of the terms in the left column with the BEST definition in the right column by placing the letter of that definition in the space next to the term. Each definition may be used once or not at all.

_A_ 1. Kehr's sign

_D_ 2. rebound

_F_ 3. guarding

_C_ 4. peritonitis

_E_ 5. tenderness

A. Pain in the shoulder caused by the phrenic nerve being in contact with blood

B. Pain in the back resulting from inflammation of the gall bladder

C. Inflammation of the membrane that lines the abdominal cavity

D. Pain that occurs when the peritoneal surfaces are rubbed together

E. Demonstrating an increased sensitivity to touch

F. Contraction of the abdominal wall musculature, either reflexively or consciously

Multiple-Choice Items

Read each question carefully. For each item, select the answer that BEST completes the statement or answers the question, and place the letter of that answer in the space provided.

_d_ 1. Abdominal structures are classified into the following groups:
   a. digestive, excretory, and endocrine.
   b. solid, digestive, and hollow.
   c. digestive, excretory, and hollow.
   d. solid, hollow, and vascular.

___C___ 2. Solid organs include all of the following EXCEPT the:
- a. liver.
- b. spleen.
- c. stomach.
- d. kidneys.

___d___ 3. The vascular structures of primary importance are the:
- a. renal and femoral arteries.
- b. superior vena cava and the renal arteries.
- c. iliac and femoral arteries.
- d. inferior vena cava and the aorta.

___a___ 4. Rib fractures often associated with splenic rupture are fractures of the:
- a. eighth, ninth, and tenth ribs on the left side.
- b. eighth, ninth, and tenth ribs on the right side.
- c. fourth, fifth, and sixth ribs on the left side.
- d. fourth, fifth, and sixth ribs on the right side.

___d___ 5. All of the following are indications of splenic rupture EXCEPT:
- a. trauma to the left lower rib cage.
- b. hypotension.
- c. Kehr's sign.
- d. bradycardia.

___b___ 6. One of the most frequently injured abdominal structures is the:
- a. spleen.
- b. liver.
- c. aorta.
- d. diaphragm.

___d___ 7. Clinical manifestations of injury to the liver include all of the following EXCEPT:
- a. rebound.
- b. hypotension.
- c. referred pain to the right shoulder.
- d. hypertension.

___d___ 8. Assessment of the patient with a colonic injury may reveal:
- a. tenderness.
- b. rebound.
- c. involuntary guarding.
- d. all of the above.

___b___ 9. Injuries to the small intestine produce:
- a. intense blood loss.
- b. peritonitis.
- c. respiratory distress.
- d. no clinical significance.

_C_ 10. Gastric injury is significantly more frequent with:
   a.   blunt trauma than with penetrating trauma.
   b.   the stomach full than with it empty.
   c.   penetrating trauma than with blunt trauma.
   d.   children than with adults.

_a_ 11. Auscultation of the abdomen in trauma cases should be:
   a.   omitted because it provides limited information.
   b.   carried out on every patient.
   c.   used because it can provide valuable information.
   d.   carried out on the scene prior to transport.

_C_ 12. Pneumatic anti-shock garments should:
   a.   never be used in abdominal trauma.
   b.   be used only as a last resort.
   c.   be used when clinical signs of hypovolemia are present.
   d.   none of the above.

_b_ 13. In cases of abdominal evisceration, the protruding organ should:
   a.   have a saline gauze placed over it.
   b.   be sealed with an occlusive dressing.
   c.   be left alone and the patient transported immediately.
   d.   have the pneumatic anti-shock garment applied.

_C_ 14. In abdominal trauma, intravenous access should be established with:
   a.   one 18-gauge catheter.
   b.   one 16-gauge catheter.
   c.   one, and possibly two, 14- or 16-gauge catheters.
   d.   any IV line possible; this is not a high priority.

_a_ 15. Definitive treatment of abdominal injuries usually requires:
   a.   rapid transport to an appropriate facility.
   b.   little surgical intervention.
   c.   a wait-and-see intervention at the hospital.
   d.   transport to any facility that has an operating room.

CHAPTER 18

Musculoskeletal Injuries

STUDY GUIDE ASSIGNMENT 18-1

- Anatomy and Physiology of the Muscular System
- Anatomy and Physiology of the Skeletal System

Reading Assignment: pages 350-365

Matching Items

Match each of the terms in the left column with the BEST definition in the right column by placing the letter of that definition in the space next to the term. Each definition may be used once or not at all.

B 1. skeletal muscle
G 2. smooth muscle
C 3. cardiac muscle
J 4. tendon
L 5. diaphysis
F 6. epiphyses
H 7. axial skeleton
K 8. appendicular skeleton
E 9. articulation
M 10. fibrous joint
I 11. cartilaginous joint
A 12. synovial joint

A. Freely movable joint; synovial cavity and articular cartilage present

B. All muscle that is predominantly under voluntary control

C. Muscle found only in the heart

D. Freely movable joint; no synovial cavity or articular cartilage present

E. Joint

F. Found at each end of a long bone

G. All muscle that is predominantly involuntary

H. The 80 bones that form the upright axis of the body

I. Slightly movable joint; no synovial cavity; bones held together by cartilage

J. Tough, whitish cord at the end of most voluntary muscles, by which they are attached to the bones that they move

K. From the appendages to the axial skeleton

L. Main shaft-like portion of a bone

M. Immovable joint; no synovial cavity; bones held together by fibrous tissue

Labeling Items

Read each question carefully and place your answer in the space provided.

1. Label the five sections of the vertebral column identified in the drawing by filling in the blank next to each letter, which corresponds with the same letter in the drawing. The five sections are to be selected from the words that follow the blanks. Each answer may be used once or not at all.

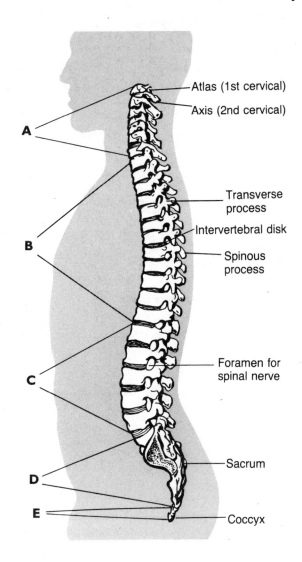

A. _____   D. _____

B. _____   E. _____

C. _____

| cervical | thoracic | coccygeal |
| lumbar | sacral | sternal |

2. Label the ten parts of the right upper extremity identified in the drawing by filling in the blank next to each letter, which corresponds with the same letter in the drawing. The ten parts are to be selected from the words that follow the blanks. Each answer may be used once or not at all.

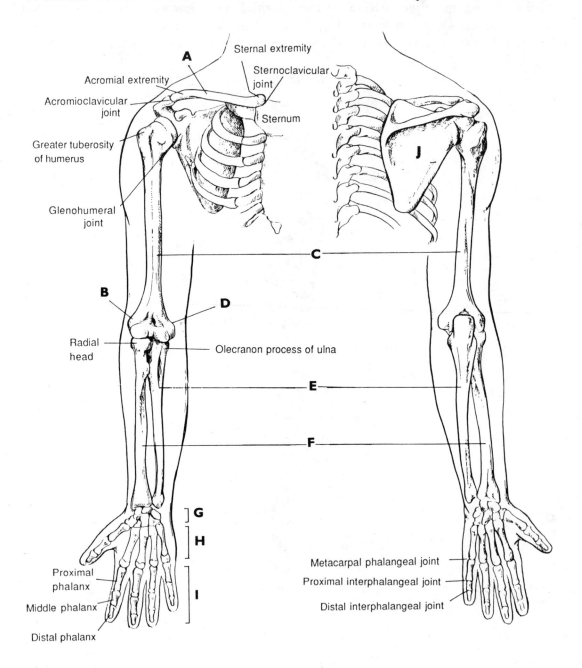

A. _____   F. _____

B. _____   G. _____

C. _____   H. _____

D. _____   I. _____

E. _____   J. _____

humerus   carpals   metacarpals
ulna   radius   phalanges
clavicle   scapula   medial humeral condyle
tarsals   lateral humeral condyle

3. Label the thirteen parts of the right lower extremity identified in the drawing by filling in the blank next to each letter, which corresponds with the same letter in the drawing. The thirteen parts are to be selected from the words that follow the blanks. Each answer may be used once or not at all.

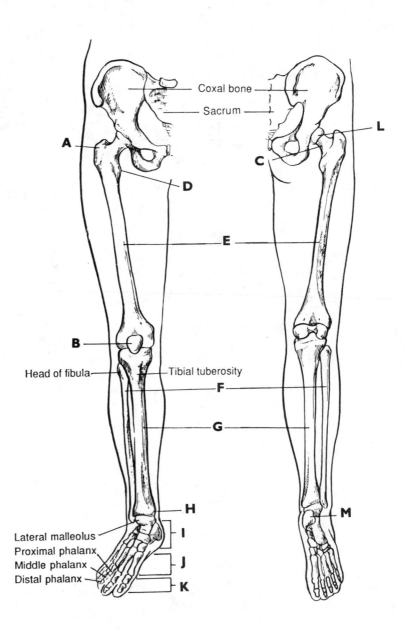

A. _____   H. _____

B. _____   I. _____

C. _____   J. _____

D. _____   K. _____

E. _____   L. _____

F. _____   M. _____

G. _____

head of femur	tarsals	lesser trochanter
tibia	medial trochanter	medial malleolus
fibula	metatarsals	calcaneus
patella	femur	greater trochanter
phalanges	neck of femur	

Multiple-Choice Items

Read each question carefully. For each item, select the answer that BEST completes the statement or answers the question, and place the letter of that answer in the space provided.

_d_ 1. The function of muscle tissue is to:
   a. facilitate movement.
   b. produce body heat.
   c. maintain posture.
   d. all of the above.

_a_ 2. _____ muscle is primarily involuntary and comprises most of the muscular tissue of the digestive tract, bronchi, urinary bladder, and blood vessels.
   a. Smooth
   b. Cardiac
   c. Skeletal
   d. Striated

_c_ 3. Muscles are attached to the skeleton by means of:
   a. cartilage.
   b. ligaments.
   c. tendons.
   d. subcutaneous fatty tissue.

_b_ 4. _____ serve(s) as a protective barrier for delicate structures of the body, such as the organ systems, glands, blood vessels, and veins.
   a. Ligaments
   b. Fascia
   c. Cartilage
   d. Muscles

131

_d_ 5.   _____ muscle has the unique property of automaticity and is innervated by both sympathetic and parasympathetic nerve fibers.
a.   Smooth
b.   Visceral
c.   Skeletal
d.   Cardiac

_c_ 6.   Energy is needed for muscles to do their work. Approximately _____ of this energy is released in the form of heat.
a.   1/2
b.   1/3
c.   2/3
d.   3/4

_a_ 7.   The layer of tissue that covers surfaces of the epiphysises is called:
a.   articular cartilage.
b.   diaphysis.
c.   periosteum.
d.   endosteum.

_d_ 8.   Which of the following statements is true of the intervertebral disc?
a.   It is a fluid-filled pad of tough cartilage.
b.   It acts as a shock absorber.
c.   It is extremely susceptible to injury.
d.   All of the above are correct.

_d_ 9.   The most frequently injured area(s) of the spine is(are) the _____ vertebra.
a.   cervical
b.   thoracic
c.   lumbar
d.   a and c

_c_ 10.   The front ends of the last two pairs of ribs hang free and are called _____ ribs.
a.   true
b.   false
c.   floating
d.   articulating

_c_ 11.   The proximal end of the humerus articulates with the scapula to form a _____ joint.
a.   saddle
b.   hinge
c.   ball and socket
d.   condyloid

_b_ 12.   The largest and uppermost bone of the pelvic girdle is the:
a.   ischium.
b.   ilium.
c.   pubis.
d.   symphysis pubis.

_C_ 13. The longest and heaviest bone in the body is the:
   a. fibula.
   b. tibia.
   c. femur.
   d. humerus.

_a_ 14. The knee joint is made up of which bones?
   a. Tibia and femur
   b. Tibia and fibula
   c. Fibula and femur
   d. Fibula, femur, and patella

_b_ 15. Fibrous joints are characterized by:
   a. no synovial fluid with bones held together by cartilage.
   b. no synovial fluid with bones held together by fibrous tissue.
   c. a synovial capsule with articular cartilage present.
   d. none of the above.

_d_ 16. A _____ joint presents with a spool-shaped process that fits into a concave socket.
   a. saddle
   b. pivot
   c. gliding
   d. hinge

_c_ 17. Movable joints allow change of position and motion. Movement that moves a bone away from the midline is called:
   a. flexion.
   b. extension.
   c. abduction.
   d. adduction.

_a_ 18. Movement that turns the forearm so that the palm of the hand faces anterior or superior is called:
   a. supination.
   b. pronation.
   c. gliding.
   d. circumduction.

STUDY GUIDE ASSIGNMENT 18-2

- Injuries to Muscle
- Injuries to Bone

Reading Assignment: pages 365-373

Matching Items

Match each of the terms in the left column with the BEST definition in the right column by placing the letter of that definition in the space next to the term. Each definition may be used once or not at all.

D 1. strain
C 2. sprain
G 3. fracture
A 4. Le Fort's fracture
E 5. greenstick fracture
I 6. comminuted fracture
B 7. transverse fracture
H 8. dislocation

A. Midface fracture

B. Fracture line is more or less at right angles to the long axis of the bone

C. Injury in which ligaments are stretched or even partially torn

D. Soft-tissue injury or muscle spasm that occurs around a joint anywhere in the musculature

E. An incomplete fracture by a compression force in the long axis of the bone; common among children

F. A twisting motion causes part of the bone to be pulled away by a ligament or tendon

G. Break in the continuity of a bone that may be either open or closed

H. Displacement of a bone end from its articular surface, sometimes with associated tearing of the ligaments that normally hold the bone end in place

I. Produced by a severe direct force; there are three or more fragments

Multiple-Choice Items

Read each question carefully. For each item, select the answer that BEST completes the statement or answers the question, and place the letter of that answer in the space provided.

b 1. A _____ is a soft-tissue injury that occurs around a joint anywhere in the musculature. It is characterized by pain on active movement. The muscle fibers involved may be stretched or partially torn.
  a. spasm
  b. strain
  c. sprain
  d. dislocation

c 2. A _____ is an injury in which ligaments are stretched or even partially torn.
  a. spasm
  b. strain
  c. sprain
  d. dislocation

134

_d_ 3. The management of a patient with a suspected sprain includes the "RICE" care. These management techniques assist the patient by:
a. easing the pain and swelling.
b. facilitating healing.
c. preventing further aggravation.
d. all of the above.

_b_ 4. Fractures that are caused by diseases of the bone, such as osteoporosis and bone tumors, are referred to as:
a. oblique.
b. pathological.
c. spiral.
d. comminuted.

_c_ 5. Consider an incomplete fracture by a compression force in the long axis of the bone. Usually, the convex surface breaks while the concave surface remains intact. This type of fracture is known as:
a. transverse.
b. epiphyseal.
c. greenstick.
d. comminuted.

_a_ 6. The primary symptom of a fracture is:
a. pain.
b. deformity.
c. discoloration.
d. paresthesia.

_d_ 7. The management of musculoskeletal injuries includes:
a. dressing all open wounds.
b. straightening all severely angulated fractures.
c. immobilizing the joint above and below the fracture site.
d. all of the above.

_c_ 8. A _____ is the displacement of a bone end from its articular surface.
a. fracture
b. sprain
c. dislocation
d. strain

CHAPTER **19**

Respiratory Emergencies

STUDY GUIDE ASSIGNMENT 19-1

▪ Anatomy and Physiology of the Respiratory System
Reading Assignment: pages 378-385

Matching Items

Match each of the terms in the left column with the BEST definition in the right column by placing the letter of that definition in the space next to the term. Each definition may be used once or not at all.

J   1. bronchi
D   2. bronchioles
H   3. alveoli
B   4. hypoxia
K   5. pleurae
C   6. diaphragm
G   7. inspiration
N   8. expiration
E   9. total lung capacity
L   10. tidal volume
M   11. inspiratory reserve volume
I   12. expiratory reserve volume
A   13. vital capacity

A. Largest volume measured during complete expiration after the deepest inspiration

B. Inadequate oxygenation of the blood

C. Muscular structure that separates the thoracic and abdominal cavities

D. The final generation of airways before the alveoli are reached

E. Volume of air in the lungs after a maximum inhalation

F. Inadequate carbon dioxide in the lungs

G. Process by which air enters the lungs through the nose or mouth

H. Delicate, thin-walled chambers within the lungs where the exchange of oxygen and carbon dioxide between the air and blood takes place

I. Maximum volume of air that can be exhaled after a normal exhalation

J. Largest airways of the lungs

K. Membranes that cover the thoracic musculature and the lungs

L. Volume of air normally inhaled or exhaled during each respiratory cycle

M. Maximum volume of air that can be inhaled after a normal inhalation

N. Passive activities of elastic recoil that create an increase in intrathoracic pressure

Labeling Items

Read each question carefully and place your answer in the space provided.

1. Label the ten structures of the lower airway identified in the drawing by filling in the blank next to each letter, which corresponds with the same letter in the drawing. The ten structures are to be selected from the words that follow the blanks. Each answer may be used once or not at all.

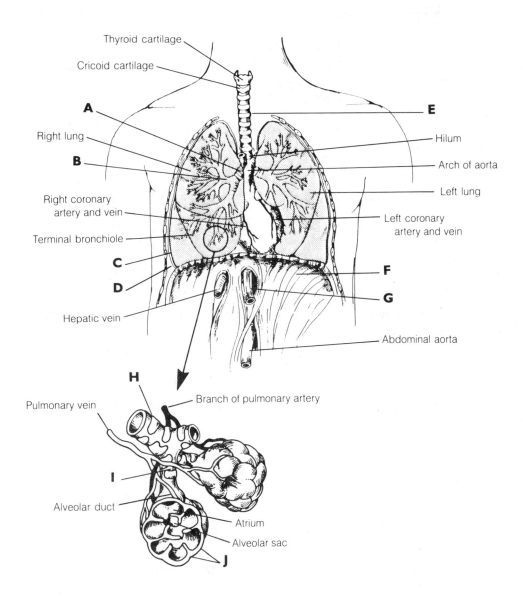

A. _____   F. _____

B. _____   G. _____

C. _____   H. _____

D. _____   I. _____

E. _____   J. _____

diaphragm   parietal pleura   alveoli
bronchiole   trachea   visceral pleura
terminal bronchiole   esophagus   respiratory bronchiole
trachealis muscle   right bronchus

Multiple-Choice Items

Read each question carefully. For each item, select the answer that BEST completes the statement or answers the question, and place the letter of that answer in the space provided.

b 1. The primary method for removal of foreign particles from the respiratory tract is:
  a. manual removal.
  b. mucus and ciliary action.
  c. bronchiole motility.
  d. alveolar movement.

a 2. The substance known as surfactant is important for which one of the following reasons?
  a. It prevents the alveoli from collapsing.
  b. It keeps the interstitial space narrow.
  c. It prevents swelling of the alveolar walls.
  d. It dilates the pulmonary capillary bed.

d 3. The body tissue(s) most affected by hypoxia is(are) which of the following?
   I. Brain
  II. Lungs
 III. Liver
  IV. Heart
     a. I
     b. I and II
     c. I, II, and IV
     d. I, II, III, and IV

c 4. The simple act of hyperventilation, in a patient with normal lungs, can boost the level of arterial oxygen as high as _____ mm Hg.
  a. 80
  b. 100
  c. 120
  d. 140

138

b 5. An easily observable clinical sign of respiratory decompensation is:
  a. increased metabolism.
  b. use of accessory muscles.
  c. hyperventilation.
  d. peripheral cyanosis.

c 6. A natural action that the body probably uses to re-expand atelectatic areas is a:
  a. sneeze.
  b. cough.
  c. sigh.
  d. hiccup.

c 7. Trauma patients who sustain injury to the spinal cord below C-5 are MOST likely to experience which one of the following effects?
  a. Interference with movement of the diaphragm
  b. Altered respiratory rate
  c. Interference with rib cage expansion
  d. Altered alveolar and bronchiolar function

d 8. The MOST prominent factor exerting control over the respiratory center is:
  a. pH of the cerebrospinal fluid.
  b. $PaCO_2$.
  c. PaO_2.
  d. a and b

a 9. When a COPD patient is said to be operating under "hypoxic drive," the patient's respiratory rate and depth respond to:
  a. PaO_2 levels below 60 mm Hg.
  b. $PaCO_2$ levels above 40 mm Hg.
  c. PaO_2 levels above 60 mm Hg.
  d. $PaCO_2$ levels below 40 mm Hg.

STUDY GUIDE ASSIGNMENT 19-2

- Assessment of the Patient in Respiratory Distress
- Respiratory Disorders

Reading Assignment: pages 385-403

Matching Items

Match each of the terms in the left column with the BEST definition in the right column by placing the letter of that definition in the space next to the term. Each definition may be used once or not at all.

B 1. eupnea
L 2. dyspnea
A 3. pleural friction rub
K 4. cyanosis
F 5. wheezes
D 6. stridor

A. Described as the creaking sound of old leather, it often accompanies pleuritis

B. Normal respiratory rate

C. During inspiration, a weakening of the pulse and a blood pressure drop of greater than 10 mm Hg

_G_ 7. rhonchi

_C_ 8. pulsus paradoxus

_J_ 9. chronic obstructive pulmonary disease (COPD)

_H_ 10. pneumonia

_I_ 11. pulmonary embolism

D. Harsh-sounding respirations due to airway obstruction

E. During inspiration, a weakening of the pulse and a blood pressure drop of greater than 20 mm Hg

F. High-pitched musical sounds that indicate narrowing of the airways from any cause

G. Abnormal coarse, rattling breath sound caused by fluid in the large airways

H. An infectious disease of the lungs

I. A serious condition that is caused by a foreign body that lodges in the pulmonary capillary bed

J. Disease processes that cause decreased ventilatory function of the lungs

K. Slightly bluish or purplish discoloration of the skin and mucous membranes as a result of hypoxia

L. Shortness of breath

Multiple-Choice Items

Read each question carefully. For each item, select the answer that BEST completes the statement or answers the question, and place the letter of that answer in the space provided.

_b_ 1. Dyspnea that occurs on exertion and goes away at rest may be:
   a. an indicator of chronic obstructive pulmonary disease.
   b. cardiac in origin.
   c. a sign of a neuromuscular disorder.
   d. an indicator of early-onset pneumonia.

_d_ 2. Characteristics of chronic obstructive pulmonary diseases include which of the following?
   I. Loss of elastic recoil
   II. Formation of blebs
   III. Reversible right-sided heart failure
   IV. Pulsus paradoxus
      a. I, II, and III
      b. II, III, and IV
      c. I, II, and IV
      d. I, II, III, and IV

_b_ 3. If it is necessary to give epinephrine down the endotracheal tube for a patient with a primary respiratory problem, it is best to give an adult a 1:10,000 solution of 0.3 to 0.5 mg and to:
   a. rapidly hyperventilate to distribute the drug more evenly.
   b. hold the lungs inflated for several seconds to enhance drug distribution.
   c. slowly ventilate with shallow volumes to enhance absorption.
   d. elevate the head of the cot to enhance even distribution.

_a_ 4. Airway burns are suspected when which of the following are present?
  I. Singed eyebrows or mustache
  II. Facial burns
  III. Swollen pharynx
  IV. An explosion was involved
    a. I, II, and III
    b. II, III, and IV
    c. I, II, and IV
    d. I, III, and IV

_c_ 5. Hyperventilation syndrome is a conclusion based on a rapid respiratory rate and:
    a. presence of carpopedal spasms.
    b. dizziness and numbness of hands and feet.
    c. elimination of more serious conditions.
    d. carpopedal spasms with seizures.

_a_ 6. Cardinal signs of respiratory distress assessed during the chief complaint include dyspnea, chest pain, cough, wheezing, and:
    a. fever, chills, or sweats.
    b. swollen ankles and sweating.
    c. hot flashes and dizziness.
    d. rash, headache, and fever.

_b_ 7. In chronic respiratory diseases, the most accurate indicator of acuity available is based on:
    a. the time of onset.
    b. a comparison with other episodes.
    c. the duration of the episode.
    d. presence of chest pain.

_c_ 8. On an acute basis, toxicity is generally NOT a problem with:
    a. theophylline preparations.
    b. sympathomimetics.
    c. corticosteroids.
    d. cromolyn sodium.

_d_ 9. Knowledge of any history of cardiac problems, seizures, or diabetes is especially important in respiratory emergencies, because:
    a. these conditions may make respiratory problems worse.
    b. drug dosages for respiratory problems are reduced when such a history exists.
    c. overdoses as a result of treatment are common.
    d. medications given for a respiratory emergency may interfere with medications for these problems.

_c_ 10. Confusion, agitation, or combativeness, in the presence of respiratory distress, is frequently associated with:
    a. medication overdose.
    b. peripheral cyanosis.
    c. hypoxemia.
    d. diaphoresis.

a 11. Retractions are caused by:
   a. breathing against an obstruction.
   b. increased intrathoracic pressure.
   c. cardiac involvement.
   d. hypoxemia.

d 12. Signs of an airway obstruction include:
   a. nasal flaring, tracheal tugging, and clubbing.
   b. tracheal tugging, clubbing, and intercostal retractions.
   c. clubbing, intercostal retractions, and nasal flaring.
   d. intercostal retractions, nasal flaring, and tracheal tugging.

b 13. The patient with hypoxia due to respiratory distress most often has:
   a. bradycardia.
   b. tachycardia.
   c. a normal pulse rate.
   d. an irregular pulse.

c 14. It is preferable to listen to breath sounds:
   a. anteriorly.
   b. laterally.
   c. posteriorly.
   d. midaxillary.

b 15. Early wheezes usually occur:
   a. during inspiration.
   b. during expiration.
   c. during both phases.
   d. after expiration.

a 16. Late stages of wheezing include wheezes:
   a. during inspiration.
   b. during expiration.
   c. during both phases.
   d. after expiration.

d 17. Stridor is caused by narrowing of the:
   a. bronchi.
   b. bronchioles.
   c. trachea.
   d. upper airway.

b 18. The best way to distinguish between rales and rhonchi is to determine:
   a. when the sound occurs in the respiratory cycle.
   b. whether or not the sound is continuous.
   c. whether the sound is wet or dry.
   d. whether the sound is associated with wheezes.

d 19. Obstructive lung disease includes:
   a. pneumonia, emphysema, and chronic bronchitis.
   b. emphysema, chronic bronchitis, and pulmonary emboli.
   c. chronic bronchitis, pulmonary emboli, and asthma.
   d. asthma, emphysema, and chronic bronchitis.

_a_ 20. A feature common to all obstructive lung diseases is:
   a. air trapping.
   b. mucus production.
   c. airway edema.
   d. bronchospasm.

_c_ 21 Effects of theophylline preparations include:
   a. vasoconstriction, tachycardia, and muscle tremors.
   b. diuresis, bradycardia, muscle tremors, and hypotension.
   c. tachycardia, tremors, diuresis, and bronchodilation.
   d. vasoconstriction, bradycardia, and hypertension.

_d_ 22. Common results of pneumonia include:
   a. atelectasis, pleuritis, and blebs.
   b. pleuritis, blebs, and sepsis.
   c. lebs, sepsis, and atelectasis.
   d. atelectasis, pleuritis, and sepsis.

_a_ 23. Your 34-year-old male patient was found in a smoke-filled room. He is now conscious but confused. There are no burns present about his face, but he is coughing sooty sputum. Breath sounds reveal wheezes in the bases. Appropriate treatment includes:
   a. high-flow oxygen, IV access, and bronchodilators.
   b. high-flow oxygen, IV access, and cricothyroidotomy.
   c. low-flow oxygen, monitor, and rapid transport.
   d. low-flow oxygen, IV access, and cricothyroidotomy.

CHAPTER 20

Cardiovascular Emergencies

STUDY GUIDE ASSIGNMENT 20-1

▪ Anatomy and Physiology of the Cardiovascular System
Reading Assignment: pages 407-416

Matching Items

Match each of the terms in the left column with the BEST definition in the right column by placing the letter of that definition in the space next to the term. Each definition may be used once or not at all.

_____ 1. arterioles
_____ 2. atria
_____ 3. capillaries
_____ 4. cardiac output
_____ 5. diastole
_____ 6. mitral valve
_____ 7. semilunar valves
_____ 8. stroke volume
_____ 9. systole
_____ 10. tricuspid valve
_____ 11. ventricles

A. Amount of blood ejected by the left ventricle with each contraction of the heart

b. Amount of blood ejected by the right ventricle with each contraction of the heart

C. Three-cusp valve located between the right atrium and right ventricle of the heart

D. Bicuspid valve located between the left atrium and left ventricle of the heart

E. Two thick-muscled lower chambers of the heart

F. Portion of the cardiac cycle during which the heart is contracting

G. Stroke volume times heart rate per minute; the amount of blood pumped by the heart each minute

H. Smallest arteries

I. Found at the termination of arterioles; connect the arterial and venous systems

J. Relaxation phase of the cardiac cycle when the ventricles are filling

K. Aortic valve located between the left ventricle and aorta and the pulmonic valve located between the right ventricle and pulmonary artery

L. Two superior chambers of the heart

Matching Items

Match each of the terms in the left column with the BEST definition in the right column by placing the letter of that definition in the space next to the term. Each definition may be used once or not at all.

_____ 12. automaticity
_____ 13. atrioventricular (AV) node
_____ 14. bundle of His
_____ 15. bundle branches
_____ 16. conductivity
_____ 17. depolarization
_____ 18. excitability
_____ 19. internodal and interatrial tracts
_____ 20. Purkinje system
_____ 21. sinoatrial (SA) or sinus node

A. Normal dominant pacemaker of the heart

B. Ability to generate an electrical impulse independently of outside stimulation

C. Ability of cells to respond to electrical stimulation, resulting in fiber contraction

D. Two conduction paths that split from the bundle of His

E. Slows conduction, creating a slight delay before electrical impulses are carried to the ventricles

F. Ability to pass, or propagate, an electrical impulse from cell to cell through the heart

G. Electrical conduction system in the interventricular septum that conducts impulses from the AV junction to the right and left bundle branches

H. Destruction of polarity that stimulates muscle fibers to contract

I. Receives electrical impulses from the bundle of His and distributes them throughout the ventricular myocardium

J. Three conduction paths that split from the bundle of His

K. Thought to route electrical impulses between the SA and AV nodes and to spread impulses across the atrial muscle

Labeling Items

Read each question carefully and place your answer in the space provided.

1. Label the fourteen structures of the heart identified in the drawing by filling in the blank next to each letter, which corresponds with the same letter in the drawing. The fourteen structures are to be selected from the words that follow the blanks. Each answer may be used once or not at all.

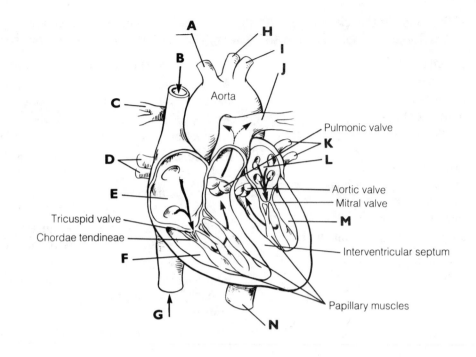

Labeled in the figure: A, H, B, I, J, Aorta, C, K, D, Pulmonic valve, E, L, Tricuspid valve, Aortic valve, Mitral valve, Chordae tendineae, M, F, Interventricular septum, Papillary muscles, G, N

A. _____	H. _____
B. _____	I. _____
C. _____	J. _____
D. _____	K. _____
E. _____	L. _____
F. _____	M. _____
G. _____	N. _____

left coronary artery	left subclavian artery	descending thoracic aorta
left pulmonary veins	left atrium	left common carotid artery
left ventricle	brachiocephalic artery	superior vena cava
right atrium	right pulmonary veins	left pulmonary artery
right ventricle	inferior vena cava	right pulmonary artery

2. Label the six structures of the electrical conduction system identified in the drawing by filling in the blank next to each letter, which corresponds with the same letter in the drawing. The six structures are to be selected from the words that follow the blanks. Each answer may be used once or not at all.

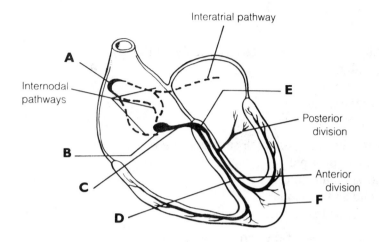

A. _____   D. _____

B. _____   E. _____

C. _____   F. _____

automatic node   AV node   right bundle branch
left bundle branch   Purkinje fibers   bundle of His
sinus node

Multiple-Choice Items

Read each question carefully. For each item, select the answer that BEST completes the statement or answers the question, and place the letter of that answer in the space provided.

_____ 1. Arteries, by definition, are blood vessels that carry blood _____ the heart.
    a.   away from
    b.   through
    c.   to
    d.   b and c

_____ 2. The innermost lining of an artery is the:
    a.   adventitia.
    b.   externa.
    c.   intima.
    d.   media.

_____ 3. The heart is located in the chest in a cavity called the:
   a. endometrium.
   b. mediastinum.
   c. periosteum.
   d. platypodia.

_____ 4. Surrounding the heart is a protective sac called the:
   a. endocardium.
   b. myocardium.
   c. pericardium.
   d. subendocardium.

_____ 5. Which of the following are both semilunar valves?
   a. Aortic and bicuspid
   b. Aortic and pulmonic
   c. Bicuspid and pulmonic
   d. Tricuspid and pulmonic

_____ 6. The contraction phase of the cardiac cycle is called:
   a. diastole.
   b. milieu.
   c. systole.
   d. tocus.

_____ 7. The relaxation phase of the cardiac cycle is called:
   a. diastole.
   b. milieu.
   c. systole.
   d. tocus.

_____ 8. Stoke volume may be defined as the:
   a. amount of blood ejected from either ventricle with a single contraction.
   b. amount of blood ejected from the heart within one minute.
   c. number of cardiac contractions in one minute.
   d. relative strength of the ventricular contraction.

_____ 9. Sympathetic stimulation has what effect on the heart?
   a. Decreased rate and less forceful contraction
   b. Decreased rate and more forceful contraction
   c. Increased rate and less forceful contraction
   d. Increased rate and more forceful contraction

_____ 10. Automaticity describes the heart's ability to:
   a. generate an electrical impulse independently of any external stimulus.
   b. respond to electrical stimulation.
   c. transmit electrical impulses from cell to cell through the heart.
   d. vary the speed and force at which the heart muscle cells shorten during systole.

_____ 11. The dominant or "natural" pacemaker of the heart is the:
   a. atrial internodal pathways.
   b. atrioventricular (AV) node.
   c. Purkinje system of the ventricles.
   d. sinoatrial (SA) node.

_____ 12. The inherent or intrinsic pacing rate of the AV node is _____ beats per minute.
   a. 20-40
   b. 40-60
   c. 70-80
   d. 60-100

STUDY GUIDE ASSIGNMENT 20-2

- Patient Assessment for Cardiac-related Problems
- Cardiovascular Disease States: Recognition and Management
- Other Acquired and Congenital Diseases of the Cardiovascular System
Reading Assignment: pages 416-430

Matching Items

Match each of the terms in the left column with the BEST definition in the right column by placing the letter of that definition in the space next to the term. Each definition may be used once or not at all.

_____ 1. angina
_____ 2. arteriosclerosis
_____ 3. atherosclerosis
_____ 4. cardiogenic shock
_____ 5. congestive heart failure
_____ 6. electromechanical dissociation
_____ 7. myocardial infarction
_____ 8. left ventricular failure
_____ 9. pericarditis
_____ 10. pulmonary edema
_____ 11. right ventricular failure

A. Chronic disease that involves thickening and hardening of vessel walls, resulting in a loss of elasticity

B. Tissue necrosis of a portion of the heart

C. Chest pain that is the result of coronary artery spasm or occlusion

D. Inflammation of the pericardial sac that surrounds the heart

E. Localized deposits of lipid material within the intimal surface of blood vessels

F. Localized deposits of protein material within the intimal surface of blood vessels

G. Inability of the left ventricle to pump blood into the systemic circulation adequately

H. Circulatory congestion that occurs in heart failure with resulting fluid retention and edema formation

I. Inability of the right side of the heart to pump blood effectively

J. Extreme form of pump failure in which the left ventricle cannot adequately perfuse body tissue

K. Serous fluid in the alveoli and interstitial tissue of the lungs

L. Any organized EKG rhythm that has an adequate rate but produces no palpable pulse

Multiple-Choice Items

Read each question carefully. For each item, select the answer that BEST completes the statement or answers the question, and place the letter of that answer in the space provided.

_____ 1. The most common chief complaint in patients with heart disease is:
  a. chest pain.
  b. dyspnea.
  c. palpitations.
  d. syncope.

_____ 2. Atherosclerosis affects which arterial wall layer?
  a. Adventitia
  b. Externa
  c. Intima
  d. Medica

_____ 3. Whereas most body tissues extract about 25% of the oxygen from the blood supplied to it, the heart extracts about _____% of the oxygen from the blood supplied to it.
  a. 10
  b. 33
  c. 50
  d. 70

_____ 4. A deficiency of blood supply to the heart to meet myocardial oxygen needs results in a condition called:
  a. cardiomegaly.
  b. myocardial infarction.
  c. myocardial ischemia.
  d. ventricular hypertrophy.

_____ 5. Angina is due to an imbalance in:
  a. catecholamines in the blood.
  b. hemoglobin in the blood.
  c. oxygen in the blood.
  d. supply and demand for oxygenated blood.

_____ 6. In angina, is there death of heart muscle?
  a. Yes, always.
  b. Yes, sometimes.
  c. No, usually not.
  d. No, never.

_____ 7. The duration of exertional angina is usually _____ minutes.
  a. 1-2
  b. 3-5
  c. 10-15
  d. 30-60

_____ 8. In myocardial infarction, is there death of heart muscle tissue?
  a. Yes, always.
  b. Yes, sometimes.
  c. No, usually not.
  d. No, never.

_____ 9. The earliest and most common cause of death in heart attack is the development of:
   a. cardiac arrhythmias.
   b. cardiac tamponade.
   c. cardiogenic shock.
   d. pump failure.

_____ 10. The most commonly presenting symptom seen in a heart attack is:
   a. chest pain.
   b. dyspnea.
   c. palpitations.
   d. shoulder pain.

_____ 11. Which of the following is the most common life-threatening arrhythmia seen in a heart attack victim and requires immediate intervention?
   a. Paroxysmal supraventricular tachycardia (PSVT)
   b. Ventricular asystole
   c. Ventricular fibrillation
   d. Ventricular tachycardia

_____ 12. A 48-year-old man is sitting in his office when he feels a sudden crushing pain in his chest. The pain has persisted with some fluctuation for the last 30 minutes. He is sweaty and complains of weakness and shortness of breath. Which of the following would be appropriate medical management procedures for this patient?
   I. Calm and reassure the patient
   II. Cardiac monitor
   III. IV, D_5W, KVO
   IV. Medications (nitroglycerin or morphine) per protocol
   V. Oxygen administration
   VI. Semireclining position (30-degree head elevation)
      a. I, II, III, and V
      b. I, III, V, and VI
      c. I, II, III, IV, V, and VI
      d. II, III, and V

_____ 13. Most commonly, in pulmonary edema, the:
   a. coronary arteries become congested with blood.
   b. left ventricle becomes an inefficient pump.
   c. right atria becomes an ineffective pump.
   d. ventricles empty too slowly.

_____ 14. The signs and symptoms of left heart failure include which of the following?
   I. Enlarged and tender liver
   II. Hemoptysis with pink, frothy sputum
   III. Jugular vein distention
   IV. Orthopnea
   V. Paroxysmal nocturnal dyspnea
   VI. Rales, rhonchi, or wheezes
      a. I, II, III, and IV
      b. I, III, V, and VI
      c. II, III, IV, and V
      d. II, IV, V, and VI

15. A 63-year-old man is having all the typical signs and symptoms of left pump failure. Which of the following are appropriate medical management procedures?
    I. Furosemide, 40 mg, slow IV push
    II. IV, normal saline, KVO
    III. Nitroglycerin, 0.4 mg, sublingual
    IV. Place in supine position
    V. Positive-pressure ventilation with 100% oxygen
        a. I, II, and III
        b. I, III, and V
        c. II, III, and IV
        d. II, III, and V

16. All of the following are causes of isolated right heart failure (right pump failure with no evidence of left heart failure) EXCEPT:
    a. acute pulmonary embolism.
    b. chronic obstructive pulmonary disease.
    c. infarction of the right ventricle.
    d. obstruction of the left coronary artery.

17. How should the cardiogenic shock patient be positioned?
    a. Fowler's (semi-sitting; 45-degree head elevation)
    b. Semi-reclining (30-degree head elevation)
    c. Supine
    d. Trendelenburg position

18. "Sudden death" due to atherosclerotic heart disease is defined as death within ____ hour(s) of the onset of symptoms.
    a. 1
    b. 3
    c. 8
    d. 24

19. _____ is the arrythmia responsible for the majority (60-70%) of cardiac arrests.
    a. Atrial fibrillation
    b. Third-degree AV block
    c. Ventricular fibrillation
    d. Ventricular tachycardia

20. Potential causes of electromechanical dissociation include all the following EXCEPT:
    a. cardiac tamponade.
    b. chronic obstructive pulmonary disease.
    c. hypovolemia.
    d. tension pneumothorax.

21. Signs and symptoms of cardiac tamponade may include which of the following?
    I. Dyspnea
    II. Hypertension
    III. Hypotension
    IV. Jugular vein distention
    V. Narrow pulse pressure
    VI. Wide pulse pressure

a. I, II, IV, and V
b. I, III, IV, and V
c. II, IV, and V
d. II, IV, and VI

_____ 22. Pulsus paradoxus describes another finding seen in cardiac tamponade. With pulsus paradoxus, the blood pressure _____ with inspiration.
   a. falls at least 10 mm Hg
   b. falls at least 30 mm Hg
   c. rises at least 20 mm Hg
   d. rises at least 40 mm Hg

STUDY GUIDE ASSIGNMENT 20-3

■ Prehospital Interventions for Specific Cardiac Conditions
Reading Assignment: pages 430-434

Matching Items

Match each of the terms in the left column with the BEST definition in the right column by placing the letter of that definition in the space next to the term. Each definition may be used once or not at all.

_____ 1. dopamine
_____ 2. epinephrine
_____ 3. furosemide
_____ 4. morphine sulfate
_____ 5. nitroglycerin
_____ 6. nitrous oxide
_____ 7. oxygen
_____ 8. sodium bicarbonate
_____ 9. theophylline ethylenediamine

A. Relaxes vascular smooth muscle, decreasing venous return to the heart; also produces coronary artery dilation

B. Stimulation of dopamine receptors in renal and mesenteric arteries

C. Decreases urine excretion

D. Primarily a bronchodilator

E. Analgesic gas

F. Potent narcotic analgesic

G. Acts directly on beta and alpha receptors in blood vessels to increase systemic vascular resistance

H. Odorless, tasteless gas necessary for all cellular life

I. Promotes urine excretion

J. Alkalinizing agent

Multiple-Choice Items

Read each question carefully. For each item, select the answer that BEST completes the statement or answers the question, and place the letter of that answer in the space provided.

_____ 1. A 39-year-old man is complaining of chest pain and shows premature ventricular complexes on the monitor. Which of the following medical management procedures is MOST indicated for this patient?
   a. Furosemide
   b. Morphine

    c. Oxygen

    d. Procainamide

_____ 2. Your patient is a 65-year-old woman who is complaining of chest pain which began while she was doing aerobic exercises in her home. For pain relief, you should give:
    a. morphine sulfate.
    b. nifedipine.
    c. nitroglycerine.
    d. nitrous oxide.

_____ 3. A 56-year-old bartender complains of chest pain and shortness of breath. Breath sounds reveal significant rales in the lung bases bilaterally. Vital signs are BP 144/90, pulse 132, respirations 32. Which of the following agents is MOST indicated for this patient?
    a. Atropine
    b. Lidocaine
    c. Morphine
    d. Theophylline ethylenediamine

_____ 4. The initial drug of choice in treating cardiogenic shock is:
    a. atropine.
    b. dopamine.
    c. epinephrine.
    d. norepinephrine.

_____ 5. A 38-year-old man is found in cardiac arrest at a golf course. The monitor shows ventricular asystole, which is confirmed in two leads. CPR has been started and an IV line has been placed. What is the first line drug to be given?
    a. Atropine
    b. Bretylium
    c. Epinephrine
    d. Lidocaine

_____ 6. Sodium bicarbonate is generally not given during the first ___ minute(s) of cardiac arrest management.
    a. 1
    b. 2
    c. 5
    d. 10

STUDY GUIDE ASSIGNMENT 20-4

▪ Arrhythmias: Interpretation and Therapeutic Intervention
  Basic Concepts of EKG Monitoring
  P Wave, QRS Complex, and T Wave
  Rhythm Strip Analysis
  Etiology and Mechanism of Arrhythmias
Reading Assignment: pages 434-442

Matching Items

Match each of the terms in the left column with the **BEST** definition in the right column by placing the letter of that definition in the space next to the term. **Each definition may be used once or not at all.**

_____	1.	PR interval
_____	2.	P wave
_____	3.	QRS complex
_____	4.	Q wave
_____	5.	R wave
_____	6.	ST segment
_____	7.	S wave
_____	8.	T wave

A. Isoelectric line

B. On an EKG, the first downward (negative) deflection after the P wave

C. First negative deflection after the R wave

D. First electrical wave seen on an EKG

E. Rounded wave that follows, and is usually in the same direction as, the QRS complex; it indicates ventricular repolarization

F. Distance between the beginning of the P wave and the beginning of the QRS complex on an EKG

G. Portion of an EKG tracing that represents depolarization of the ventricles

H. Distance between the S wave of the QRS complex and the beginning of the T wave on an EKG

I. First positive deflection after the P wave

Multiple-Choice Items

Read each question carefully. For each item, select the answer that BEST completes the statement or answers the question, and place the letter of that answer in the space provided.

Use this rhythm strip for questions 1-3.

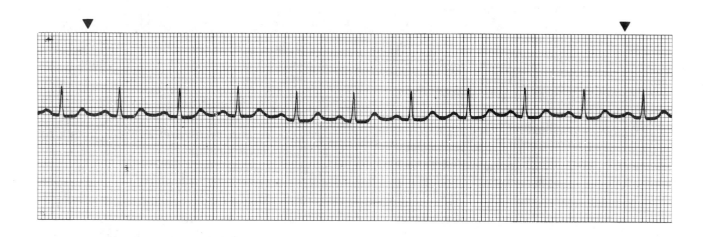

____ 1. A 21-year-old female complains of lower abdominal pain and vaginal spotting. The cardiac monitor displays the rhythm shown here, which can be described as:

    a. normal sinus rhythm.

    b. sinus rhythm with two premature atrial complexes.

    c. sinus arrhythmia.

    d. wandering atrial pacemaker.

_____ 2.   The EKG pattern shown before question 1 usually produces which of the following signs/symptoms in patients?
 a.   Shortness of breath
 b.   Chest pain
 c.   Syncope
 d.   None of the above

_____ 3.   The patient with the EKG pattern shown before question 1 may be treated with:
 a.   atropine.
 b.   epinephrine.
 c.   no specific prehospital arrhythmia management.
 d.   sodium bicarbonate.

STUDY GUIDE ASSIGNMENT 20-5

▪ Arrhythmias: Interpretation and Therapeutic Intervention
   Arrhythmias That Originate in the SA Node
   Arrhythmias That Originate in the Atria
Reading Assignment: pages 443-461

Matching Items

Match each of the terms in the left column with the BEST definition in the right column by placing the letter of that definition in the space next to the term. Each definition may be used once or not at all.

_____ 1.   atrial fibrillation
_____ 2.   atrial flutter
_____ 3.   multifocal atrial tachycardia
_____ 4.   paroxysmal supraventricular tachycardia
_____ 5.   premature atrial complex
_____ 6.   sinus arrest
_____ 7.   sinus arrhythmia
_____ 8.   sinus bradycardia
_____ 9.   sinus tachycardia
_____ 10. wandering atrial pacemaker
_____ 11. Wolff-Parkinson-White syndrome

A.   Cardiac arrhythmia in which the atrial impulses occur at a rate of 250-350 per minute

B.   Sudden appearance and cessation of rapid atrial rhythm with a rate between 150 and 250 beats per minute

C.   Rapid, erratic electrical discharge from multiple atrial foci or from multiple reentry circuits within the atria, generating 350-600 impulses per minute

D.   Rhythm that results when the discharge rate of the SA node decreases to less than 40 per minute

E.   Early or premature discharge of an ectopic focus located somewhere in the atria other than the SA node

F.   Preexcitation syndrome that occurs when the atria uses accessory conduction pathways to stimulate the ventricles earlier than is expected from the normal conduction syndrome

G.   Disorder of automaticity characterized by atrial rates greater than 100 per minute, P waves of at least three different morphologies in the same lead, and irregular P to P, PR, and R to R intervals

H.   Failure of the SA node to discharge, manifested by the absence of an electrical activity on the EKG

I.   Cardiac arrhythmia that occurs when the

pacemaker site shifts from the SA node to other foci in the atria and AV junction and then moves back to the SA node

J. An increase in the discharge rate of the SA node to greater than 100 per minute

K. Rhythm that results when the discharge rate of the SA node decreases to less than 60 per minute

L. Rhythm that results from an irregular discharge rate of the SA node

Multiple-Choice Items

Read each question carefully. For each item, select the answer that BEST completes the statement or answers the question, and place the letter of that answer in the space provided.

Use this rhythm strip for questions 1-3.

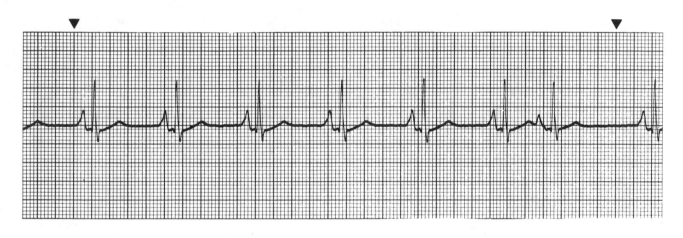

_____ 1. A 20-year old-female college student is complaining of anxiety, shortness of breath, and "sticky" chest pain. The cardiac monitor displays the rhythm shown here, which can be described as:
   a. normal sinus rhythm.
   b. sinus arrhythmia.
   c. sinus rhythm with an episodes of sinus arrest.
   d. sinus rhythm with one premature atrial complex (PAC).

_____ 2. The patient with the EKG pattern shown before question 1 may complain of:
   a. jaw pain and/or congestion.
   b. palpitations and/or crushing substernal chest pain.
   c. palpitations, or perhaps no additional complaints at all.
   d. syncope and/or crushing substernal chest pain.

_____ 3. The patient with the EKG pattern shown before question 1 may be treated with:
   a. atropine.
   b. bretylium.
   c. no specific prehospital arrhythmia management.
   d. lidocaine.

Use this rhythm strip for questions 4-5.

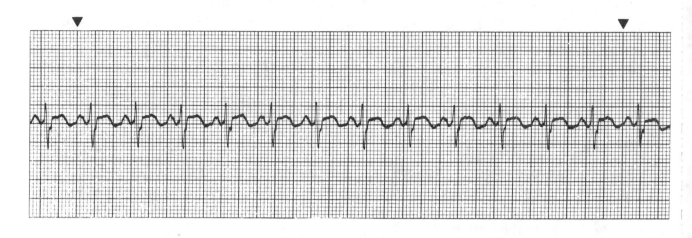

_____ 4. A 12-year-old boy is complaining of influenza type symptoms. His oral temperature is 103 degrees Fahrenheit. The cardiac monitor displays the rhythm shown here, which can be described as:
- a. atrial flutter.
- b. paroxysmal supraventricular tachycardia.
- c. sinus tachyarrhythmia.
- d. sinus tachycardia.

_____ 5. The patient with the EKG pattern shown before question 4 may be treated:
- a. with atropine.
- b. with carotid sinus massage.
- c. by treating the underlying cause.
- d. with lidocaine.

Use this rhythm strip for questions 6-8.

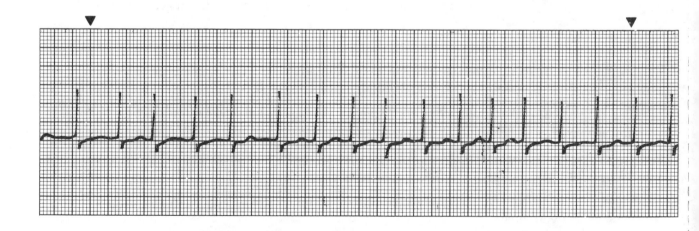

____ 6. A well-known national politician complains of sustained shortness of breath and palpitations following a tennis match. She denies chest pain and offers no other complaints. Her skin reveals pallor and her blood pressure is 96/54. The cardiac monitor displays the rhythm shown here, which can be described as:
a. sinus rhythm with multiple PACs.
b. sinus rhythm with PJC trigeminy.
c. sinus arrhythmia.
d. uncontrolled atrial fibrillation.

____ 7. The EKG pattern shown before question 6 is associated with:
a. a dramatic increase in cardiac output.
b. a slight increase in cardiac output.
c. a reduction in cardiac output.
d. no change in cardiac output.

____ 8. The patient with the EKG pattern shown before question 6 may be treated with:
a. atropine.
b. lidocaine.
c. verapamil.
d. none of the above.

Use this rhythm strip for questions 9-11.

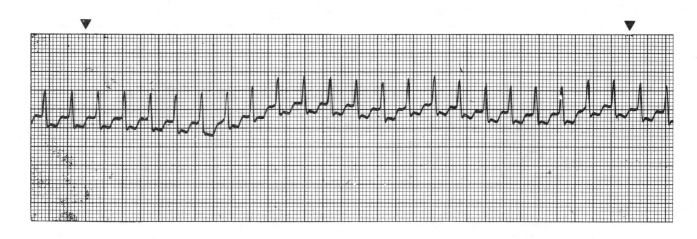

____ 9. A 24-year-old female complains of a "racing heart," which began while she was jogging but failed to abate with rest. The cardiac monitor displays the rhythm shown here, which can be described as:
a. paroxysmal supraventricular tachycardia.
b. sinus tachycardia.
c. uncontrolled atrial fibrillation.
d. ventricular tachycardia.

____ 10. After administering oxygen and placing an IV line, the first line therapy one should give to patients with the EKG pattern shown before question 9 is:
a. cardioversion.
b. digoxin.

c. vagal stimulation.

d. verapamil.

_____ 11. The second line therapy for patients with the EKG pattern shown before question 9 is:

a. cardioversion.

b. digoxin.

c. vagal stimulation.

d. verapamil.

Use this rhythm strip for questions 12-13.

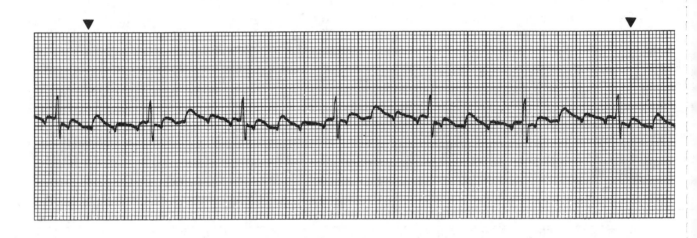

_____ 12. A 32-year-old music teacher is giving a piano lesson when he feels his heart racing. The cardiac monitor displays the rhythm shown here, which can be described as:

a. atrial fibrillation.

b. atrial flutter.

c. sinus rhythm with artifact.

d. wandering atrial pacemaker.

_____ 13. The EKG pattern shown before question 12 is consistent with an irritable focus in the:

a. atrial conduction system.

b. AV junctional tissue.

c. sinus node.

d. ventricular Purkinje system.

STUDY GUIDE ASSIGNMENT 20-6

▪ Arrhythmias: Interpretation and Therapeutic Intervention
  Arrhythmias That Originate in the AV Junction
  Arrhythmias That Originate in the Ventricles
Reading Assignment: pages 462-482

Matching Items

Match each of the terms in the left column with the BEST definition in the right column by placing the letter of that definition in the space next to the term. Each definition may be used once or not at all.

_____ 1. accelerated idioventricular rhythm

_____ 2. accelerated junctional rhythm

_____ 3. asystole

_____ 4. junctional escape complexes and rhythms

_____ 5. paroxysmal junctional tachycardia

_____ 6. premature junctional complex

_____ 7. premature ventricular complex

_____ 8. torsade de pointes

_____ 9. ventricular escape complexes and rhythms

_____ 10. ventricular fibrillation

_____ 11. ventricular tachycardia

A. Decreased automaticity of the AV junction

B. Absence of electrical activity in the heart

C. Ventricular pacemaker sites that discharge faster than the inherent ventricular rate

D. Idioventricular rhythm that occurs when the ventricle takes over as pacemaker for the heart and creates an escape complex or rhythm at a rate of 20-40 per minute

E. Cardiac arrhythmia that occurs when the AV junction stimulates the ventricles at a rate of 100-180 per minute

F. Occurs when an ectopic focus in either ventricle creates an impulse before the next expected sinus beat

G. Continuous broad, rapid ventricular complexes

H. Increased automaticity of the AV junction

I. Quivering and twitching of the heart as a result of disorganized electrical activity in the ventricles

J. Condition in which the polarity of the complexes on the EKG constantly shifts, giving the rhythm strip a twisted appearance

K. Occurs during sinus rhythm earlier than the next expected sinus beat and is created by premature discharge of an ectopic focus in the AV junctional tissue

L. Cardiac complexes or rhythms as a result of the AV junction that functions as the heart's pacemaker for one or more cardiac cycles

Multiple-Choice Items

Read each question carefully. For each item, select the answer that BEST completes the statement or answers the question, and place the letter of that answer in the space provided.

Use this rhythm strip for questions 1-3.

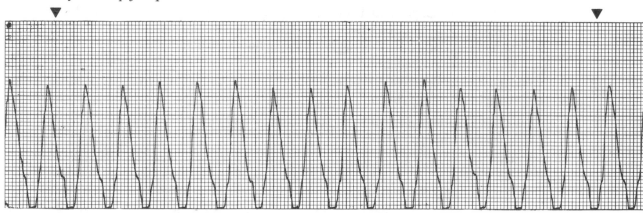

_____ 1. A 44-year-old school teacher complains of feeling weak and dizzy. The patient is conscious and has no hypotension or pulmonary edema. The cardiac monitor displays the rhythm shown here, which can be described as:
   a. atrial flutter.
   b. paroxysmal supraventricular tachycardia.
   c. torsade de pointes.
   d. ventricular tachycardia.

_____ 2. The patient with the EKG pattern shown before question 1 may be treated with:
   a. diazepam and cardiovert at 50 joules.
   b. lidocaine 1 mg/kg.
   c. precordial thump.
   d. unsynchronized cardioversion at 50 joules.

_____ 3. If the patient (see question 1) does not respond to your initial step but remains stable, you should next try:
   a. diazepam and cardiovert at 50 joules.
   b. lidocaine 0.5 mg/kg.
   c. precordial thump.
   d. unsynchronized cardioversion at 50 joules.

Use this rhythm strip for questions 4-6.

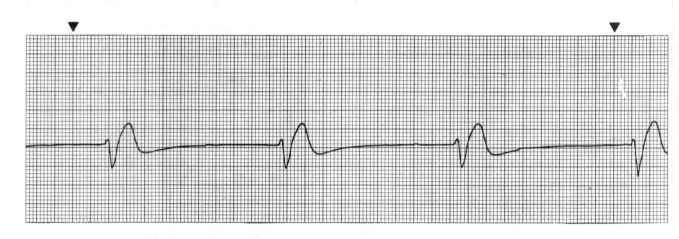

_____ 4. A 53-year-old man is found unconscious outside of a neighborhood bar. The pulse is not palpable and the patient is not breathing. The cardiac monitor displays the rhythm shown here, which can be described as:
   a. slow atrial fibrillation with wide QRS.
   b. third-degree AV block.
   c. type II second-degree AV block.
   d. ventricular escape rhythm.

_____ 5. How would you initially treat the patient with the EKG pattern shown before question 4?
   a. Atropine 1 mg IV
   b. CPR
   c. Defibrillate at 200 joules
   d. Epinephrine 0.5-1.0 mg IV

_____ 6. After first line therapy has been given, an IV line has been placed. What would you do NEXT in treating the patient with the EKG pattern shown before question 4?
   a. Atropine 1 mg IV
   b. CPR
   c. Defibrillate at 200 joules
   d. Epinephrine 0.5-1.0 mg IV

Use this rhythm strip for questions 7-8.

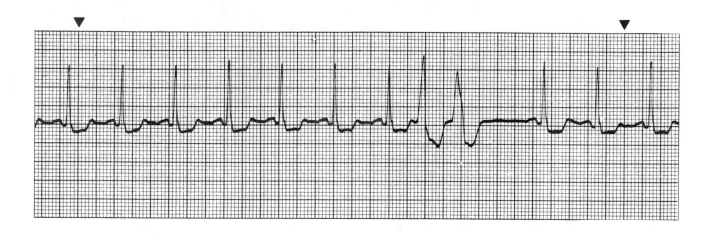

_____ 7. A 38-year-old construction worker experiences some weakness, nausea, and shortness of breath after eating a large lunch. The cardiac monitor displays the rhythm shown here, which can be described as:
   a. sinus tachyarrhythmia with couplet PJCs.
   b. sinus rhythm with couplet PVCs.
   c. sinus tachycardia with bigeminal PVCs.
   d. sinus tachycardia with couplet PVCs.

_____ 8. The patient with the EKG pattern shown before question 7 may be treated with:
   a. carotid sinus massage.
   b. bretylium.
   c. lidocaine.
   d. no specific prehospital arrhythmia management.

Use this rhythm strip for questions 9-10.

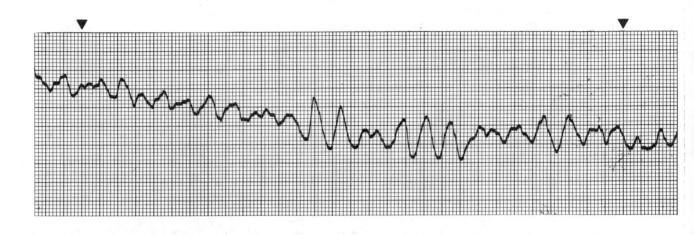

_____ 9. A 14-year-old drowning victim has just been pulled from the pool. Time of submersion is unknown. The cardiac monitor displays the rhythm shown here, which can be described as:
   a. agonal rhythm.
   b. ventricular asystole.
   c. ventricular escape rhythm.
   d. ventricular fibrillation.

_____ 10. What is the first line drug which can be given to make the rhythm shown before question 9 easier to convert?
   a. Atropine
   b. Dopamine
   c. Epinephrine
   d. Lidocaine

Use this rhythm strip for questions 11-12.

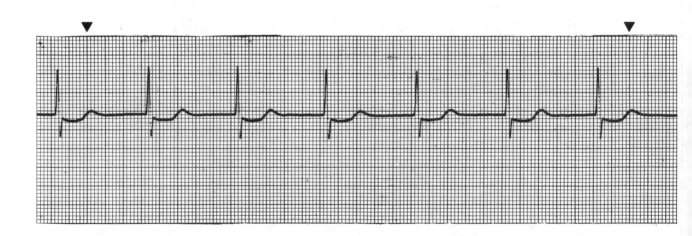

_____ 11. A 60-year-old taxi driver is complaining of weakness, dizziness, and nausea. He states that he has had some chest pain but that it is absent at the moment. Vital signs are within normal limits. The cardiac monitor displays the foregoing rhythm, which can be described as:
   a. junctional escape rhythm.
   b. sinus bradycardia.
   c. slow atrial fibrillation.
   d. ventricular escape rhythm.

_____ 12. The patient with the EKG pattern shown before question 11 may be treated with:
   a. atropine.
   b. bretylium.
   c. isoproterenol.
   d. no specific prehospital arrhythmia management.

Use this rhythm strip for questions 13-14.

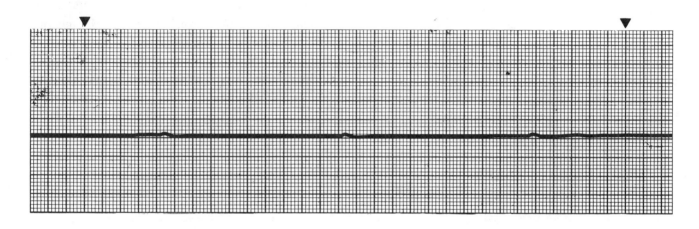

_____ 13. An 80-year-old nursing home patient could not be roused from sleeping by the nursing staff. She does not respond to verbal or pain stimuli. The cardiac monitor displays the rhythm shown here, which can be described as:
   a. third-degree AV block.
   b. ventricular asystole.
   c. ventricular escape rhythm.
   d. ventricular fibrillation.

_____ 14. The patient with the EKG pattern shown before question 13 should initially be treated with:
   a. CPR.
   b. defibrillation.
   c. epinephrine.
   d. precordial thump.

STUDY GUIDE ASSIGNMENT 20-7

- Arrhythmias: Interpretation and Therapeutic Intervention
  Arrhythmias That Are Disorders of Conduction
  Artificial Pacemaker Rhythms

Reading Assignment: pages 483-501

Matching Items

Match each of the terms in the left column with the BEST definition in the right column by placing the letter of that definition in the space next to the term. Each definition may be used once or not at all.

_____ 1. artificial cardiac pacemaker
_____ 2. first-degree AV block
_____ 3. Mobitz I
_____ 4. Mobitz II
_____ 5. third-degree block

A. Implantable device used to stimulate the heart electronically in place of the heart's natural pacemaker or conduction systems

B. Type I second-degree AV block

C. Type III second-degree AV block

D. Complete heart block; total absence of conduction between atria and ventricles as a result of complete electrical block at or below the AV node

E. Condition characterized by a delay in conduction of impulses through the AV junction

F. Type II second-degree AV block

Multiple-Choice Items

Read each question carefully. For each item, select the answer that BEST completes the statement or answers the question, and place the letter of that answer in the space provided.

Use this rhythm strip for questions 1-3.

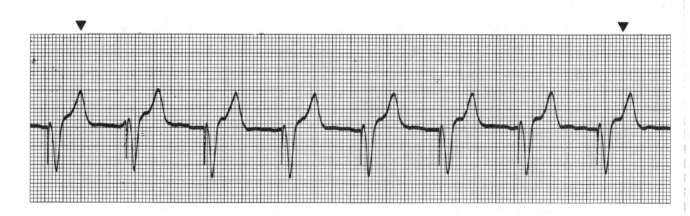

_____ 1. A 60-year-old female complains of lower-back pain and joint pain. She has a history of rheumatoid arthritis. Her only medication is aspirin. The cardiac monitor displays the rhythm shown here, which can be described as:
   a. accelerated idioventricular rhythm.
   b. artificial pacemaker rhythm.

c.   sinus rhythm with wide QRS.

d.   slow ventricular tachycardia.

____ 2.   The patient with the EKG pattern shown before question 1 would usually present with:

a.   chest pain.

b.   palpitations.

c.   shortness of breath.

d.   none of the above.

____ 3.   The patient with the EKG pattern shown before question 1 should be treated with:

a.   bretylium.

b.   lidocaine.

c.   no specific prehospital arrhythmia management.

d.   procainamide.

Use this rhythm strip for questions 4-6.

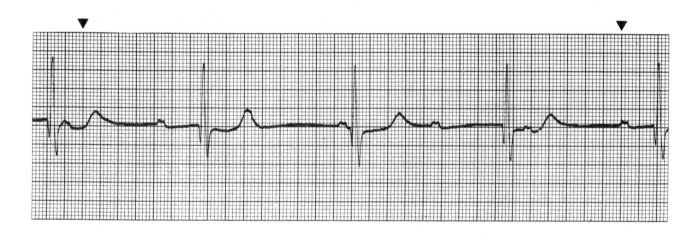

____ 4.   A 73-year-old grandmother complains of weakness, shortness of breath, and profuse sweating, which began while she was sitting on her porch. She denies chest pain. The cardiac monitor displays the rhythm shown here, which can be described as:

a.   slow atrial fibrillation with wide QRS.

b.   type II second-degree AV block.

c.   third-degree AV block.

d.   ventricular escape rhythm.

____ 5.   Given the patient presentation, which of the following conditions is MOST likely to be the cause of this patient's complaints?

a.   Cardiac tamponade

b.   Pulmonary embolism

c.   Silent myocardial infarction

d.   Spontaneous pneumothorax

____ 6.   If left untreated, the EKG pattern shown before question 4 could degenerate into:

a.   sinus arrest.

b.   third-degree AV block.

c.   ventricular asystole.
d.   ventricular escape rhythm.

Use this rhythm strip for questions 7-8.

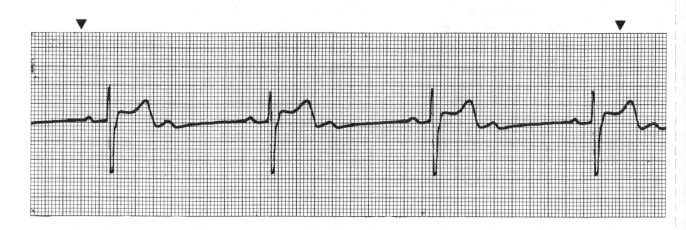

_____ 7.   A worker in a dry cleaning plant complains of chest pain and shortness of breath. The cardiac monitor displays the rhythm shown here, which can be described as:
a.   sinus bradycardia.
b.   type I (Wenckebach) second-degree AV block.
c.   type II second-degree AV block.
d.   third-degree AV block.

_____ 8.   The patient with the EKG pattern shown before question 7 may be treated with:
a.   atropine.
b.   epinephrine.
c.   lidocaine.
d.   vagal stimulation.

Use this rhythm strip for questions 9-10.

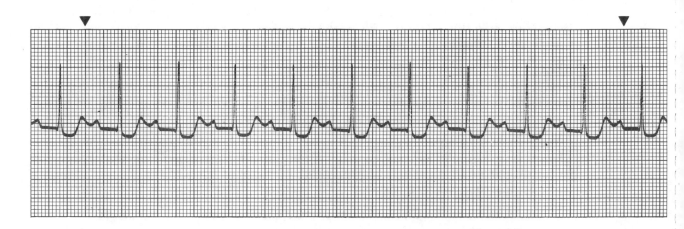

_____ 9. You have been called to a dermatologist's office where a file clerk is experiencing lower abdominal tenderness with non-menstrual vaginal bleeding. The cardiac monitor displays the rhythm shown here, which can be described as:
   a. normal sinus rhythm.
   b. sinus arrhythmia.
   c. sinus rhythm with first-degree AV block.
   d. wandering atrial pacemaker.

_____ 10. The patient with the EKG pattern shown before question 9 may be treated with:
   a. atropine.
   b. epinephrine.
   c. lidocaine.
   d. no specific prehospital arrhythmia management.

STUDY GUIDE ASSIGNMENT 20-8

▪ Arrhythmias: Interpretation and Therapeutic Intervention
  Prehospital Intervention: EKG Monitoring
  Prehospital Intervention for Arrhythmias That Result from Increased Automaticity or Reentry
  Skill 20-1. Defibrillation and Synchronized Cardioversion
Reading Assignment: pages 501-519

Matching Items

Match each of the terms in the left column with the BEST definition in the right column by placing the letter of that definition in the space next to the term. Each definition may be used once or not at all.

_____ 1. bretylium tosylate
_____ 2. atropine sulfate
_____ 3. carotid sinus massage
_____ 4. defibrillation
_____ 5. isoproterenol
_____ 6. lidocaine
_____ 7. precordial thump
_____ 8. synchronized cardioversion
_____ 9. Valsalva's maneuver
_____ 10. verapamil

A. "Bearing down" action that is a form of reflex vagal stimulation
B. Generates a small amount of electrical current
C. Potent beta stimulating drug
D. Used to increase vagal tone
E. Possesses both direct cardiac effects and effects on the autonomic nervous system
F. Calcium-channel blocking agent
G. Suppresses most atrial arrhythmias
H. First line drug used to suppress beats and rhythms of ventricular origin
I. A shock to the heart that is timed to the heart's existing electrical activity
J. Involves passing sufficient electrical current through the heart to depolarize fibrillating cells
K. Potent parasympathetic (vagal) blocking agent

STUDY GUIDE ASSIGNMENT 20-9

▪ Arrhythmia Interpretation

The following EKG tracings are actual strips from cardiac patients. Above each rhythm strip is a 6-second indicator for rapid rate calculation. Below each rhythm strip are specific areas to be completed (such as rate, rhythm, P wave, and so on). Fill in all blanks for each rhythm strip.

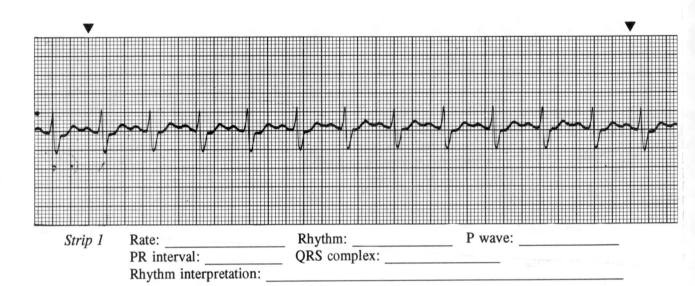

Strip 1   Rate: _____   Rhythm: _____   P wave: _____
PR interval: _____   QRS complex: _____
Rhythm interpretation: _____

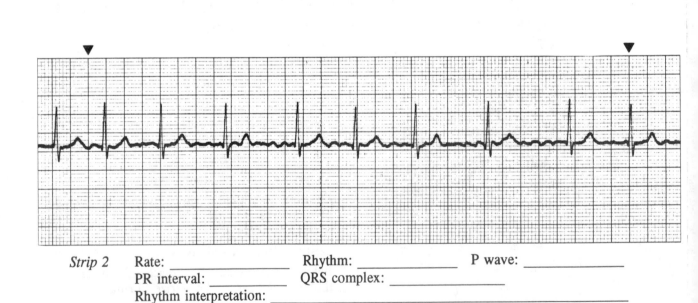

Strip 2   Rate: _____   Rhythm: _____   P wave: _____
PR interval: _____   QRS complex: _____
Rhythm interpretation: _____

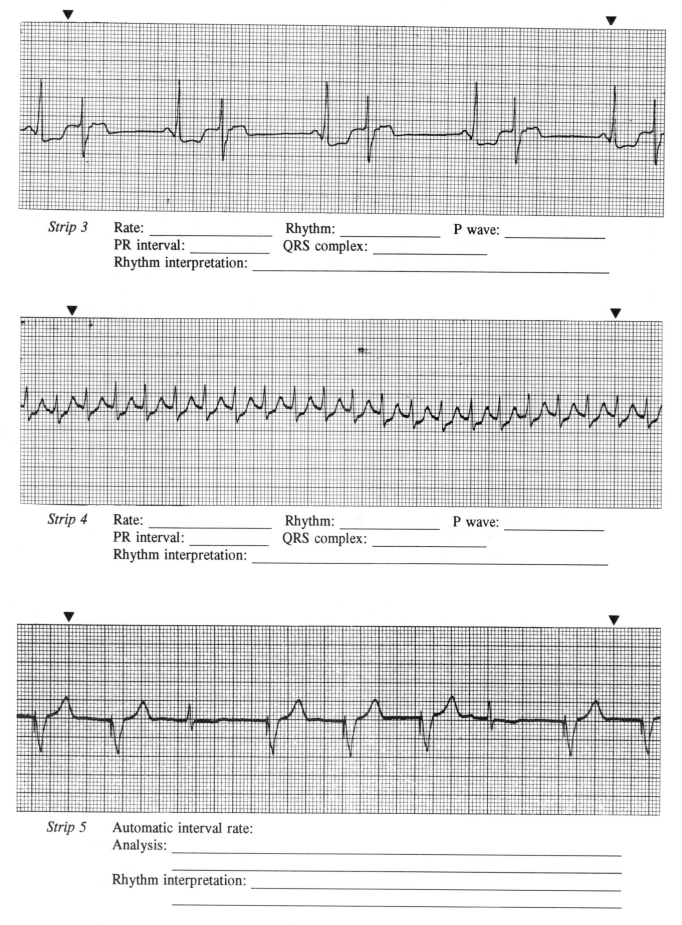

Strip 3   Rate: _____   Rhythm: _____   P wave: _____
              PR interval: _____   QRS complex: _____
              Rhythm interpretation: _____

Strip 4   Rate: _____   Rhythm: _____   P wave: _____
              PR interval: _____   QRS complex: _____
              Rhythm interpretation: _____

Strip 5   Automatic interval rate:
              Analysis: _____
              _____
              Rhythm interpretation: _____
              _____

Strip 6   Rate: _____   Rhythm: _____   P wave: _____
PR interval: _____   QRS complex: _____
Rhythm interpretation: _____

Strip 7   Rate: _____   Rhythm: _____   P wave: _____
PR interval: _____   QRS complex: _____
Rhythm interpretation: _____

Strip 8   Rate: _____   Rhythm: _____   P wave: _____
PR interval: _____   QRS complex: _____
Rhythm interpretation: _____

Strip 9   Rate: _____   Rhythm: _____   P wave: _____
PR interval: _____   QRS complex: _____
Rhythm interpretation: _____

Strip 10   Rate: _____   Rhythm: _____   P wave: _____
PR interval: _____   QRS complex: _____
Rhythm interpretation: _____

Strip 11   Rate: _____   Rhythm: _____   P wave: _____
PR interval: _____   QRS complex: _____
Rhythm interpretation: _____

Strip 12   Rate: _____   Rhythm: _____   P wave: _____
PR interval: _____   QRS complex: _____
Rhythm interpretation: _____

Strip 13   Rate: _____   Rhythm: _____   P wave: _____
PR interval: _____   QRS complex: _____
Rhythm interpretation: _____

Strip 14   Rate: _____   Rhythm: _____   P wave: _____
PR interval: _____   QRS complex: _____
Rhythm interpretation: _____

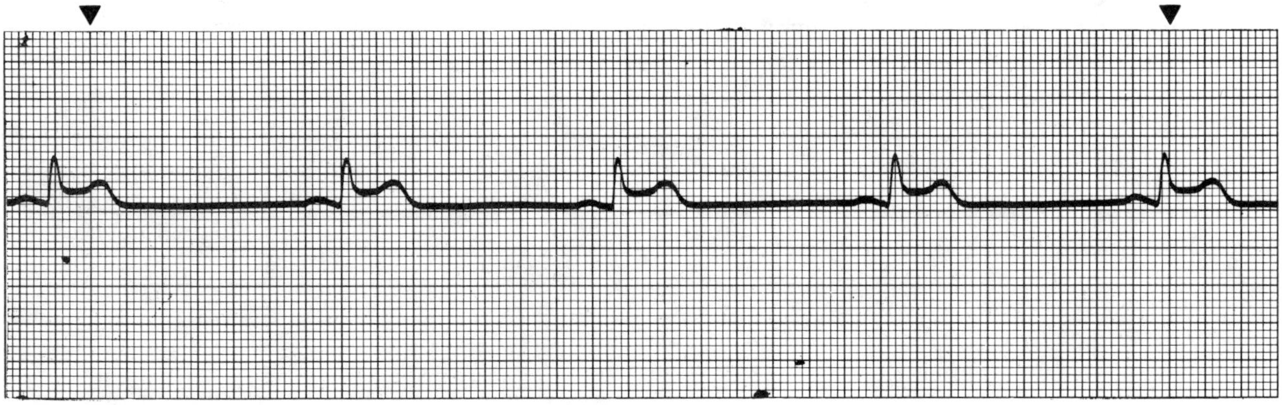

Strip 15   Rate: _____   Rhythm: _____   P wave: _____

PR interval: _____   QRS complex: _____

Rhythm interpretation: _____

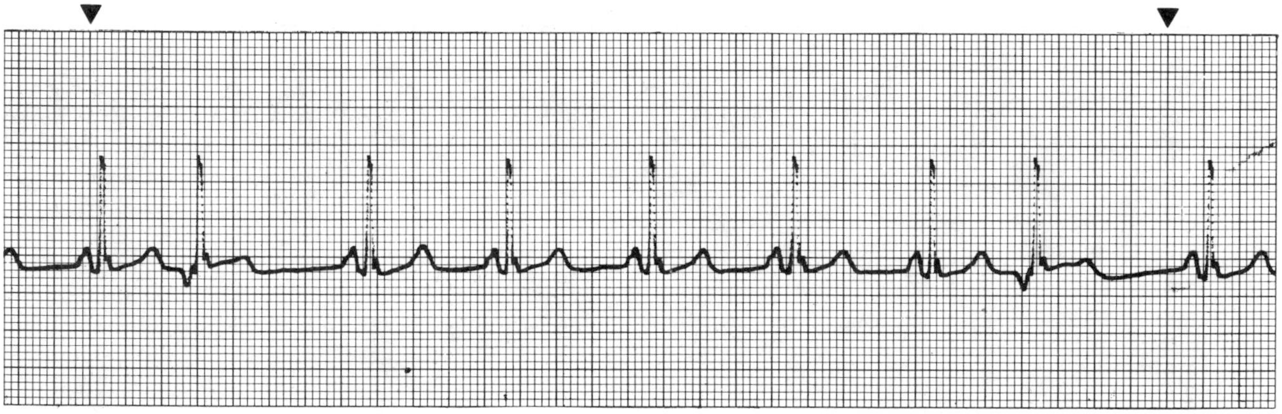

Strip 16   Rate: _____   Rhythm: _____   P wave: _____

PR interval: _____   QRS complex: _____

Rhythm interpretation: _____

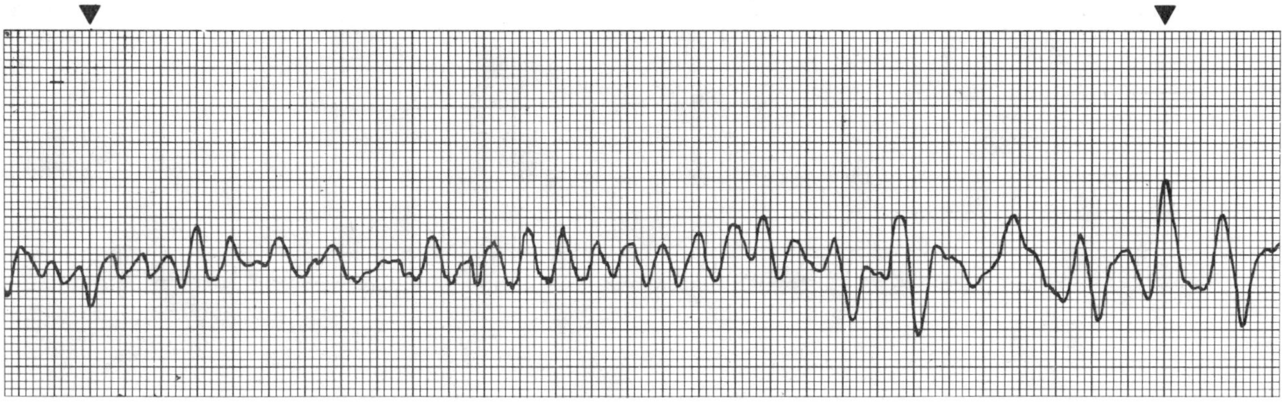

Strip 17   Rate: _____   Rhythm: _____   P wave: _____

PR interval: _____   QRS complex: _____

Rhythm interpretation: _____

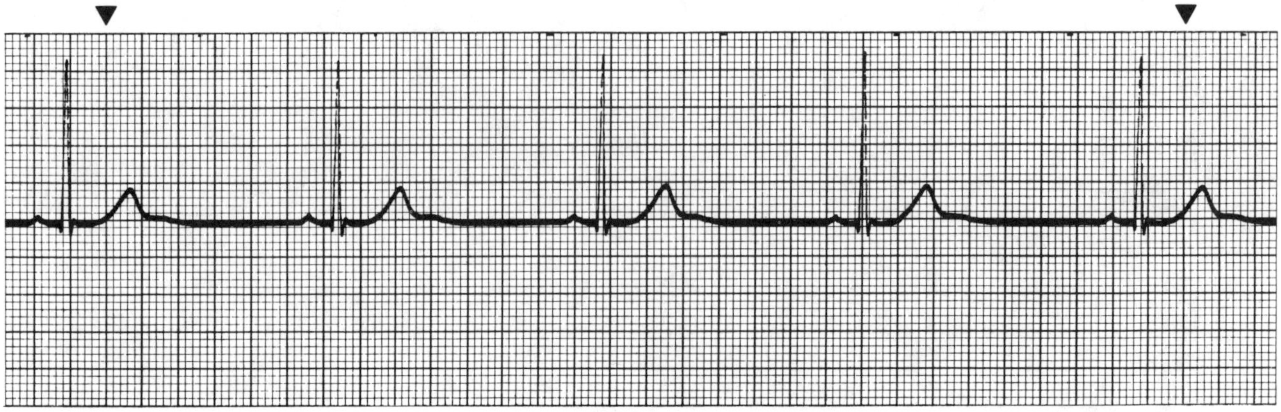

Strip 18 Rate: _____ Rhythm: _____ P wave: _____

PR interval: _____ QRS complex: _____

Rhythm interpretation: _____

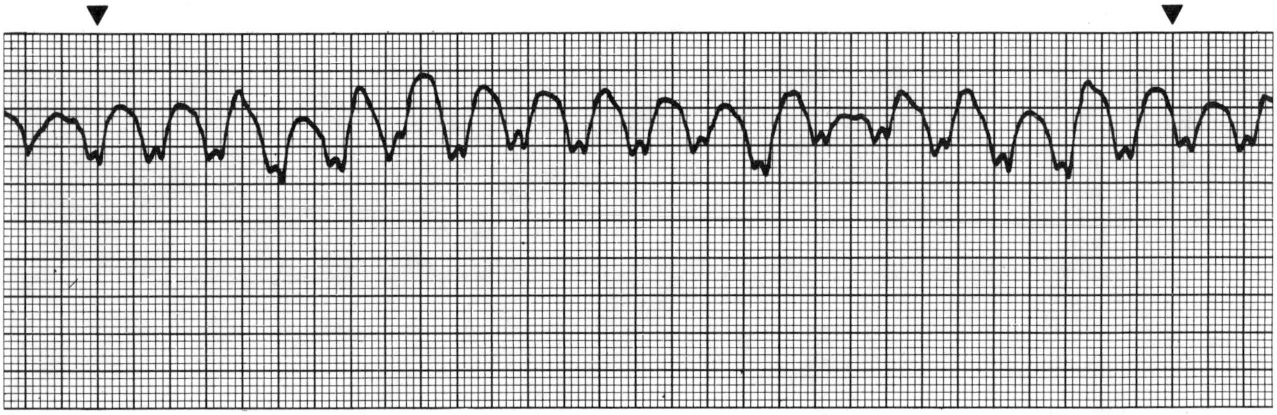

Strip 19 Rate: _____ Rhythm: _____ P wave: _____

PR interval: _____ QRS complex: _____

Rhythm interpretation: _____

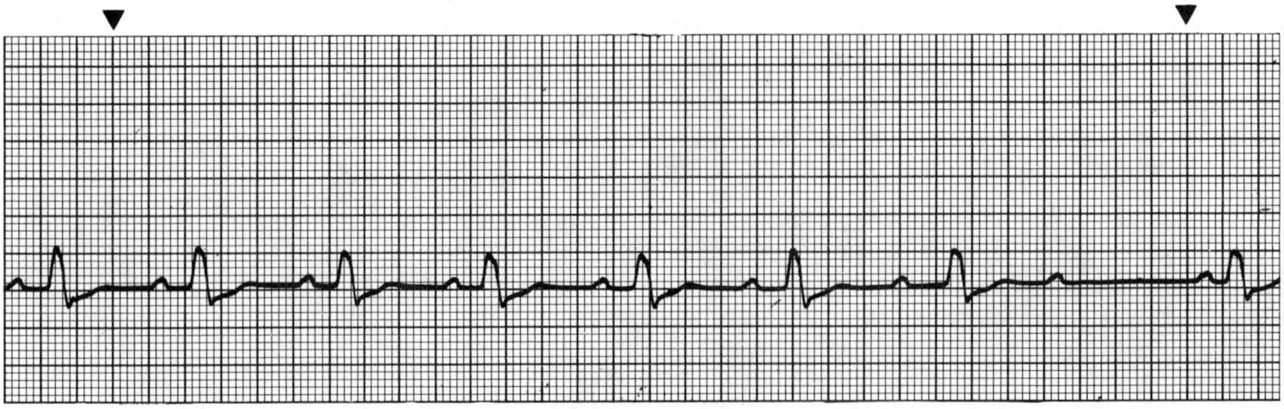

Strip 20 Rate: _____ Rhythm: _____ P wave: _____

PR interval: _____ QRS complex: _____

Rhythm interpretation: _____

Strip 21 Rate: _____ Rhythm: _____ P wave: _____
PR interval: _____ QRS complex: _____
Rhythm interpretation: _____

Strip 22 Rate: _____ Rhythm: _____ P wave: _____
PR interval: _____ QRS complex: _____
Rhythm interpretation: _____

Strip 23 Rate: _____ Rhythm: _____ P wave: _____
PR interval: _____ QRS complex: _____
Rhythm interpretation: _____

Strip 24 Rate: _____ Rhythm: _____ P wave: _____
PR interval: _____ QRS complex: _____
Rhythm interpretation: _____

Strip 25 Rate: _____ Rhythm: _____ P wave: _____
PR interval: _____ QRS complex: _____
Rhythm interpretation: _____

Strip 26 Rate: _____ Rhythm: _____ P wave: _____
PR interval: _____ QRS complex: _____
Rhythm interpretation: _____

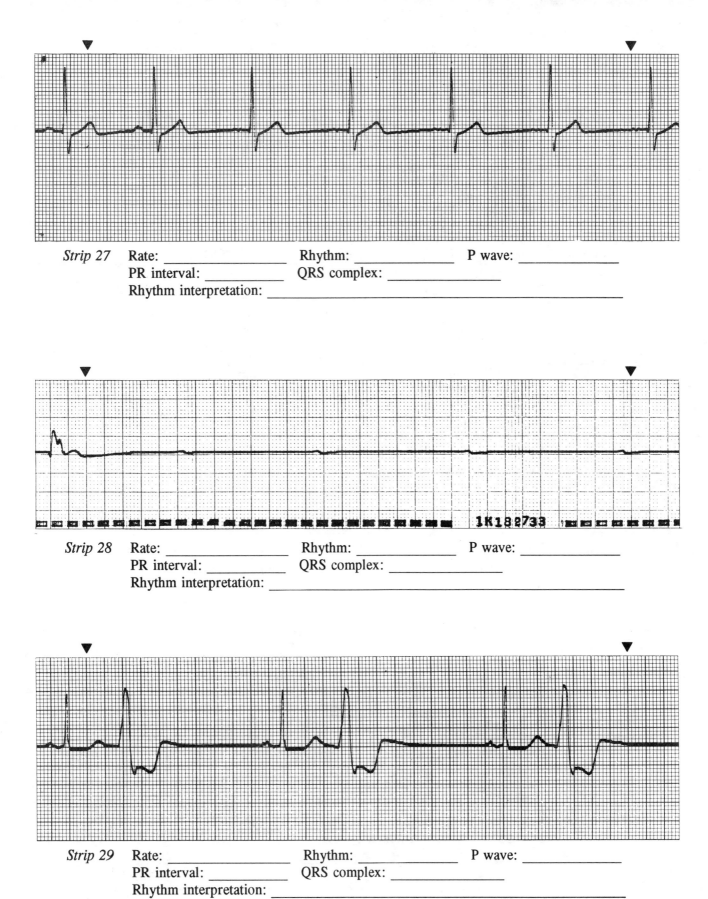

Strip 27   Rate: _____   Rhythm: _____   P wave: _____
           PR interval: _____   QRS complex: _____
           Rhythm interpretation: _____

Strip 28   Rate: _____   Rhythm: _____   P wave: _____
           PR interval: _____   QRS complex: _____
           Rhythm interpretation: _____

Strip 29   Rate: _____   Rhythm: _____   P wave: _____
           PR interval: _____   QRS complex: _____
           Rhythm interpretation: _____

179

Strip 30 Rate: _____ Rhythm: _____ P wave: _____
PR interval: _____ QRS complex: _____
Rhythm interpretation: _____

Strip 31 Rate: _____ Rhythm: _____ P wave: _____
PR interval: _____ QRS complex: _____
Rhythm interpretation: _____

Strip 32 Rate: _____ Rhythm: _____ P wave: _____
PR interval: _____ QRS complex: _____
Rhythm interpretation: _____

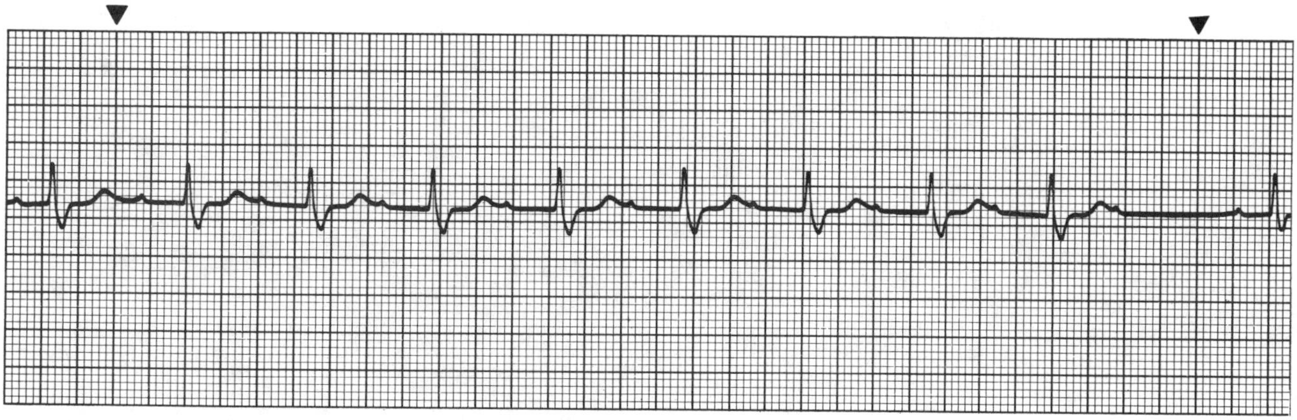

Strip 33   Rate: _____   Rhythm: _____   P wave: _____
            PR interval: _____   QRS complex: _____
            Rhythm interpretation: _____

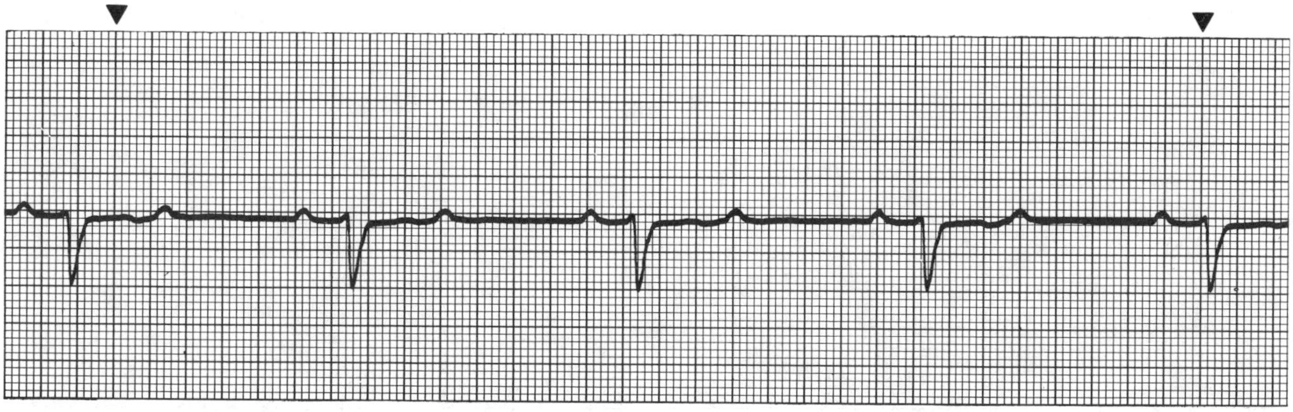

Strip 34   Rate: _____   Rhythm: _____   P wave: _____
            PR interval: _____   QRS complex: _____
            Rhythm interpretation: _____

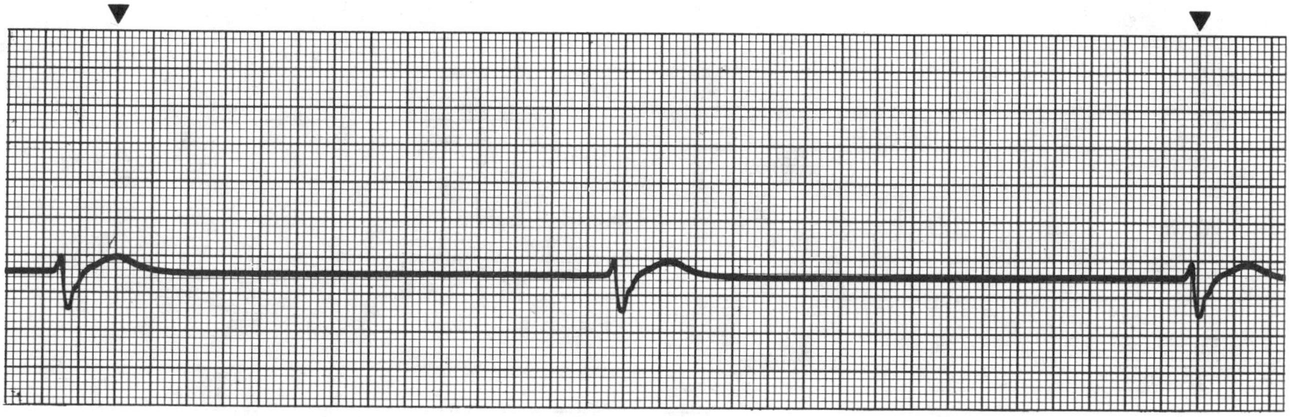

Strip 35   Rate: _____   Rhythm: _____   P wave: _____
            PR interval: _____   QRS complex: _____
            Rhythm interpretation: _____

181

Strip 36   Rate: _____   Rhythm: _____   P wave: _____
PR interval: _____   QRS complex: _____
Rhythm interpretation: _____

Strip 37   Rate: _____   Rhythm: _____   P wave: _____
PR interval: _____   QRS complex: _____
Rhythm interpretation: _____

Strip 38   Rate: _____   Rhythm: _____   P wave: _____
PR interval: _____   QRS complex: _____
Rhythm interpretation: _____

182

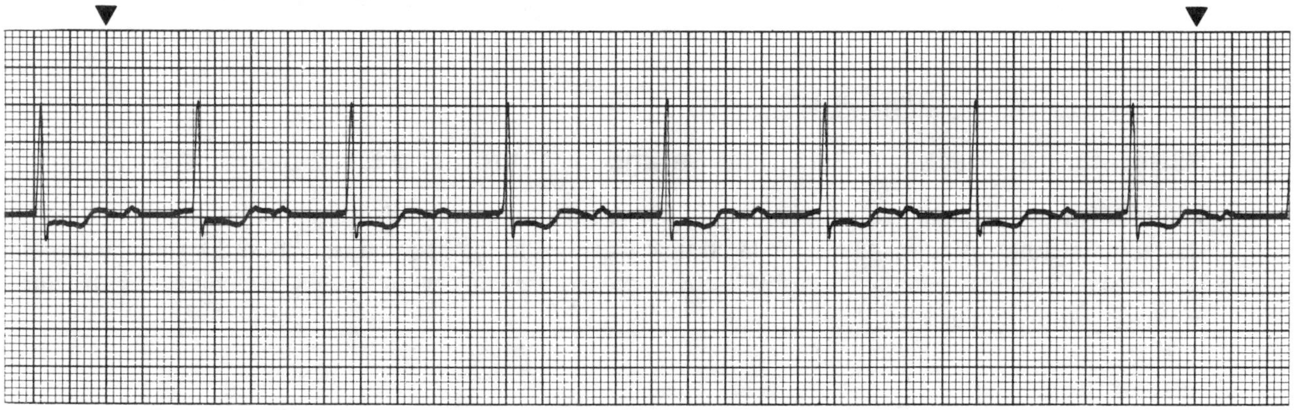

Strip 39   Rate: _____   Rhythm: _____   P wave: _____
           PR interval: _____   QRS complex: _____
           Rhythm interpretation: _____

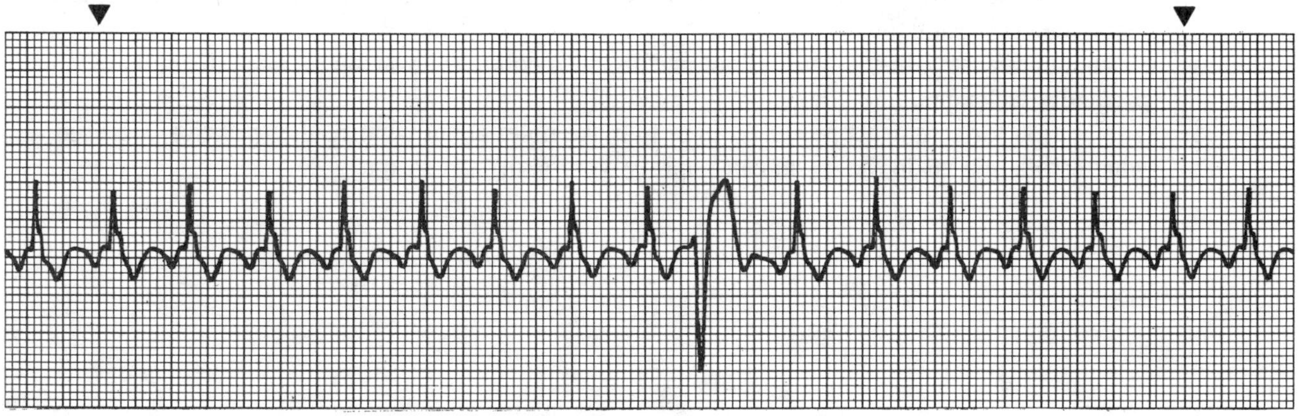

Strip 40   Rate: _____   Rhythm: _____   P wave: _____
           PR interval: _____   QRS complex: _____
           Rhythm interpretation: _____

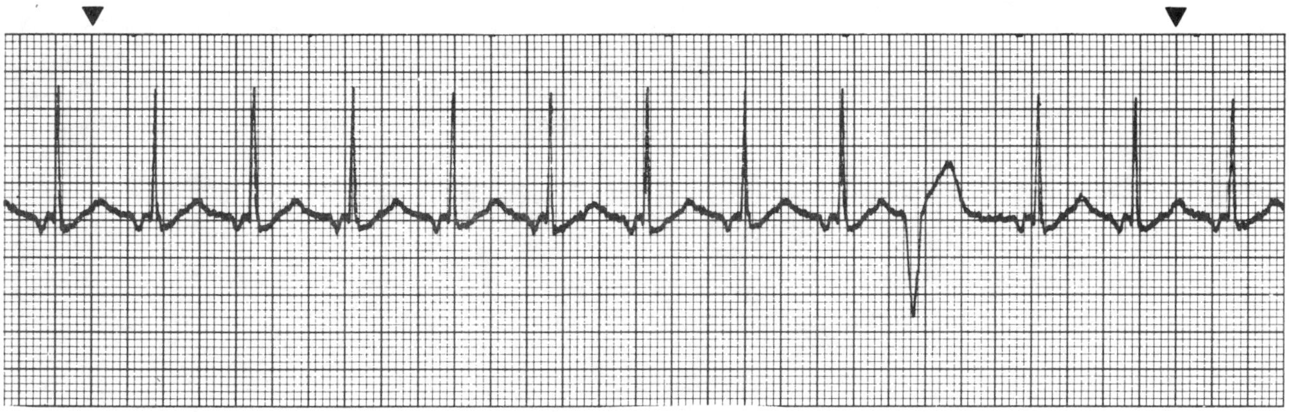

Strip 41   Rate: _____   Rhythm: _____   P wave: _____
           PR interval: _____   QRS complex: _____
           Rhythm interpretation: _____

183

STUDY GUIDE ASSIGNMENT 20-10

Performance Checklist: Defibrillation and Synchronized Cardioversion

The following skill should be practiced until you reach competency. Practice can be done in classroom settings using manikins, or in clinical rotations in the hospital or out on the ambulance or rescue unit. You may evaluate yourself, work with another student, or have a preceptor or instructor evaluate you using this form.

Instructions

1. Place a check mark in the "C" ("competent") column if you used the recommended technique the first time you performed each activity.
2. Place a check mark in the "A" ("acceptable") column if you used the recommended technique but it took you several times to perform each activity.
3. Place a check mark in the "U" ("unsatisfactory") column if you used some but not all of each recommended technique.
4. Place a check mark in the "NP" ("not performed") column if you forgot to perform that particular technique.
5. The section for comments provides space to make notes about what further practice you need, what errors you made, how you can improve your skill, and so on.

Performance Checklist: Defibrillation and Synchronized Cardioversion

C	A	U	NP	C = competent; A = acceptable; U = unsatisfactory; NP = not performed
☐	☐	☐	☐	Check responsiveness
☐	☐	☐	☐	Check airway
☐	☐	☐	☐	Check breathing
☐	☐	☐	☐	Check circulation
☐	☐	☐	☐	Assemble and check:

Primary equipment
- Monitor-defibrillator
- Electrode paste or defibrillation pads

Accessory equipment and supplies
- Gloves

C	A	U	NP	
☐	☐	☐	☐	Establish rhythm diagnosis
☐	☐	☐	☐	Determine need for defibrillation or cardioversion
☐	☐	☐	☐	Prepare defibrillator
☐	☐	☐	☐	Prepare patient
☐	☐	☐	☐	Reassess pulse
☐	☐	☐	☐	Reassess EKG
☐	☐	☐	☐	State "All clear"
☐	☐	☐	☐	Defibrillate or cardiovert
☐	☐	☐	☐	Reassess pulse
☐	☐	☐	☐	Reassess EKG

OUTCOME: ☐ Pass ☐ Fail ☐ Retest

Comments:

Student's Signature _____ Date _____

Instructor's Signature _____ Date _____

CHAPTER 21

Endocrine Emergencies

STUDY GUIDE ASSIGNMENT 21-1

- Anatomy and Physiology of the Endocrine System
Reading Assignment: pages 522-529

Matching Items

Match each of the terms in the left column with the BEST definition in the right column by placing the letter of that definition in the space next to the term. Each definition may be used once or not at all.

I	1.	adrenocorticotropin (ACTH)
B	2.	antidiuretic hormone (ADH)
J	3.	diabetes mellitus
A	4.	follicle-stimulating hormone (FSH)
N	5.	growth hormone (GH)
O	6.	hyperthyroidism
L	7.	hyperparathyroidism
F	8.	hypoparathyroidism
M	9.	hypothyroidism
K	10.	insulin
C	11.	luteinizing hormone (LH)
D	12.	oxytocin
H	13.	prolactin
G	14.	thyroid-stimulating hormone (THS)

A. Stimulates growth of ovarian follicles and testes

B. Hormone secreted by the posterior pituitary that acts primarily in the kidney

C. Controls ovulation and menstruation in women

D. Hormone secreted by the posterior pituitary that stimulates milk ejection and causes muscular contraction in the uterus

E. Stimulates liver to release glucose

F. Condition caused by lack of parathyroid secretion, resulting in reduced plasma calcium level and increased plasma phosphate level

G. Hormone that promotes growth of the thyroid and increased synthesis and release of thyroid hormones

H. Hormone that enhances milk production during pregnancy

I. Stimulates the adrenal cortex to produce cortical hormones

J. Disorder of carbohydrate, fat, and protein metabolism that results from a relative or absolute deficiency of insulin

K. Hormone secreted by the pancreas that is essential for the proper regulation of blood sugar

L. Condition caused by excessive secretion of parathyroid hormone, resulting in a high plasma calcium level and a decreased plasma phosphate level

M. Deficiency of thyroid hormone that results in a hypometabolic state

N. Promotes growth of all body tissues

O. Excess secretion of thyroid hormone that results in a hypermetabolic state

Matching Items

Match each of the terms in the left column with the BEST definition in the right column by placing the letter of that definition in the space next to the term. Each definition may be used once or not at all.

_E_ 15. hypothalamus

_G_ 16. pancreas

_F_ 17. parathyroid glands

_D_ 18. pituitary gland

_C_ 19. thyroid gland

_A_ 20. adrenal glands

A. Small, pyramid-shaped organs located retroperitoneally in close association with the upper part of each kidney

B. Aids in transport of electrolytes

C. Endocrine gland that regulates metabolism, growth, and development

D. Located at the base of the brain; secretes hormones that regulate many bodily processes

E. Portion of the diencephalon functionally related to the pituitary gland

F. Four pea-shaped glands situated in the neck in close proximity to the thyroid gland

G. Soft, oblong gland behind the stomach that secretes digestive enzymes, glucagon, and insulin

Multiple-Choice Items

Read each question carefully. For each item, select the answer that BEST completes the statement or answers the question, and place the letter of that answer in the space provided.

_C_ 1. Amines, polypeptides, glycoproteins, and steroids are:
   a. effector hormones.
   b. tropic hormones.
   c. chemical classes of hormones.
   d. specific hormones of the adrenal glands.

_D_ 2. A tropic hormone is BEST defined as a hormone that:
   a. stimulates release of other hormones from the various endocrine glands.
   b. is responsible for producing biologic effects in the organism itself.
   c. inhibits release of other hormones from other endocrine glands.
   d. stimulates or inhibits release of other hormones from other endocrine glands.

_B_ 3. An effector hormone is BEST defined as a hormone that:
   a. stimulates release of other hormones from the various endocrine glands.
   b. is responsible for producing biologic effects in the organism itself.
   c. inhibits release of other hormones from other endocrine glands.
   d. stimulates or inhibits release of other hormones from other endocrine glands.

_A_ 4. The biggest difference between endocrine and exocrine glands is that endocrine glands:
   a. do not possess ducts but secrete directly into the circulation.
   b. possess ducts that secrete directly into the target organ.
   c. do not possess ducts but secrete directly into the target organ.
   d. possess ducts that secrete directly into the circulation.

_B_ 5. Where is the pituitary gland located?
   a. In front and to either side of the trachea
   b. In a small depression in the sphenoid bone
   c. Just on top of the kidneys
   d. Retroperitoneally behind the stomach

_A_ 6. The link between the central nervous system and the endocrine system is the:
   a. pituitary gland.
   b. "fight or flight" response.
   c. sella turcica.
   d. hypothalamus.

_C_ 7. The posterior pituitary is unique in that it:
   a. synthesizes and secretes only two hormones.
   b. synthesizes and secretes six tropic hormones.
   c. stores two hormones synthesized by the hypothalamus.
   d. secretes hormones that will stimulate other hormones.

_B_ 8. Knowledge of which gland(s) is critical to cases in which emergency airway management calls for a cricothyroidotomy?
   a. Parathyroid glands
   b. Thyroid gland
   c. Thymus gland
   d. Pituitary gland

_B_ 9. A rescue squad may be summoned for a person suffering from hypoparathyroidism due to:
   a. an acute onset of paranoia.
   b. seizures with EKG changes.
   c. an acute onset of hypertension.
   d. acute depression with bradycardia.

_C_ 10. The adrenal glands are located:
   a. in front and to either side of the trachea.
   b. in a small depression in the sphenoid bone.
   c. just on top of the kidneys.
   d. retroperitoneally behind the stomach.

_C_ 11. The adrenal medulla secretes catecholamines, which are also known as:
   a. mineralocorticoids.
   b. dexamethasone and decadron.
   c. epinephrine and norepinephrine.
   d. aldosterone and renin.

D 12. Release of catecholamines primarily results in:
  a. lowered heart rate, lowered blood pressure, and increased peristalsis.
  b. increased salivation, increased GI motility, and increased urine production.
  c. lowered blood sugar, increased fat deposits, and lowered heart rate.
  d. increased heart rate, increased blood pressure, and increased cardiac output.

A 13. Adrenocortical insufficiency can be life-threatening and can cause the patient to present in a state of:
  a. hypovolemic shock.
  b. hypertensive emergency.
  c. acute paranoia.
  d. generalized edema.

D 14. Where is the pancreas located?
  a. In front and to either side of the trachea
  b. In a small depression in the sphenoid bone
  c. Just on top of the kidneys
  d. Retroperitoneally behind the stomach

B 15. The overall effect of glucagon is to:
  a. lower blood sugar levels.
  b. raise blood sugar levels.
  c. lower insulin levels.
  d. raise insulin levels.

C 16. Normally, insulin production is stimulated by:
  a. glucagon.
  b. glycogen.
  c. eating.
  d. fasting.

B 17. The clinical results of insulin production include:
  a. lowered blood glucose, decreased muscle protein synthesis, and decreased fat deposition.
  b. lowered blood glucose, increased muscle protein synthesis, and increased fat deposition.
  c. elevated blood glucose, decreased muscle protein synthesis, and decreased fat deposition.
  d. elevated blood glucose, increased muscle protein synthesis, and increased fat deposition.

B 18. The onset of diabetes in early adulthood, with almost no insulin production and the tendency to develop ketosis, is known as:
  a. adult-onset diabetes.
  b. type I diabetes.
  c. non-insulin-dependent diabetes.
  d. type II diabetes.

C 19. Secondary diabetes is diabetes that results from:
  a. no readily identifiable cause.
  b. extreme dieting.
  c. a preexisting condition.
  d. surgical removal of the pancreas.

STUDY GUIDE ASSIGNMENT 21-2

▪ Assessment of Endocrine Emergencies
▪ Diabetic Emergencies
Reading Assignment: pages 529-533

Matching Items

Match each of the terms in the left column with the BEST definition in the right column by placing the letter of that definition in the space next to the term. Each definition may be used once or not at all.

_B_ 1. diabetic ketoacidosis

_A_ 2. hypoglycemia

_C_ 3. hyperosmolar hyperglycemic nonketotic coma

A. Low blood glucose concentration

B. Complication of diabetes mellitus in which hyperglycemia, ketonemia, and acidosis occur

C. Clinical entity principally characterized by severe hyperosmolality, often secondary to extreme hyperglycemia

D. Clinical entity principally characterized by severe hyperosmolality, often secondary to extreme hypoglycemia

Multiple-Choice Items

Read each question carefully. For each item, select the answer that BEST completes the statement or answers the question, and place the letter of that answer in the space provided.

_A_ 1. The two hallmark biochemical features of diabetic ketoacidosis, hyperglycemia and hyperketonemia, can be detected in the field by the presence of:
   I. dehydration.
   II. hypotension.
   III. Kussmaul's respirations.
   IV. history of weight loss.
      a. I, II, and III
      b. II, III, and IV
      c. I, II, and IV
      d. I, III, and IV

_B_ 2. The presence of infection in the insulin-dependent diabetic can potentially precipitate severe:
   a. hypertension.
   b. diabetic ketoacidosis.
   c. hypoglycemia.
   d. hypovolemic shock.

_D_ 3. Which of the following signs and symptoms are MOST typical of a patient with diabetic ketoacidosis?
  I. Warm, dry skin
  II. Abdominal pain and tenderness
  III. Tachycardia
  IV. Deep, rapid, and labored respirations
    a. I, II, and III
    b. II, III, and IV
    c. I, III, and IV
    d. I, II, III, and IV

_B_ 4. In a known diabetic with an altered level of consciousness, why would the treatment of choice be 50% dextrose?
    a. 50% dextrose is never harmful.
    b. Hypoglycemia, which may be life-threatening, may be present.
    c. Diabetic ketoacidosis also responds to dextrose.
    d. 50% dextrose may prevent dehydration.

_C_ 5. Type II diabetics who are older and suffer a CVA, infection, or trauma are much more likely to develop:
    a. insulin shock.
    b. diabetic ketoacidosis.
    c. hyperosmolar hyperglycemic nonketotic coma.
    d. severe hypertension.

_D_ 6. Even though it may sometimes be difficult to tell the difference, hypoglycemia may present differently from diabetic ketoacidosis. Which of the following descriptions is more typical of the hypoglycemic patient?
    a. Warm, dry skin; rapid, deep respirations; the odor of acetone; abdominal pain
    b. Rapid, deep respirations; the odor of acetone; abdominal pain; tachycardia
    c. The odor of acetone; abdominal pain; tachycardia; cool, pale, and diaphoretic skin
    d. Tachycardia; cool, pale, and diaphoretic skin; rapid, shallow respirations

CHAPTER 22

Neurologic Emergencies

STUDY GUIDE ASSIGNMENT 22-1

▪ Anatomy and Physiology of the Nervous System
Reading Assignment: pages 536-548

Matching Items

Match each of the terms in the left column with the BEST definition in the right column by placing the letter of that definition in the space next to the term. Each definition may be used once or not at all.

_____ 1. afferent neuron
_____ 2. arachnoid
_____ 3. autonomic nervous system
_____ 4. axon
_____ 5. brain stem
_____ 6. central nervous system
_____ 7. cerebellum
_____ 8. cerebrum
_____ 9. dendrites
_____ 10. diencephalon
_____ 11. dura mater
_____ 12. efferent neuron
_____ 13. interneuron
_____ 14. neuron
_____ 15. parasympathetic division
_____ 16. peripheral nervous system
_____ 17. pia mater
_____ 18. spinal cord
_____ 19. sympathetic division

A. Contains the thalamus and the hypothalamus

B. Plays an essential role in maintaining homeostatic levels

C. Connecting neuron

D. Brain and spinal cord; functions as the body's communication control center; directly responsible for all aspects of cognitive and voluntary nervous function

E. Division of the autonomic nervous system; provides systemic effects that result in the "fight or flight" phenomenon

F. Two-way path for conducting impulses to and from the brain

G. Process of a neuron that carries the impulse away from the cell body

H. Sensory neuron

I. Three-way path for conducting impulses to and from the brain

J. Maintains and regulates insulin release, pupil constriction, and salivary and digestive gland secretion

K. Innermost layer of the meninges that directly covers the brain

L. Includes all nerve fibers outside the brain and spinal cord

M. Delicate membrane that lies between the dura mater and pia mater

N. Inferior to the cerebrum and anterior to the cerebellum; controls motor, sensory and reflex functions

O. Largest portion of the brain; controls sensory and motor functions

P. Fibers that extend from the cell body of the neuron

Q. Outermost of the three meninges that protect the brain

R. Primarily involved in regulating voluntary muscle activity

S. Motor neuron

T. Individual nerve cell

Labeling Items

Read each question carefully and place your answer in the space provided.

1. Label the six meningeal layers and their potential spaces identified in the drawing by filling in the blank next to each letter, which corresponds with the same letter in the drawing. The six layers and potential spaces are to be selected from the words that follow the blanks. Each answer may be used once or not at all.

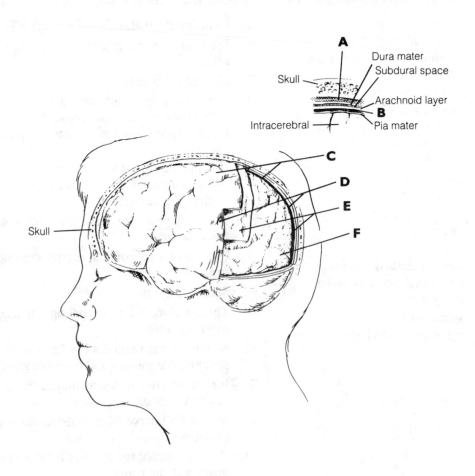

A. _____   D. _____

B. _____   E. _____

C. _____   F. _____

pia mater   epidural space   subdural space
cortex   subarachnoid space   arachnoid mater
dura mater

2. Label the six divisions of the brain identified in the drawing by filling in the blank next to each
    letter, which corresponds with the same letter in the drawing. The six divisions are to be selected
    from the words that follow the blanks. Each answer may be used once or not at all.

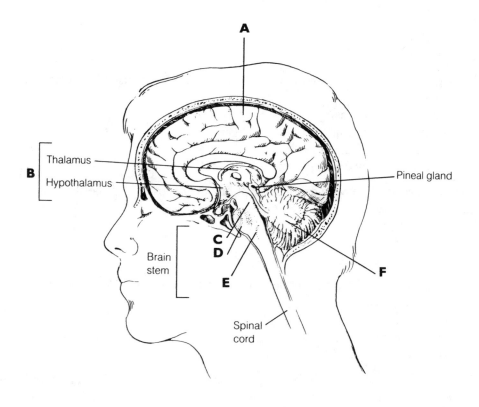

A. _____   D. _____

B. _____   E. _____

C. _____   F. _____

diencephalon   medulla oblongata   cerebrum
cerebellum   circle of Willis   midbrain
pons

Multiple-Choice Items

Read each question carefully. For each item, select the answer that BEST completes the statement or answers the question, and place the letter of that answer in the space provided.

_A_ 1. Components of the central nervous system include the:
   I.   brain.
   II. spinal cord.
   III. cranial nerves.
   IV. spinal nerves.
      a. I and II
      b. II and III
      c. III and IV
      d. I, II, and IV

_D_ 2. The basic unit of the nervous system is the:
      a. ganglion.
      b. axon.
      c. dendrite.
      d. neuron.

_D_ 3. Damage to the nerves within the central nervous system is usually permanent because those nerves lack:
      a. dendrites and axons.
      b. axons and neurilemma.
      c. neurilemma and dendrites.
      d. myelin sheath and neurilemma.

_A_ 4. The potential space between the dura mater and the periosteum of the skull is referred to as the:
      a. epidural space.
      b. subdural space.
      c. epiarachnoid space.
      d. subarachnoid space.

_B_ 5. The potential space between the dura mater and the arachnoid membrane is known as the:
      a. epidural space.
      b. subdural space.
      c. epiarachnoid space.
      d. subarachnoid space.

_D_ 6. The potential space below the arachnoid membrane but above the pia mater is referred to as the:
      a. epidural space.
      b. subdural space.
      c. epiarachnoid space.
      d. subarachnoid space.

_D_ 7. The major portion of the blood supply to the brain comes from the _____ arteries.
      a. inominant and brachial
      b. clavicular and inominant
      c. brachial and carotid
      d. vertebral and carotid

B 8. A vascular structure found in the base of the brain maintains perfusion of the brain if an occlusion occurs in one of the vessels supplying the brain. This structure is called the:
   a. pia mater.
   b. circle of Willis.
   c. pons.
   d. brain stem.

A 9. The main function of the cerebrum is to:
   a. control sensory and motor functions, speech, thought processes, and emotion.
   b. function as a "relay station" for sensory impulses en route to the cortex.
   c. register emotions.
   d. function as a bridge between the nervous system and the endocrine system.

D 10. The main function of the hypothalamus is to:
   a. control sensory and motor functions, speech, thought processes, and emotion.
   b. function as a "relay station" for sensory impulses en route to the cortex.
   c. register emotions.
   d. function as a bridge between the nervous system and the endocrine system.

C 11. The area of the brain that controls body temperature is located in the:
   a. cerebrum.
   b. thalamus.
   c. hypothalamus.
   d. diencephalon.

D 12. The portion of the brain that controls coordinated skeletal muscle movement is the:
   a. cerebrum.
   b. hypothalamus.
   c. brain stem.
   d. cerebellum.

C 13. The pneumotaxic centers, pupillary reflex coordination, and cardiac and vasomotor centers are located in the:
   a. cerebrum.
   b. hypothalamus.
   c. brain stem.
   d. cerebellum.

B 14. The spinal cord has two main functions, to act as a two-way path for conducting impulses and to act as a:
   a. control center.
   b. reflex center.
   c. synergistic center.
   d. relay center.

C 15. How many vertebra are located in the cervical spine?
   a. 4
   b. 5
   c. 7
   d. 12

_B_ 16. Your patient has loss of sensation that begins at the nipple line. This indicates cord damage at which level of the spine?
   a. C-5 to C-7
   b. T-4
   c. T-10
   d. L-1 to L-5

_C_ 17. Your paraplegic patient has no feeling below the umbilicus. This indicates cord damage at which level of the spine?
   a. C-5 to C-7
   b. T-4
   c. T-10
   d. L-1 to L-5

_C_ 18. Many signs and symptoms of patients in the field are effects of which part of the nervous system?
   a. Peripheral
   b. Central
   c. Autonomic
   d. Somatic

_B_ 19. The body's reaction known as the "fight or flight syndrome" is primarily controlled by which part of the nervous system?
   a. Somatic
   b. Sympathetic
   c. Peripheral
   d. Parasympathetic

_C_ 20. The primary nerve of the parasympathetic system is the vagal nerve, which controls certain actions of the:
   a. lungs, liver, and heart.
   b. liver, heart, and stomach.
   c. heart, stomach, and GI tract.
   d. stomach, GI tract, and lungs.

STUDY GUIDE ASSIGNMENT 22-2

▪ Assessment of Nervous System Emergencies
▪ Types of Nervous System Disorders
Reading Assignment: pages 548-556

Matching Items

Match each of the following terms with the BEST definition by placing the letter of that definition in the blank space next to the term. Each definition may be used once or not at all.

_E_ 1. AVPU   A. Recurrent seizures from an unknown cause, thought to be irreversible

_G_ 2. coma

_D_ 3. Cushing's reflex   B. Epileptic attacks in rapid succession with no regaining of consciousness

_I_ 4. decerebrate posturing

K	5.	decorticate posturing
A	6.	epilepsy
H	7.	Glasgow Coma Scale
J	8.	seizure
B	9.	status epilepticus
C	10.	stroke

C. Sudden interruption in blood flow to the brain with resultant neurologic deficits

D. Threefold phenomenon associated with increasing intracranial pressure

E. Acronym for responsiveness

F. Twofold phenomenon associated with increasing intracranial pressure

G. Deep state of unconsciousness; cannot be aroused by external stimuli

H. Guide to assess baseline degree of brain dysfunction

I. Upper extremities extend and rotate inward with palms facing lateral, and lower extremities extend and are rigid

J. Manifestation of a massive electrical discharge of one or more groups of neurons in the brain

K. Flexion of the upper extremities, with the lower extremities rigid and extended

Multiple-Choice Items

Read each question carefully. For each item, select the answer that BEST completes the statement or answers the question, and place the letter of that answer in the space provided.

D 1. In the neurologic patient, the MOST serious concerns are:
a. responsiveness and pupil reaction.
b. pupil reaction and pulse rate.
c. pulse rate and respiratory status.
d. respiratory status and responsiveness.

D 2. Abnormal respiratory patterns that result from neurologic impediments include which of the following?
 I. Cheyne-Stokes respiration
 II. Shallow tachypnea
 III. Central neurogenic hyperventilation
 IV. Ataxic breathing
   a. I, II, and III
   b. II, III, and IV
   c. I, II, and IV
   d. I, III, and IV

B 3. Cardiac arrhythmias that result from increasing intracranial pressure are BEST treated by:
a. using the appropriate drug for a given arrhythmia.
b. aggressive hyperventilation.
c. correcting the associated hypotension.
d. correcting the associated hypertension.

C 4. Patient assessment findings that may indicate a neurological problem include the level of consciousness, pupil size and reaction, and:
I. the position in which the patient was found.
II. speech patterns.
III. pulse regularity.
IV. posturing.
   a. I, II, and III
   b. II, III, and IV
   c. I, II, and IV
   d. I, III, and IV

A 5. For a coma to occur, which part or parts of the brain are involved?
   a. Cerebral cortex or reticular activating system
   b. Cerebral cortex or cerebellum
   c. Cerebellum or brain stem
   d. Brain stem or reticular activating system

C 6. A patient whose coma was preceded by fever, slow onset, and symmetrical findings in the secondary exam is probably suffering from a coma due to:
   a. structural lesions.
   b. reticular activating system dysfunction.
   c. metabolic causes.
   d. trauma.

B 7. As a general rule, structural lesions that affect the reticular activating system include:
   a. infection.
   b. subdural bleed.
   c. overdose.
   d. uremia.

B 8. Appropriate pharmacologic therapy for the comatose patient may include 50% dextrose, and:
I. diazepam.
II. naloxone.
III. thiamine.
IV. sodium bicarbonate.
   a. I, II, and III
   b. II, III, and IV
   c. II and III
   d. I and IV

C 9. Which of the following definitions of seizure is MOST accurate?
   a. Seizure is a disease resulting in uncontrollable, bizarre muscle movements with a complete loss of consciousness during the episode.
   b. Seizure consists of recurrent episodes of massive electrical discharges of one or more groups of neurons in the brain.
   c. Seizure is a manifestation of a massive electrical discharge of one or more neurons in the brain and is a symptom of an underlying disorder.
   d. Seizure is a disease that is manifested by abnormal activity of the neurons in the brain, and is thought to be caused by an irreversible underlying condition.

_C_ 10. A 24-year-old male seizure patient who appears conscious but repeats a single word over and over, smacks his lips, and repeatedly taps his knee with his hand is MOST likely to be having a(an):
   a. general complex seizure.
   b. Jacksonian seizure.
   c. partial complex seizure.
   d. hysterical seizure.

_D_ 11. Complications from status epilepticus include:
   a. brain damage, aspiration, hypoxia, and bowel obstruction.
   b. aspiration, hypoxia, bowel obstruction, and dehydration.
   c. hypoxia, bowel obstruction, dehydration, and brain damage.
   d. dehydration, brain damage, hypoxia, and aspiration.

_D_ 12. With a patient suffering from status epilepticus, one of the most common causes is:
   a. head trauma.
   b. stroke.
   c. brain tumors.
   d. not taking medication.

_D_ 13. Appropriate drugs to administer to the seizuring patient include:
   a. diazepam, phenytoin, and naloxone.
   b. phenytoin, naloxone, and thiamine.
   c. naloxone, thiamine, and 50% dextrose.
   d. 50% dextrose, phenytoin, and diazepam.

_C_ 14. The two general causes of strokes are:
   a. thrombosis and embolism.
   b. embolism and cerebrovascular hemorrhage.
   c. cerebrovascular hemorrhage and vascular obstruction.
   d. vascular obstruction and thrombosis.

CHAPTER 23

Gastrointestinal, Urinary, and Reproductive System Emergencies

STUDY GUIDE ASSIGNMENT 23-1

- Anatomy and Physiology of the Gastrointestinal System
- Anatomy and Physiology of the Abdomen
- Anatomy and Physiology of the Urinary System
- Anatomy and Physiology of the Reproductive Systems
- The Acute Abdomen
- Pathophysiology of the Urinary System
- Pathophysiology of Reproductive System Disorders

Reading Assignment: pages 558-569

Matching Items

Match each of the terms in the left column with the BEST definition in the right column by placing the letter of that definition in the space next to the term. Each definition may be used once or not at all.

B	1.	acute abdomen	A. Hollow, narrow tube with a closed end, located at the lower end of the colon
D	2.	appendicitis	
A	3.	appendix	B. Abdominal disorder that develops quickly and is severe in nature
J	4.	cholecystitis	
F	5.	colic	C. Lesion or sore of the duodenal mucosa resulting from the action of gastric juice
I	6.	diverticulitis	
C	7.	duodenal ulcers	D. Inflammation of the appendix
H	8.	epididymitis	E. Inflammation of the liver
G	9.	epiglottis	F. Spasm of the smooth muscle lining of the intestinal tract
			G. Protects the lower airways from foreign bodies

H. Inflammation or infection of the epididymis, which travels via the vas deferens

I. Inflammation of the diverticula in the intestinal tract, especially in the colon

J. Inflammation of the gall bladder

Multiple-Choice Items

Read each question carefully. For each item, select the answer that BEST completes the statement or answers the question, and place the letter of that answer in the space provided.

_C_ 1. The _____ are portions of the small intestine.
   a. ascending colon, transverse colon, and descending colon
   b. splenic fixture, ileocecal valve, and pyloric sphincter
   c. duodenum, jejunum, and ileum
   d. cecum, appendix, and rectum

_B_ 2. Saliva, a product of the salivary glands, begins the digestion of:
   a. lipids.
   b. carbohydrates.
   c. proteins.
   d. all of the above.

_C_ 3. The organ responsible for the secretion of digestive enzymes, glucagon, and insulin is the:
   a. liver.
   b. gallbladder.
   c. pancreas.
   d. stomach.

_A_ 4. The gallbladder is located in the _____ quadrant.
   a. right upper
   b. left upper
   c. right lower
   d. left lower

_A_ 5. The outer layer of the membranous sac that lines the abdominal cavity is the:
   a. parietal peritoneum.
   b. parietal pleura.
   c. visceral peritoneum.
   d. visceral pleura.

_C_ 6. Examples of solid abdominal organs include the:
   I. spleen.
   II. gallbladder.
   III. uterus.
   IV. liver.
   V. kidneys.
      a. I, II, and III
      b. I, III, and V
      c. I, IV, and V
      d. II, III, and IV

D 7. Hollow organs contained within the urinary system include the:
   a. stomach.
   b. intestines.
   c. kidneys.
   d. urinary bladder.

B 8. The kidneys are located:
   a. in the retroperitoneal space from approximately the 5th thoracic to the 11th thoracic vertebrae.
   b. on either side of the spinal column from approximately the 12th thoracic to the 3rd lumbar vertebrae.
   c. on the right side of the spinal column from approximately the 1st lumbar to the 4th sacral vertebrae.
   d. within the confines of the small intestines from approximately the 1st to the 5th intercostal spaces.

D 9. The _____ houses sperm cells until they reach maturity.
   a. glans penis
   b. ductus deferens
   c. seminal vesicle
   d. epididymis

C 10. The male reproductive gland that secretes an alkaline fluid which neutralizes seminal fluid and increases sperm motility is the:
   a. prepuce.
   b. seminal duct.
   c. prostate.
   d. testis.

D 11. Which of the following statements is true of the ovaries in the female reproductive system?
   a. They house the fertilized ovum.
   b. They produce and release eggs.
   c. They secrete sex hormones.
   d. Both b and c are correct.

C 12. The general causes of gastrointestinal disorders include:
   I. inflammation.
   II. infection.
   III. overdose.
   IV. obstruction.
   V. hemorrhage.
      a. I, II, and III
      b. II, IV, and V
      c. I, II, IV, and V
      d. I, II, III, IV, and V

B 13. _____ is the irritation and inflammation of the abdominal cavity lining as a result of the spillage of gastrointestinal contents.
   a. Diverticulitis
   b. Peritonitis

c. Cholecystitis

d. Pleuritis

C 14. The most frequent complaint elicited from a patient experiencing an acute abdominal disorder is:

a. hemorrhage.

b. anorexia.

c. pain.

d. nausea.

A 15. Symptoms of intestinal obstruction include:

a. cramping and nausea.

b. sharp pain in the suprapubic region.

c. abdominal distention.

d. left lower quadrant pain.

D 16. The onset of pain associated with duodenal ulcers occurs:

a. in the early morning immediately upon arising.

b. several hours after engaging in exercise.

c. after consuming fried, greasy, or spicy foods.

d. approximately 1 hour after meals.

C 17. Cholecystitis occurs primarily in middle-aged women as a result of:

a. overuse of diuretics earlier in life.

b. blockage by a bone fragment or fruit seed.

c. eating fried, greasy, or spicy foods.

d. b and c.

C 18. If perforation occurs in a case of appendicitis, the patient is likely to experience:

I. a decrease in pain.

II. severe peritonitis.

III. an increase in pain.

IV. shock.

a. I and IV

b. II and IV

c. I, II, and IV

d. I, III, and IV

D 19. Physical examination of the abdomen of the patient with an abdominal aortic aneurysm may reveal:

a. a tender left flank.

b. severe distention.

c. umbilical cyanosis.

d. a pulsating mass.

C 20. The stool of a patient experiencing bleeding in the stomach, duodenum, or small bowel appears:

a. dark red.

b. bright red.

c. black and tarry.

d. normal.

D 21. Management of the patient who is experiencing an acute abdominal disorder should include:
   I. oxygen by nasal cannula.
   II. IV D$_5$W at a keep-open rate.
   III. monitoring of vital signs and EKG.
   IV. high-flow oxygen.
   V. large-bore IV of lactated Ringer's.
      a. I, II, and III
      b. I, III, and V
      c. II, III, and IV
      d. III, IV, and V

B 22. The patient exhibits yellow-tinted skin with frosty crystals. She has pitting edema of the ankles with very thin arms and legs. A family member states that this condition has been developing for prolonged period of time. The paramedic should suspect:
   a. acute dehydration.
   b. chronic renal failure.
   c. formation of renal calculi.
   d. urinary tract infection.

A 23. The formation of kidney stones is the result of:
   a. calcium deposits in the kidneys.
   b. prolonged chronic renal failure.
   c. eating fried, greasy, or spicy foods.
   d. injury to one or both kidneys.

C 24. The signs and symptoms of a urinary tract infection include:
   I. polyuria.
   II. dysuria.
   III. hyperthermia.
   IV. hematuria.
      a. I, II, and III
      b. I, III, and IV
      c. II, III, and IV
      d. I, II, III, and IV

B 25. In the event of a severing of a portion of a shunt in a traumatized hemodialysis patient, the paramedic should:
   a. quickly remove the damaged shunt tube.
   b. quickly clamp the damaged tube.
   c. not touch the damaged tube.
   d. inject heparin into the damaged tube.

C 26. In general, management of disorders of the male reproductive system should include:
   a. stopping internal bleeding by packing 4x4 pads into the opening of the penis.
   b. a recommendation that the patient contact the family physician within a week.
   c. supportive care, including reassessment of airway status, and monitoring of vital signs.
   d. a and b.

_B_ 27. The site of most ectopic pregnancies is the:
   a. ovaries.
   b. fallopian tubes.
   c. uterus.
   d. abdominal wall.

_D_ 28. Management of the patient with a non-traumatic disorder of the female reproductive system may include:
   I. frequent reassessment of the airway.
   II. establishment of an IV life-line.
   III. general supportive care, including monitoring of vital signs.
   IV. use of the pneumatic anti-shock garment.
   V. transport in a comfortable position.
      a. I and III
      b. II, III, and V
      c. I, III, and V
      d. I, II, III, IV, and V

Labeling Items

Read each question carefully and place your answer in the space provided.

1.   Label the fourteen parts of the gastrointestinal system identified in the drawing by filling in the blank next to each letter, which corresponds with the same letter in the drawing. The fourteen parts are to be selected from the words that follow the blanks. Each answer may be used once or not at all.

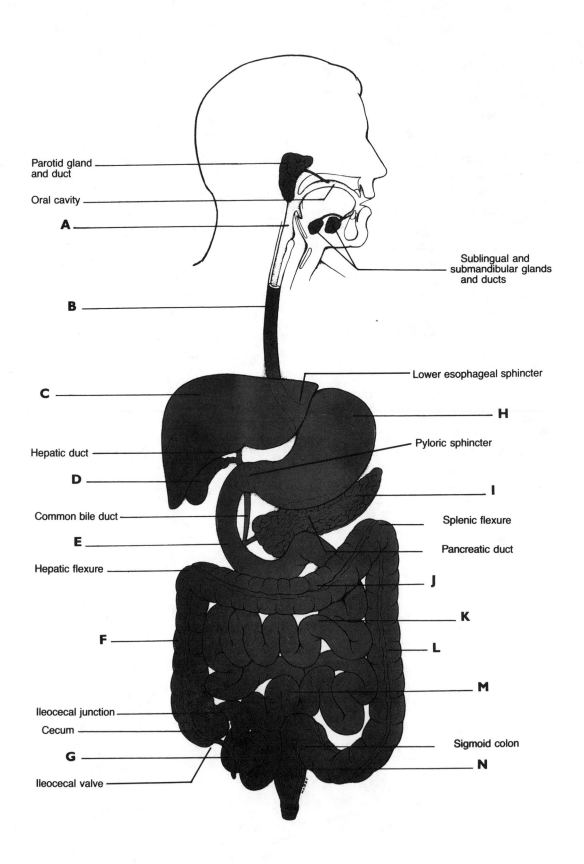

Parotid gland
and duct

Oral cavity

A

Sublingual and
submandibular glands
and ducts

B

Lower esophageal sphincter

C

H

Pyloric sphincter

Hepatic duct

D

I

Common bile duct

Splenic flexure

E

Pancreatic duct

Hepatic flexure

J

K

F

L

M

Ileocecal junction

Cecum

Sigmoid colon

G

N

Ileocecal valve

A. _____

B. _____

C. _____

D. _____

E. _____

F. _____

G. _____

H. _____

I. _____

J. _____

K. _____

L. _____

M. _____

N. _____

stomach	jejunum	esophagus
duodenum	rectum	pharynx
appendix	ascending colon	liver
pancreas	gallbladder	descending colon
transverse colon	ileum	

2. Label the eight parts of the reproductive system identified in the drawing by filling in the blank next to each letter, which corresponds with the same letter in the drawing. The eight parts are to be selected from the words that follow the blanks. Each answer may be used once or not at all.

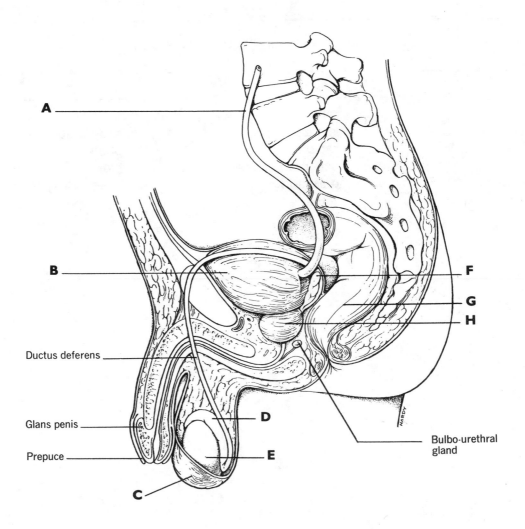

A. _____   E. _____

B. _____   F. _____

C. _____   G. _____

D. _____   H. _____

bladder   seminal vesicle   epididymis
testis   prostate   ureter
scrotum   rectum   appendix

CHAPTER 24

Allergic and Anaphylactic Reactions

STUDY GUIDE ASSIGNMENT 24-1

- Concepts and Terminology
- Common Allergens
- Pathophysiology
- Assessment of the Anaphylactic Patient
- Management of Allergic and Anaphylactic Reactions
- Prevention and Patient Education

Reading Assignment: pages 572-577

Matching Items

Match each of the terms in the left column with the BEST definition in the right column by placing the letter of that definition in the space next to the term. Each definition may be used once or not at all.

F	1.	allergy
A	2.	allergic reaction
H	3.	anaphylaxis
B	4.	anaphylactic reaction
J	5.	antibody
D	6.	antigen
G	7.	histamine
E	8.	immunity
I	9.	sensitization

A. Oversensitive and harmful response to a foreign substance

B. Acute generalized allergic reaction that has systemic signs and symptoms

C. Protective hormone formed in the body as a result of contact with an antigen

D. Foreign substance that induces the formation of antibodies

E. The body's natural resistance to poisons and foreign substances

F. Abnormal and individual hypersensitivity to substances that are ordinarily harmless

G. Substance normally present in the body that exerts a pharmacologic action when tissue damage occurs

H. Acute generalized allergic reaction

I. Exposure to allergens and the resulting production of antibodies

J. Protective protein substance formed in the body as a result of contact with an antigen

211

Multiple-Choice Items

Read each question carefully. For each item, select the answer that BEST completes the statement or answers the question, and place the letter of that answer in the space provided.

B 1. The number of anaphylactic deaths from insect stings in the United States per year is estimated to be at least:
   a. 20.
   b. 50.
   c. 1000.
   d. 50,000.

D 2. The immune response is designed to:
   a. provide "fight or flight" capabilities when the organism is stressed.
   b. regulate metabolic functions during exercise.
   c. create a negative adaptive response to allergens.
   d. guard the body against dangerous foreign substances.

C 3. Immunity requires that the body be able to distinguish between:
   a. adaptation and reaction.
   b. bacteria and viruses.
   c. self and non-self.
   d. histamine and antihistamine.

D 4. Antigens induce the formation of:
   a. bacteria.
   b. immunoglobulins.
   c. antibodies.
   d. b and c.

A 5. Allergy is:
   a. an abnormal sensitivity to a substance that is harmless to most persons.
   b. a gradual exposure to a foreign substance in order to stimulate formation of antibodies.
   c. the body's ability to repel foreign substances by the development of immune bodies.
   d. a sensitivity to substances to which most people exhibit sensitivity.

B 6. An acute generalized allergic reaction beginning within minutes to hours after exposure to a foreign substance is called:
   a. sensitization.
   b. anaphylaxis.
   c. antigenesis.
   d. immunity.

D 7. An allergen may be introduced into the body by:
   I. injection.
   II. ingestion.
   III. absorption.
   IV. inhalation.
      a. I and II
      b. II and III

c. III and IV

d. I, II, III, and IV

C 8. A person allergic to penicillin is also likely to be allergic to:

a. aspirin.

b. IV pyelogram dye.

c. ampicillin.

d. tetanus vaccine.

D 9. A patient who has previously been stung by a bumblebee may thereafter have an increased allergic response to:

a. a spider bite.

b. fire ant bites.

c. a wasp sting.

d. a yellow jacket sting.

A 10. The antigen-antibody reaction occurs on the surface of:

a. mast cells and basophils.

b. hemoglobin in the red blood cells.

c. immune or T-cells.

d. secondary platelets.

B 11. Signs and symptoms of anaphylactic reactions include:

I. urticaria.

II. rhinitis.

III. constipation.

IV. cardiac arrhythmias.

V. paresthesias.

a. I, III, and V

b. I, II, and IV

c. II, IV, and V

d. II, III, and IV

D 12. The primary cause of death in anaphylaxis is:

a. cardiovascular collapse.

b. hypovolemia.

c. seizures.

d. airway obstruction.

D 13. History taking in the patient with suspected anaphylaxis should include:

I. determination of time between exposure and onset of signs and symptoms.

II. detailing of other medical problems, especially heart problems and asthma.

III. determination of any similar occurrences in the past.

IV. observing the scene for evidence of epinephrine or similar medications.

a. I, II, and III

b. I, III, and IV

c. II, III, and IV

d. I, II, III, and IV

_B_ 14. The physical examination of a patient with suspected anaphylaxis should include a thorough assessment of circulatory function. This assessment should include:
 I. capillary refill test.
 II. pulse rate and regularity.
 III. pulse quality.
 IV. blood pressure.
  a. I, II, and III
  b. I, II, III, and IV
  c. II, III, and IV
  d. I, II, and IV

_B_ 15. Your pediatric patient is experiencing respiratory involvement following a beesting. Treatment of this patient should include the administration of _____ epinephrine 1:1000.
 a. 0.01 mg
 b. 0.01 mg/kg
 c. 0.5 mg
 d. 0.5 mg/kg

_D_ 16. If your anaphylactic patient continues to experience bronchospasm despite the administration of diphenhydramine, the paramedic should administer:
 a. Benadryl.
 b. D₅0.9 NaCl.
 c. lactated Ringer's.
 d. theophylline ethylenediamine.

_A_ 17. The use of epinephrine is effective in anaphylaxis because:
 a. it causes vasoconstriction and bronchial dilation.
 b. it prevents further release of histamine.
 c. it raises blood pressure, preventing hypotension.
 d. it prevents development of cardiac irritability.

_D_ 18. Side effects of rapid or high-dose theophylline administration include:
 a. dry mouth.
 b. nausea and vomiting.
 c. cardiac arrhythmias.
 d. b and c.

_D_ 19. An individual who is susceptible to allergic reactions induced by insect stings may minimize the probability of being stung by:
 a. avoiding brightly colored clothing.
 b. wearing shoes when outdoors.
 c. not wearing floral perfumes.
 d. all of the above.

CHAPTER 25

Toxicology and Drug and Alcohol Abuse

READING ASSIGNMENT 25-1

■ Poisoning and Overdose
Reading Assignment: pages 580-584

Multiple-Choice Items

Read each question carefully. For each item, select the answer that BEST completes the statement or answers the question, and place the letter of that answer in the space provided.

___C___ 1. Which of the following BEST describes cutaneous absorption?
    a. Rapid absorption.
    b. Most absorption occurs in the gastrointestinal tract.
    c. Slowest absorption.
    d. Immediate absorption.

___D___ 2. Hypoxia may develop after an inhalation exposure from which of the following?
    a. Displacement of air by gases
    b. Noxious fumes
    c. Asphyxiation by dusts
    d. All of the above

___A___ 3. Following a poison ingestion, the paramedic expects most of the poison to be absorbed through the:
    a. small intestine.
    b. large intestine.
    c. stomach.
    d. all of the above.

___C___ 4. Which of the following statements is(are) true about the respiratory status of poisoning victims?
    a. Pulmonary edema results from an overhydration phenomenon in the vascular space.
    b. Emesis is rare because of the decreased muscular tension.

c. A patient who has ingested a hydrocarbon and is coughing can be assumed to have aspirated.

d. All of the above.

_B_ 5. Altered levels of consciousness may be treated with pharmacological agents. Which of the following drugs might be utilized?

a. Valium

b. Naloxone

c. Benadryl

d. All of the above

_C_ 6. When a patient is grossly contaminated with a dry chemical, the paramedic should first:

a. flush with copious amounts of sterile saline.

b. flush with copious amounts of water.

c. brush off the excess.

d. disrobe the patient completely.

_C_ 7. Syrup of ipecac is effective because it stimulates vomiting by:

a. gastric stimulation.

b. duodenal stimulation.

c. triggering the region of the brain stem that controls vomiting.

d. none of the above.

_B_ 8. The appropriate dosage of syrup of ipecac for a child age 1 to 5 years is:

a. 10 ml.

b. 15 ml.

c. 15-30 ml.

d. 30 ml.

_D_ 9. Syrup of ipecac should NOT be given in cases of:

a. coma.

b. seizure.

c. caustic ingestion.

d. all of the above.

STUDY GUIDE ASSIGNMENT 25-2

- Specific Toxicologic Problems and Management
- Drug Abuse Emergencies
- Alcoholism

Reading Assignment: pages 584-599

Multiple-Choice Items

Read each question carefully. For each item, select the answer that BEST completes the statement or answers the question, and place the letter of that answer in the space provided.

_D_ 1. When managing a patient who has ingested a caustic, the paramedic should consider which of the following emergencies?

a. Esophageal perforation

b. Tissue necrosis

c. Delayed airway complications
d. All of the above

_D_ 2. The most common cause of alkali ingestion is:
a. intentional ingestion by an adult.
b. accidental ingestion by an adult.
c. intentional ingestion by a child.
d. accidental ingestion by a child.

_A_ 3. Which of the following chemicals is classified as an acid?
a. Rust remover
b. Drain opener
c. Household bleach
d. Isopropyl alcohol

_C_ 4. Ingestion of a petroleum distillate often results in wheezing from bronchospasm. Which of the following drugs would be effective in the treatment of the bronchospasm?
a. Epinephrine
b. Theophylline ethylenediamine
c. Metaproterenol
d. All of the above

_A_ 5. Methanol and ethylene glycol are often present in automotive products. Ingestion of these products often produces:
a. metabolic acidosis.
b. metabolic alkalosis.
c. respiratory acidosis.
d. respiratory alkalosis.

_C_ 6. _____ is a chemical change created by heat and may generate toxic gases.
a. Pyrogenesis
b. Pyrokenesis
c. Pyrolysis
d. Toxigenesis

_C_ 7. The initial treatment of cyanide poisoning, which includes crushing two inhalants in a gauze pad and allowing ventilation of the patient either by normal or artificial means, is accomplished by which of the following drugs?
a. Sodium thiosulfate
b. Sodium nitrite
c. Amyl nitrite
b. Sodium nitrate

_D_ 8. You respond to a local residence and find a 42-year-old female unconscious in the bathroom with diffuse wheezing and obvious difficult breathing. There are a variety of cleaning products present in the room. You suspect:
a. an underlying medical problem.
b. asthma.
c. heart disease.
d. toxic inhalation.

D 9. Organophosphate and carbamate insecticide exposures can occur via:
   a. inhalation.
   b. ingestion.
   c. skin contact.
   d. all of the above.

B 10. During organophosphate poisoning the increased salivation, lacrimation, urination, and diarrhea are caused by:
   a. increased acetylcholine.
   b. inhibition of acetylcholine.
   c. increased serotonin.
   d. inhibition of serotonin.

D 11. The pharmalogical treatment for organophosphate poisoning includes:
   a. methyl blue.
   b. epinephrine.
   c. II-Pam.
   d. atropine sulfate.

C 12. The primary treatment of victims of food poisoning is:
   a. control of nausea and vomiting.
   b. treatment of abdominal pain and cramping.
   c. management of hypovolemia.
   d. determining the source of contamination.

C 13. Which of the following statements is NOT true af the black widow spider?
   a. The bite immediately produces burning pain.
   b. There is an hourglass-shaped red mark on the spider's abdomen.
   c. It has hemotoxic venom.
   d. The venom causes muscle pain and rigidity.

D 14. Treatment of a pit viper bite includes all of the following EXCEPT:
   a. limiting the absorption of the venom.
   b. placing of a constricting band.
   c. restricting activity.
   d. placing an ice pack on the affected area.

A 15. Which of the following is NOT a sign or symptom of narcotic overdose?
   a. Pupillary dilation
   b. Pupillary constriction
   c. Decreased level of consciousness
   d. Respiratory depression

D 16. The initial adult dose of naloxone is:
   a. 0.01 mg.
   b. 0.1 mg.
   c. 0.04 mg.
   d. 0.4 mg.

_A_ 17. _____ are general central nervous system depressants. Their actions inhibit impulse conduction in the ascending reticular activating system and depress the cerebral cortex.
   a. Barbiturates
   b. Benzodiazepines
   c. Amphetamines
   d. Antipsychotics

_D_ 18. The problem with acetaminophen overdose is that, if it goes untreated or unappreciated, serious and even fatal _____ failure can occur several days later.
   a. heart
   b. kidney
   c. lung
   d. liver

_C_ 19. The immediate toxicologic problems of _____ overdose are cardiac arrhythmias and hypotension, with sinus tachycardia progressing to ventricular fibrillation.
   a. salicylate
   b. antipsychotic
   c. tricyclic antidepressant
   d. narcotic

_D_ 20. Narcotic withdrawal can present with which of the following signs and symptoms?
   a. Piloerection
   b. Flushing
   c. Irritability
   d. All of the above

_B_ 21. Patients under the influence of _____ often exhibit sensory anesthesia to pain. This presents a problem for the emergency responders, because the patient has the potential for inflicting considerable trauma.
   a. amphetamines
   b. phencyclidine
   c. phenylpropanolamine
   d. hallucinogens

_C_ 22. A suspected alcoholic patient may experience a hypoglycemic episode. Prior to administering 50% dextrose, the paramedic should consider administering:
   a. .4 mg Narcan.
   b. 5 mg Valium.
   c. 100 mg thiamine.
   d. 50 mg Benadryl.

_C_ 23. When an alcoholic stops drinking, withdrawal symptoms generally begin within _____ hours.
   a. 2-4
   b. 4-6
   c. 6-8
   d. 8-10

CHAPTER 26

Infectious Diseases

STUDY GUIDE ASSIGNMENT 26-1

- Immune System
Reading Assignment: pages 602-603

Matching Items

Match each of the terms in the left column with the BEST definition in the right column by placing the letter of that definition in the space next to the term. Each definition may be used once or not at all.

I 1. airborne transmission
D 2. communicable disease
J 3. IgA
G 4. IgE
H 5. IgG
C 6. IgM
F 7. immune system
B 8. infectious disease
E 9. vehicle transmission

A. Immunoglobulin; induces the cell to release a number of pharmacologically inactive ingredients

B. Illness caused by the invasion of an organism, be it a virus, bacterium, or fungus

C. Immunoglobulin; first to respond to the presence of a new antigen

D. Disease that can be transmitted directly or indirectly from one individual to another

E. Transmission of disease through the ingestion of infected food or matter

F. Body's protective mechanism, made up of separate cells and molecules

G. Immunoglobulin; induces the cell to release a number of pharmacologically active agents

H. Immunoglobulin; presence signifies past exposure to a disease

I. Transfer of infection from one individual to another through droplets of moisture that contain the infectious agent

J. Immunoglobulin; appears in the serum within a few days to a week after onset of certain viral illnesses

Multiple-Choice Items

Read each question carefully. For each item, select the answer that BEST completes the statement or answers the question, and place the letter of that answer in the space provided.

_C_ 1. The lymphatic system is referred to as the body's "middle man" because it:
    a. assists in the exchange of oxygen and nutrients from the red blood cells to the white blood cells.
    b. functions primarily in the middle of the body.
    c. functions to move fluids and molecules from tissue spaces to the blood.
    d. relays messages from the nervous system to the endocrine or hormonal system.

_C_ 2. Lymph nodes perform all of the following functions EXCEPT:
    a. filter the blood.
    b. produce antibodies.
    c. produce antigens.
    d. produces lymphocytes.

_A_ 3. Humoral immunity is the part of the immune system that defends the body against:
    a. bacteria.
    b. fungi.
    c. protozoa.
    d. viruses.

_B_ 4. The process in which white blood cells seek out, attack, and destroy certain antigens is known as:
    a. foveation.
    b. phagocytosis.
    c. piloerection.
    d. sicchasia.

_D_ 5. Which of the following is an example for an infectious disease that is NOT communicable?
    a. Influenza
    b. Meningoccal meningitis
    c. Staphylococcal pneumonia
    d. Viral meningitis

_C_ 6. "Vehicle transmission" describes the route of transmission that occurs by:
    a. breathing in infected airborne droplets.
    b. contact with a "vector," such as being bitten by a mosquito.
    c. eating or drinking contaminated food or water.
    d. touching an infected body area or fluid.

STUDY GUIDE ASSIGNMENT 26-2

- Communicable Diseases of Adults and Children
- Techniques of Management

Reading Assignment: pages 603-614

Matching Items

Match each of the terms in the left column with the BEST definition in the right column by placing the letter of that definition in the space next to the term. **Each definition may be used once or not at all.**

F   1. cytomegalovirus
H   2. gonorrhea
A   3. hepatitis A
J   4. hepatitis B
N   5. hepatitis C
M   6. herpes zoster
C   7. herpes simplex types 1 and 2
Q   8. herpetic whitlow
D   9. human immunodeficiency virus (HIV)
P   10. lice
O   11. meningitis
I   12. mumps
R   13. rubella
L   14. rubeola
S   15. scabies
E   16. syphilis
G   17. tuberculosis
B   18. varicella

A. Transmitted through direct contact with infected stool and urine

B. Member of the herpesvirus family and the cause of chickenpox

C. Virus that results in cold sores or fever blisters or that affects the genital area

D. Viral agent responsible for acquired immunodeficiency syndrome

E. Sexually transmitted disease; causative organism is *Treponema pallidum*

F. Virus common in immune-compromised people; member of the herpesvirus family

G. Airborne communicable disease caused by the tubercle bacillus *Mycobacterium tuberculosis*

H. Common sexually transmitted disease caused by the bacterium *Neisseria gonorrhoeae*

I. Viral disease caused by the virus *Myxovirus parotiditis;* less common than other childhood diseases

J. More insidious onset that Hepatitis A

K. Known as the "kissing" disease

L. Red measles

M. Presents as a unilateral rash that progresses to pustules; its lesions contain live chickenpox virus that is contagious through direct contact (also called shingles)

N. Transfusion-related hepatitis

O. Inflammation of the membranes of the spinal cord or brain

P. Small wingless insects that live as parasites on the outer surface of the body

Q. Viral infection of the finger or fingers; an occupational health risk for health care workers

R. Viral disease transmitted by direct contact with nasopharyngeal secretions from an infected individual

S. Highly communicable skin disease caused by arachnids, especially mites

Multiple-Choice Items

Read each question carefully. For each item, select the answer that BEST completes the statement or answers the question, and place the letter of that answer in the space provided.

C 1. Tuberculosis is a bacterial infection that produces which of the following symptoms?
 I. Disseminated rash
 II. Fever
 III. Hemoptysis
 IV. Night sweats
 V. Productive cough
 VI. Seizures
 a. I, II, III, and V
 b. I, III, V, and VI
 c. II, III, IV, and V
 d. II, III, V, and VI

D 2. Your patient is a 44-year-old male who has been diagnosed with tuberculosis. Which of the following precautions should you take?
 a. Place a face mask on the patient.
 b. Shower and change clothing after patient contact.
 c. Wear a face mask.
 d. a and c.

B 3. The most common form of viral hepatitis is:
 a. alcoholic hepatitis.
 b. hepatitis A.
 c. hepatitis B.
 d. hepatitis C.

C 4. Although some forms of hepatitis are relatively asymptomatic, when signs and symptoms occur, they are essentially the same regardless of the form of hepatitis. Signs and symptoms of hepatitis may include jaundice and:
 I. Cheyne-Stokes respiration.
 II. dark ("coffee-colored") urine.
 III. fever.
 IV. nausea and vomiting.
 V. right upper quadrant abdominal pain.
 VI. yellow vision.
 a. I, II, III, and IV
 b. I, III, IV, and VI
 c. II, III, IV, and V
 d. II, IV, V, and VI

D 5. An 8-year-old girl has been diagnosed with hepatitis A. The attending paramedic should take which of the following precautions?
 a. Wash hands after patient contact.
 b. Wear disposable gloves.
 c. Wear a face mask.
 d. a and b.

_D_ 6. A 28-year-old woman has been diagnosed with hepatitis B. The attending paramedic should take all of the following precautions EXCEPT:

a. obtain hepatitis B vaccination series.

b. take particular care in dealing with contaminated needles.

c. wear disposable gloves and wash hands after patient contact.

d. wear a face mask.

_A_ 7. Hepatitis C (formerly known as non-A, non-B hepatitis) is spread primarily through contact with:

a. blood.

b. feces.

c. respiratory secretions.

d. saliva.

_D_ 8. The signs and symptoms of viral and bacterial meningitis are essentially the same and include which of the following?

I. Dark urine

II. Difficulty swallowing

III. Fever

IV. Headache

V. Nausea and vomiting

VI. Rash

a. I, II, III, and IV

b. I, III, IV, and VI

c. II, III, IV, and VI

d. III, IV, V, and VI

_A_ 9. Which of the following statements about the communicability of meningitis is correct?

a. Bacterial meningitis is very communicable; viral meningitis is not readily communicable.

b. Viral meningitis is very communicable; bacterial meningitis is not readily communicable.

c. Both bacterial and viral meningitis are very readily communicable.

d. Both bacterial and viral meningitis are not readily communicable.

_B_ 10. A 15-year-old girl has been diagnosed with meningitis. The paramedic should take which of the following precautions?

I. Place a face mask on the patient.

II. Use artificial ventilation devices.

III. Wear disposable gloves.

IV. Wear a face mask.

V. Wear a gown or sterile apron.

VI. Wear protective eye wear when intubating or suctioning.

a. I, II, III, IV, and V

b. I, II, III, IV, and VI

c. I, III, IV, V, and VI

d. II, III, IV, V, and VI

_D_ 11. Prior to erupting as skin lesions, the herpesvirus usually lives silently in the _____ cells of the body.
   a. connective tissue
   b. epithelial tissue
   c. muscle
   d. nerve

_B_ 12. "Fever blisters" or "cold sores" are usually manifestations of:
   a. cytomegalovirus.
   b. herpes simplex 1 virus.
   c. herpes simplex 2 virus.
   d. herpes zoster virus.

_D_ 13. Your patient is a 20-year-old female college student who has been diagnosed with herpes simplex virus. Which of the following precautions would you take?
   I. Avoid contact with contaminated stretcher bedding.
   II. Wash hands after patient contact.
   III. Wear disposable gloves.
   IV. Wear a face mask when ventilating the patient.
   V. Wear a gown or sterile apron.
   VI. Wear protective eye wear.
      a. I, II, III, and IV
      b. I, II, III, and V
      c. I, II, III, and VI
      d. II, III, IV, and VI

_B_ 14. _____ is a form of herpesvirus infection that can affect health care providers. It occurs when the herpes simplex virus infects a finger or several fingers by entering the body through a cut, open sore, or torn hangnail.
   a. Cytomegalovirus
   b. Herpetic whitlow
   c. Psoriasis
   d. Rosacea

_A_ 15. _____ is an antiviral medication that can shorten the duration, and minimize the symptoms, of the herpesviruses.
   a. Acyclovir (Zovirax)
   b. Diclofenac (Volarin)
   c. Sucralfate (Carafate)
   d. Zidovudine (Retrovir)

C 16. Usual signs and symptoms of varicella (chickenpox) infection include which of the following?
   I. Fever
   II. Headache
   III. Photophobia
   IV. Sore throat
   V. Vesicular rash
   VI. White patches on tongue
      a. I, II, III, and V
      b. I, II, III, and VI
      c. I, II, IV, and V
      d. II, III, V, and VI

D 17. The paramedic who has been exposed to varicella and is not immune to the chickenpox must be:
   a. given a gamma globulin booster.
   b. placed at bedrest for the next 7 days.
   c. quarantined at home for the next 30 days.
   d. removed from duty for the 10th through the 21st day following exposure.

D 18. The danger to paramedics in caring for patients with herpes zoster (singles) is that contact with lesion drainage could cause _____ infection in the paramedic who is not immune.
   a. cytomegalovirus
   b. herpes simplex I
   c. herpes simples II
   d. varicella (chickenpox)

A 19. Cytomegalovirus is usually a latent viral infection, which produces signs and symptoms only in patients who are:
   a. immunosuppressed.
   b. of Mediterranean descent.
   c. very old.
   d. very young.

D 20. Gonorrhea may be asymptomatic, especially in women. When present, the signs and symptoms of gonorrhea include which of the following?
   I. Dark ("coffee-colored") urine
   II. Lower abdominal pain
   III. Nausea and vomiting
   IV. Pain on urination
   V. Urethral discharge
      a. I, II, and III
      b. I, III, and IV
      c. II, III, and IV
      d. II, IV, and V

_D_ 21. Your patient is a well-known "street person" with a well-known infestation with both scabies and lice. Which of the following precautions should you take?
a. Change and wash clothing that has contacted the patient.
b. Wear disposable gloves.
c. Wear a face mask and protective eye wear.
d. a and b.

_B_ 22. The MMR vaccine is a combination vaccine providing prophylaxis against which three diseases?
a. Malaria, Malta fever, and rheumatic fever
b. Measles, mumps, and rubella
c. Meningitis, measles, and rubeola
d. Moniliasis, meningitis, and rabies

_D_ 23. A 5-year-old patient is sick with the mumps, also known as infectious parotitis. As the attending paramedic, you should take all of the following precautions EXCEPT:
a. wash your hands after patient contact.
b. wear disposable gloves.
c. wear a face mask.
d. wear protective eye wear.

_D_ 24. Rubella, also known as the German measles, can be transmitted by:
a. direct contact with nasopharyngeal secretions.
b. handling fomites (contaminated articles such as clothing).
c. inhaling airborne droplets.
d. all of the above.

_D_ 25. Rubella presents a danger to women if they become infected with the virus during the first trimester of their pregnancy. The disease is associated with "congenital rubella syndrome," which could cause her infant to have:
a. cryptorchidism.
b. mental retardation.
c. multiple birth defects.
d. b and c.

_D_ 26. Koplik's spots are the:
a. purple-red spots on the skin of AIDS patients.
b. red spots on the skin of rubeola patients.
c. white blotches on the tongues of AIDS patients.
d. white spots seen inside the mouths of rubeola patients.

_D_ 27. The agent that causes acquired immunodeficiency syndrome (AIDS) is:
a. coxsackievirus.
b. cytomegalovirus.
c. Ebstein-Barr virus.
d. human immunodeficiency virus.

_D_ 28. Which of the following are known to be methods of transmitting the AIDS virus?
   I. Kissing and/or saliva contact
   II. Sharing household objects (such as drinking cups and toothbrushes)
   III. Sexual intercourse
   IV. Sharing IV needles
   V. Verticle transmission from pregnant female to fetus
      a. I, II, and III
      b. I, III, and IV
      c. II, III, and IV
      d. III, IV, and V

_A_ 29. The primary risk for paramedics in caring for AIDS patients is the danger of AIDS transmission through:
   a. accidental needle stick injury.
   b. contact with contaminated personal articles (clothing).
   c. contact with respiratory secretions (sputum).
   d. saliva contact from mouth-to-mouth ventilation.

_D_ 30. The concept that describes the approach of considering the blood and body fluids of all patients as potentially infectious for AIDS and hepatitis B is labeled by the Centers for Disease Control as _____ precautions.
   a. absolute
   b. infection control
   c. total
   d. universal

_D_ 31. The Centers for Disease Control recommends that used needles should not be:
   a. cut or bent for disposal.
   b. recapped.
   c. removed from their syringes.
   d. all of the above.

_A_ 32. Blood spills may be cleaned with a _____% sodium hypochlorite (bleach) solution.
   a. 10
   b. 25
   c. 50
   d. 100

CHAPTER 27

Environmental Emergencies and Hazardous Materials

STUDY GUIDE ASSIGNMENT 27-1

- Thermoregulation
- Disruptions of thermoregulation

Reading Assignment: pages 618-627

Matching Items

Match each of the terms in the left column with the BEST definition in the right column by placing the letter of that definition in the space next to the term. Each definition may be used once or not at all.

B   1. conduction
D   2. convection
J   3. evaporation
I   4. febrile illness
C   5. frostbite
K   6. heat stroke
H   7. heat exhaustion
E   8. hyperthermia
G   9. hypothermia
A   10. radiation

A. Process by which warmer materials emit heat to cooler ones

B. Mechanism of heat loss in which direct transfer of heat between materials of unequal temperature occurs

C. Condition that occurs when small body parts that have a high ratio of surface area to tissue mass are exposed to extreme cold

D. Transport of heat away from the skin by air movement

E. General condition of excess body heat

F. Infectious illness in which pyrogens reset the body's hypothalamic thermostat to a lower temperature

G. General condition of deficient body heat

H. A more advanced stage of the homeostatic imbalance that sometimes begins with heat cramps

I. Infectious illness in which pyrogens reset the body's hypothalamic thermostat to a higher temperature

J. Absorption of heat, by water, through the process of vaporization

K. True emergency in which the body's compensatory mechanisms such as vasodilation and sweating are exhausted or actually cause further trouble through shock and dehydration, and hypothalamic control weakens, then collapses

Multiple-Choice Items

Read each question carefully. For each item, select the answer that BEST completes the statement or answers the question, and place the letter of that answer in the space provided.

_a_ 1. A state of physiologic equilibrium in which the body adjusts in the process of maintaining temperature is known as:
   a. homeostasis.
   b. climostasis.
   c. thermoequilibrium.
   d. none of the above.

_c_ 2. The _____, the primary organ of temperature control, senses body temperature and activates mechanisms for heat gain or loss to offset changes from normal.
   a. cerebellum
   b. medulla
   c. hypothalamus
   d. parathyroid

_a_ 3. The law of nature that states that warmer materials tend to emit heat to cooler ones, in keeping with the thermal gradient principle, is known as:
   a. radiation.
   b. conduction.
   c. convection.
   d. evaporation.

_c_ 4. _____ is the transport of heat away from the skin by air movement.
   a. Radiation
   b. Conduction
   c. Convection
   d. Evaporation

_d_ 5. Which of the following statements is true about shivering?
   a. Heat is produced by friction between contracting muscle fibers.
   b. Heat production can be increased by 500%.
   c. Shivering is caused by involuntary muscle activity.
   d. All of the above.

_d_ 6. When the hypothalamus senses a need for more heat production, it stimulates the adrenal medulla to secrete epinephrine. Epinephrine causes:
   a. increased cardiac output.
   b. vasodilation.
   c. distribution of heat peripherally.
   d. all of the above.

C 7. _____ is(are) actually a chemical rather than a thermal disruption that results from profuse sweating.
a. Heat stroke
b. Heat exhaustion
c. Heat cramps
d. Hyperthermia

a 8. _____ is a true emergency in which the body's compensatory mechanisms such as vasodilation and sweating are exhausted.
a. Heat stroke
b. Heat exhaustion
c. Heat cramp
d. Hyperthermia

d 9. Following a hyperthermic event, salt tablets should be used on patients with symptoms of:
a. heat stroke.
b. heat exhaustion.
c. heat cramps.
d. none of the above.

C 10. Which of the following statements regarding the management of heat stroke is NOT true?
a. It demands rapid cooling.
b. It should concentrate on the core surface areas.
c. Overcooling is not a problem because of the seriousness of the situation.
d. None of the above; that is, all **are** true

b 11. Which of the following statements is true about hypothermia?
a. Bare skin markedly decreases the loss of heat by convection and evaporation.
b. The elderly develop hypothermia over a more gradual process of heat loss.
c. Alcohol slows heat loss by constricting blood vessels.
d. Medical conditions such as sepsis and congestive heart failure affect the heat production of the body.

C 12. _____ refers to the early stage wherein a patient is alert and physically coordinated. The body is attempting to compensate by shivering.
a. Moderate frostbite
b. Severe frostbite
c. Moderate hypothermia
d. Severe hypothermia

d 13. Severe hypothermia affects the brain and heart in which of the following ways?
a. Oxygen dissociates less readily from hemoglobin.
b. Cold acidotic blood can precipitate ventricular fibrillation.
c. Pulmonary edema begins to develop around 75°F.
d. All of the above.

a 14. Basic management of a hypothermic patient includes:
a. removing wet clothes and covering the patient.
b. giving coffee or tea to assist in the vasoconstriction process.
c. rapid warming of the peripheral, distal circulatory areas.
d. all of the above.

_b_ 15. In frostbite, the initial reaction of the body in exposure to extreme cold is that:
   a. tissues freeze and ice crystals form and grow between cells.
   b. a spasm in the small blood vessels slows or blocks circulation.
   c. the cells are deprived of water and dehydration results.
   d. all of the above.

STUDY GUIDE ASSIGNMENT 27-2

▪ Water Emergencies
Reading Assignment: pages 627-633

Matching Items

Match each of the terms in the left column with the BEST definition in the right column by placing the letter of that definition in the space next to the term. Each definition may be used once or not at all.

_B_ 1. air embolism
_A_ 2. barotrauma
_I_ 3. Boyle's law
_G_ 4. decompression sickness
_H_ 5. drowning
_E_ 6. Henry's law
_F_ 7. near drowning
_D_ 8. nitrogen narcosis

A. Pressure-related injury
B. Obstruction of a blood vessel by an air bubble
C. Syndrome of disorientation and other mental changes related to the use of oxygen when diving
D. Syndrome of disorientation and other mental changes related to the use of nitrogen when diving
E. The amount of gas that dissolves in a fluid is directly proportional to the pressure of that gas as it contacts the fluid
F. Submersion incident in which recovery occurs
G. Nitrogen bubble formation in the tissues or blood that can occur when diving (also called "the bends")
H. Death from asphyxia during an immersion episode
I. The volume of a gas varies inversely with the external pressure applied to it

Multiple-Choice Items

Read each question carefully. For each item, select the answer that BEST completes the statement or answers the question, and place the letter of that answer in the space provided.

_C_ 1. The victim of a _____ drowning is the type of patient most likely to be resuscitated following a drowning incident.
   a. salt water
   b. fresh water
   c. dry
   d. wet

a 2. Pulmonary edema is most characteristically seen in _____ drowning.
   a. salt water
   b. fresh water
   c. cold water
   d. all of the above

d 3. Most patients who have been submerged long enough to stop breathing become acidotic. The paramedic may treat these patients with:
   a. hyperventilation.
   b. 1 mEq/kg sodium bicarbonate.
   c. 1 mg/kg lidocaine.
   d. all of the above.

c 4. The amount of gas that dissolves in a fluid is directly proportional to the pressure of that gas as it contacts the fluid. This is known as:
   a. Caisson's law.
   b. Boyle's law.
   c. Henry's law.
   d. none of the above.

d 5. Which of the following statements is true about decompression sickness?
   a. The most critical period is the length of bottom time.
   b. Complete excretion of excess nitrogen takes place within 8 hours.
   c. The bubbles create platelet destruction resulting in increased bleeding.
   d. Extreme intravascular bubble formation can lead to tissue infarct.

c 6. Direct treatment for decompression sickness, prior to chamber recompression, is:
   a. 100% oxygen.
   b. an IV of 0.9% NaCl or lactated Ringer's.
   c. a and b are correct.
   d. none of the above.

STUDY GUIDE ASSIGNMENT 27-3

▪ Hazardous Materials
Reading Assignment: pages 633-645

Matching Items

Match each of the terms in the left column with the BEST definition in the right column by placing the letter of that definition in the space next to the term. Each definition may be used once or not at all.

J 1. alpha particles
H 2. beta particles
K 3. cold zone
I 4. dose
C 5. gamma rays
E 6. hazardous material

A. Emits ionizing radiation
B. In a hazardous materials incident, the area outside of the hot zone where personal protection is not required
C. Electromagnetic waves similar to x-rays
D. Common unit of radiation measurement

F	7.	hot zone
A	8.	radioactive substances
D	9.	roentgen
B	10.	warm zone

E. Any substance that jumps out of its container when something goes wrong and hurts or harms the things it touches

F. Area surrounding a hazardous materials incident that is dangerous to life and health

G. No material can protect against them

H. Light metal and possibly heavy clothing stop them

I. The amount of radiation absorbed by the body

J. Large, heavy, and slow-moving particles

K. Area close to a hazardous materials incident that is safe for agencies directly involved in the intervention

Multiple-Choice Items

Read each question carefully. For each item, select the answer that BEST completes the statement or answers the question, and place the letter of that answer in the space provided.

b 1. Individuals who respond to releases or potential releases of hazardous substances and are part of the initial response to the site for the purposes of protecting nearby persons and properties, and who respond in a defensive fashion without trying to stop the release, should be trained to the:
  a. first responder awareness level.
  b. first responder operations level.
  c. technician level.
  d. specialist level.

d 2. Proper identification of a hazardous material depends on:
  a. container shape.
  b. placards and labels.
  c. shipping papers.
  d. all of the above.

a 3. The NFPA 704 system is used to identify hazardous materials in:
  a. fixed facilities.
  b. railroad tank cars.
  c. over-the-road truck transports.
  d. all of the above.

b 4. The four-digit identification number found in the center of a placard is:
  a. required on all placards.
  b. used to identify a product in the Emergency Response guidebook.
  c. used to recognize the hazard class of the substance.
  d. all of the above.

d 5. Proper planning and preparation for a hazardous materials incident must include:
  a. appropriate vehicle equipment to protect responders and patients.
  b. access to interagency radio communication.
  c. coordinated rescue considerations.
  d. all of the above.

c 6. The area that surrounds a hazardous materials incident that is dangerous to life and health is known as the:
   a. cold zone.
   b. warm zone.
   c. hot zone.
   d. decontamination zone.

a 7. Light materials such as clothing prevent penetration of _____ particles and their ionizing force.
   a. alpha
   b. beta
   c. gamma
   d. all of the above

d 8. A work uniform provides _____ protection. It should be worn only when no possibility of respiratory or skin exposure exists.
   a. level A
   b. level B
   c. level C
   d. level D

d 9. Which of the following statements about the management of a hazardous materials victim is true?
   a. Treatment should begin only after the patient is in the triage area.
   b. Treatment is not like conventional emergency medical treatment.
   c. Heavy gloves and other protective garments must be worn during treatment.
   d. All of the above.

CHAPTER 28

Geriatric Emergencies

STUDY GUIDE ASSIGNMENT 28-1

- Anatomy and Physiology of the Aging Process
- Assessment of the Geriatric Patient
- Respiratory Emergencies
- Cardiovascular Emergencies
- Neurologic Emergencies
- Psychiatric Disorders in the Elderly

Reading Assignment: pages 650-660

Multiple-Choice Items

Read each question carefully. For each item, select the answer that BEST completes the statement or answers the question, and place the letter of that answer in the space provided.

_d_ 1. The three leading causes of death in the elderly population are heart disease and:
   a. cerebrovascular accident and pneumonia.
   b. pneumonia and chronic obstructive pulmonary disease.
   c. chronic obstructive pulmonary disease and cancer.
   d. cancer and cerebrovascular accident.

_a_ 2. Normal changes that occur with aging may result in:
   a. inadequate ventilations and chronic hypoxia.
   b. normal ventilations but chronic hypoxia.
   c. inadequate ventilations but good compensation.
   d. normal ventilations but inadequate respiratory rates.

_b_ 3. A decrease in stroke volume and a decrease in heart rate as a result of the aging process may result in:
   a. hypertension, syncope, and falls.
   b. syncope, falls, and heart failure.
   c. falls, heart failure, and emphysema-like changes.
   d. heart failure, emphysema-like changes, and hypertension.

_a_ 4. The end result of arteriosclerosis in the elderly trauma patient may cause:
   a. inadequate tissue perfusion at a blood pressure of 100 systolic.
   b. less circulating blood volume.
   c. alveolar collapse in the lungs.
   d. decreased sensitivity to hypoxia.

_a_ 5. Nocturia is:
   a. excessive urination at night.
   b. inability to retain urine.
   c. urinary retention at night.
   d. excessively diluted urine.

_c_ 6. A good explanation for nocturia in the elderly is that:
   a. arteriosclerosis affects the renal arterioles.
   b. chronic hypertension and diabetes increase urine.
   c. the production of urine becomes the same day and night.
   d. the smaller size of the kidney increases the work load.

_c_ 7. Which of the following is affected by aging?
   I. Intelligence
   II. Ability to verbalize
   III. Long-term memory
   IV. Short-term memory
      a. I, II, and IV
      b. III and IV
      c. IV
      d. I, II, III, and IV

_d_ 8. Loss of flexibility due to changes of aging affects:
   a. response time and adaptation to a changing environment.
   b. adaptation to a changing environment and mobility.
   c. mobility, balance, and adequate strength for daily living.
   d. balance, response time, and mobility.

_b_ 9. The site of the most common distress in the elderly is which one of the following body systems?
   a. Nervous
   b. Gastrointestinal
   c. Cardiac
   d. Renal

_d_ 10. Experiencing heartburn after meals in the elderly is BEST explained by:
   a. the increasing secretion of stomach acids and enzymes.
   b. slowing of peristalsis and movement of food.
   c. reduction of blood flow to the intestines.
   d. relaxation of muscles in the walls of the esophagus.

_a_ 11. Which of the following are particularly pertinent to the physical exam of the elderly?
   a. Many layers of clothing may indicate a sensitivity to the cold.
   b. Many layers of clothing may indicate a fear of loss of belongings or paranoia.
   c. The elderly may have a lower pain threshold and may concentrate on and maximize small discomforts.
   d. Necrotic toes are readily noticed and may be the focus of all their attention.

b 12. Elderly patients with hemoptysis of a volume approaching several hundred milliliters is usually the result of epistaxis, anticoagulants, or:
a. repeated minor trauma.
b. use of aspirin.
c. rupture of bronchial vessels.
d. vascular aneurysm.

c 13. Symptoms of bronchial asthma in the elderly differ from symptoms of asthma at a younger age because:
a. coughing and wheezing decrease in intensity with age.
b. coughing and wheezing increase in intensity with age.
c. nocturnal episodes of asthma increase with age.
d. precipitating factors increase with age.

d 14. Precipitating factors for pulmonary embolism in the elderly include:
a. advancing age, atrial fibrillation, and arthritis home medication (aspirin).
b. atrial fibrillation, arthritis home medication (aspirin), and incidence of COPD.
c. arthritis home medication (aspirin), incidence of COPD, and advancing age.
d. incidence of congestive heart failure, advancing age, and atrial fibrillation.

a 15. In an elderly patient suffering from an acute exacerbation of COPD, the drugs of choice include:
a. metaproterenol and albuterol.
b. albuterol and epinephrine.
c. aminophylline and morphine.
d. morphine and furosemide.

b 16. The signs and symptoms of an acute myocardial infarction in an elderly person may differ from those of that condition in other age groups in which of the following ways?
a. Severe chest pain with mild shortness of breath.
b. Mild chest pain with significant shortness of breath.
c. Severe indigestion and pain radiating to the left arm.
d. Angina prior to shortness of breath and weakness.

c 17. Orthopnea is BEST defined as:
a. a condition related to pulmonary edema.
b. shortness of breath.
c. difficulty breathing related to body position.
d. nausea and weakness.

d 18. In a myocardial infarction without pain, a common first sign is:
a. nausea and vomiting.
b. acute shortness of breath.
c. irregular heart rate.
d. syncope.

b 19. Your elderly patient suffered a syncopal episode when the patient reached up to change a ceiling light bulb. The BEST explanation for this is:
a. hypoglycemia.
b. atherosclerotic carotid arteries.

238

     c.   silent myocardial infarction.

     d.   pooling of blood in the body.

_d_ 20.   The difference between the cause of a coma in an elderly person and the cause of a coma in a younger person is that in the elderly, the coma is usually caused by:

     a.   atherosclerotic changes.

     b.   medication.

     c.   a single factor.

     d.   multiple factors.

_a_ 21.   One of the most common causes of seizures in the elderly is:

     a.   a cerebral vascular accident.

     b.   hypoxia.

     c.   Stokes-Adams syndrome.

     d.   an accidental overdose of medication.

_C_ 22.   Which of the following is more indicative of dementia than of "normal" forgetfulness?

     a.   Losing the check book.

     b.   Forgetting to comb one's hair.

     c.   Forgetting how to balance the check book.

     d.   Forgetting a neighbor's name.

_C_ 23.   In the management of neurologic emergencies in the elderly, an IV of _____ is reasonable.

     a.   normal saline, 50% dextrose, and naloxone.

     b. D_5W, 50% dextrose, and naloxone.

     c.   lactated Ringer's, thiamine, and naloxone.

     d. D_5W, thiamine, and naloxone.

STUDY GUIDE ASSIGNMENT 28-2

- Musculoskeletal Problems
- Gastrointestinal Emergencies
- Trauma in the Elderly
- Pharmacology in Geriatrics
- Environmental Emergencies
- Geriatric Abuse

Reading Assignment: pages 660-665

Multiple-Choice Items

Read each question carefully. For each item, select the answer that BEST completes the statement or answers the question, and place the letter of that answer in the space provided.

_C_ 1.   To accommodate for decreased fat stores in the elderly, splints must be:

     a.   conformed to the fracture site.

     b.   not placed on joints.

     c.   well padded.

     d.   secured with paper tape.

b 2. The most common cause of upper gastrointestinal bleeding in the nonalcoholic elderly person is:
a. esophageal varices.
b. peptic ulcers.
c. Mallory-Weiss syndrome.
d. gastritis.

d 3. Relatively large amounts of bright red rectal bleeding with minimal abdominal pain should be suspected of coming from:
a. hemorrhoids.
b. peptic ulcers.
c. ischemic colitis.
d. diverticula.

b 4. Rib fractures are considered significant in the elderly because of the:
a. frequency of lacerated pleura.
b. high risk of pneumonia.
c. frequency of lung contusion.
d. high risk of tension pneumothorax.

d 5. In comparison to younger patients, shock due to blood loss predisposes the elderly to:
a. hypothermia.
b. pneumonia.
c. restlessness.
d. myocardial infarction.

a 6. Signs and symptoms of hypothermia in the elderly may be missed because these signs and symptoms can:
I. mimic a stroke.
II. mimic a diabetic emergency.
III. be a part of early pneumonia.
IV. cause an early rise in temperature.
a. I, II, and III
b. II, III, and IV
c. I, II, and IV
d. I, III, and IV

c 7. Factors that predispose the elderly to hyperthermia include:
I. chronic disease.
II. medications.
III. dementia.
IV. fatigue.
a. I, II, and III
b. II, III, and IV
c. I, II, and IV
d. I, III, and IV

CHAPTER 29

Pediatric Emergencies

STUDY GUIDE ASSIGNMENT 29-1

- Approach to the Pediatric Patient
- Developmental Stages
- Common Pediatric Problems

Reading Assignment: pages 668-673

Multiple-Choice Items

Read each question carefully. For each item, select the answer that BEST completes the statement or answers the question, and place the letter of that answer in the space provided.

___d___ 1. Upon approaching the pediatric patient, the paramedic should immediately establish a relationship with:
   a. the child.
   b. the parent.
   c. medical command.
   d. a and b.

___C___ 2. The initial approach to the pediatric patient should be aimed at fostering cooperation and gaining the child's confidence:
   a. in all situations.
   b. only when a parent is not present.
   c. when life-threatening problems are absent.
   d. only when the parent is present.

___a___ 3. Keeping the child with a parent or caretaker:
   a. is usually beneficial and desirable, because information and cooperation can be obtained more easily.
   b. is usually detrimental to both parent and child and should be avoided whenever possible.
   c. is necessary only when the child has a life-threatening injury and permission to treat is needed.
   d. is desirable only if the child is between the ages of 6 months and 2 years.

___C___ 4. Your patient is 5 years old and weighs approximately 23 kg. She has been vomiting for the past 3 hours. Your partner records the following vital signs: BP 102/60, pulse 120, respirations 26. Your interpretation of these vital signs is that:
   a. all are within normal limits.
   b. the blood pressure is high and the pulse and respirations are slow.

c. the blood pressure is normal and the pulse and respirations are rapid.
d. the blood pressure is low and the pulse and respirations are normal.

d 5. When assessing respirations on a young infant, the BEST method of calculation is to take the respiratory rate for:
a. 10 seconds and multiply by 6.
b. 15 seconds and multiply by 4.
c. 30 seconds and multiply by 2.
d. a full 60 seconds.

c 6. The _____ are membrane-covered spaces between the incompletely ossified cranial bones of an infant.
a. ossifications
b. osseous canals
c. fontanelles
d. bone spurs

d 7. An important clinical indicator in the pediatric patient is the
a. blood pressure.
b. pulse and respirations.
c. pupillary response.
d. level of consciousness.

b 8. Stridor in the pediatric patient is an indication of upper airway obstruction that may be a caused by:
 I. edema.
 II. fatigue.
 III. foreign bodies.
 IV. infection.
 V. hypoxia.
    a. I, II, and V
    b. I, III, and IV
    c. II, III, IV, and V
    d. I, II, III, IV, and V

c 9. Development refers to:
a. an increase in body size.
b. response to stress.
c. improvement or maturation.
d. recognition of needs.

b 10. Limited language skills, a short attention span, and a testing of reality are developmental characteristics observed in the _____ age group.
a. 0-12 month
b. 1-3 year
c. 5-12 year
d. 12-19 year

d 11. The leading cause of death in children between the ages of 1 year and 15 years is:
a. sudden infant death syndrome.
b. cancer.
c. disease.
d. accidents.

STUDY GUIDE ASSIGNMENT 29-2

- Problems Specific to the Pediatric Patient
- Techniques of Management

Reading Assignment: pages 673-687

Matching Items

Match each of the terms in the left column with the BEST definition in the right column by placing the letter of that definition in the space next to the term. Each definition may be used once or not at all.

<table>
<tr><td>B</td><td>1.</td><td>asthma</td></tr>
<tr><td>D</td><td>2.</td><td>bronchiolitis</td></tr>
<tr><td>C</td><td>3.</td><td>croup</td></tr>
<tr><td>I</td><td>4.</td><td>epiglottitis</td></tr>
<tr><td>A</td><td>5.</td><td>sudden infant death syndrome</td></tr>
<tr><td>G</td><td>6.</td><td>Reye's syndrome</td></tr>
<tr><td>H</td><td>7.</td><td>septicemia</td></tr>
<tr><td>E</td><td>8.</td><td>febrile seizure</td></tr>
</table>

A. Sudden and unexpected death of an infant or young child; etiology is uncertain

B. Sudden, periodic dyspnea usually accompanied with wheezing and caused by swollen mucous membranes or bronchial tube spasms

C. Laryngotracheobronchitis, a viral infection

D. Respiratory infection characterized by wheezing

E. Caused by a high body temperature; occurs mostly in children

F. Infection of the lung

G. Rare, acute, life-threatening disease that affects all age groups; peak incidence is 4 to 15 years; etiology is unclear

H. Pathogenic bacteria in the blood

I. Hallmark is a swollen, cherry-red epiglottis

Multiple-Choice Items

Read each question carefully. For each item, select the answer that BEST completes the statement or answers the question, and place the letter of that answer in the space provided.

b 1. In sudden infant death syndrome:
I. the infant's death is expected.
II. the infant's death is unexpected.
III. a cause of death is not revealed on autopsy.
IV. evidence of child abuse is found on autopsy.
V. a rare brain abnormality is found on autopsy.
   a. I and IV
   b. II and III
   c. I and V
   d. II and IV

d 2. When dealing with a suspected case of sudden infant death syndrome:
   a. the parents should receive support from the paramedic.
   b. regardless of local protocol, CPR should be initiated even if rigor mortis has set in.
   c. the paramedic should be familiar with grief reactions and with available support services.
   d. a and c.

243

a 3. Febrile seizures usually occur in children:
a. under 6 months of age and are caused by infection.
b. over 8 years of age and often progress to status epilepticus.
c. between 6 months and 6 years of age and are self-limiting.
d. between 8 months and 8 years of age and are often a precursor to epilepsy.

d 4. Signs that may be present in a child suffering from dehydration include:
I. increased skin turgor.
II. hypertension.
III. tachycardia.
IV. orthostatic hypotension.
V. shock.
a. I, III, and V
b. I, II, and III
c. II, III, and V
d. III, IV, and V

5. Management of the pediatric patient who exhibits signs of dehydration and shock should include:
a. IV lactated Ringer's or normal saline wide open.
b. IV D₅W at a keep-open rate.
c. IV lactated Ringer's or normal saline at 20 mL/kg.
d. IV D₅W at 10 mL/kg.

d 6. _____ is an infection of the tissues that cover the brain and spinal cord.
a. Haemophilus influenzae B
b. Kernig's disease
c. Reye's syndrome
d. Meningitis

a 7. The anterior fontanelle of an infant suffering from septicemia is:
a. normal.
b. sunken.
c. swollen.
d. fractured.

c 8. Your patient is an 8-year-old female whose mother reported that she showed signs of a cold 2 days earlier. Her condition has progressively worsened. Upon examination, you find your patient comatose with decorticate posturing. The pupils are slow to react. Treatment for this patient should include:
I. maintenance of a patent airway.
II. oxygen by nasal cannula.
III. ventilatory assistance with high-flow oxygen.
IV. IV of normal saline at 40 mL/kg/hr.
V. rapid transport.
a. I, II, and IV
b. I, II, and V
c. I, III, and V
d. I, III, IV, and V

244

_d_ 9. The symptoms present in the pediatric patient with a foreign body obstruction depend on:
a. the object's size.
b. the object's location.
c. the patency of the remaining airway.
d. all of the above.

_a_ 10. Relief of bronchospasm in the pediatric patient experiencing anaphylaxis should include:
a. 0.01 mg/kg epinephrine 1:1000 SQ.
b. 0.1 mg/kg epinephrine 1:1000 IV.
c. 5 mg/kg diphenhydramine IM.
d. 6 mg/kg Aminophylline IV drip.

_a_ 11. Laryngotracheobronchitis occurs as a result of:
a. inflammation and edema in the subglottic area.
b. a bacterial infection that affects the larynx.
c. a foreign body obstruction in the lower airways.
d. a and b.

_b_ 12. Endotracheal intubation of the patient experiencing epiglottitis is:
a. never indicated under any circumstances.
b. indicated for total airway obstruction.
c. always indicated after initial oxygenation.
d. always indicated before initial oxygenation.

_c_ 13. The clinical picture of bronchiolitis may include:
I. high fever.
II. low-grade fever.
III. tachycardia.
IV. wheezing.
V. stridorous inspiration.
a. I, III, and V
b. I, III, and IV
c. II, III, and IV
d. III, IV, and V

_d_ 14. In the pediatric asthma patient, epinephrine:
a. should not be given if the heart rate exceeds 180 beats per minute.
b. should be followed by the administration of Benadryl.
c. should be administered subcutaneously at 0.01 mg/kg of a 1:1000 solution.
d. a and c.

_b_ 15. _____ are primary causes of cardiopulmonary arrest in the pediatric patient.
a. Arrhythmias and febrile seizures
b. Shock and respiratory problems
c. Trauma and congenital defects
d. a and b

d 16. Management of the pediatric patient exhibiting the signs and symptoms of shock should begin with:
a. an IV of lactated Ringer's at 20 mL/kg.
b. an IV of normal saline wide open.
c. the pneumatic anti-shock garment.
d. 100% oxygen.

d 17. A 4-year-old has sustained blunt trauma to his upper abdominal region. The paramedic should be concerned about an injury to this area because:
a. the small and large intestines are fragile and easily injured.
b. the liver is relatively large in size and is virtually unprotected.
c. injury to the spleen might have occurred.
d. b and c.

d 18. Injuries that may be seen in an abused child include:
a. wounds in various stages of healing.
b. pattern injuries, such as rope marks.
c. immersion burns on the buttocks and ankles.
d. all of the above .

b 19. The paramedic who suspects that his or her pediatric patient has been abused should:
a. assume that the police will file charges.
b. report the incident to the authorities.
c. confront the parent or suspected abuser.
d. record, but not mention, any evidence of abuse found.

b 20. Pediatric and infant resuscitation bags:
a. should be equipped with a pressure-relief valve.
b. should not be equipped with a "pop-off" valve.
c. should be capable of delivering 80% oxygen.
d. a and c.

C 21. A _____ endotracheal tube should be utilized for a 5-year-old child.
a. 2.0-3.0
b. 3.0-4.0
c. 4.0-6.0
d. 6.0-8.0

a 22. The optimum size tubing to use when infusing IV fluids into a young child is:
a. microdrip.
b. macrodrip.
c. regular.
d. not important.

b 23. To prevent fluid overload in an 8-kg infant, the paramedic should infuse fluids at a rate of _____ mL/kg.
a. 1
b. 4
c. 10
d. 20

CHAPTER 30

Gynecologic, Obstetric, and Newborn Emergencies

STUDY GUIDE ASSIGNMENT 30-1

- Anatomy and Physiology of the Female Reproductive System
- Ovulation and the Menstrual Cycle
- Pregnancy and Fetal Growth

Reading Assignment: pages 690-696

Matching Items

Match each of the terms in the left column with the BEST definition in the right column by placing the letter of that definition in the space next to the term. Each definition may be used once or not at all.

_____ 1. fallopian tubes
_____ 2. menstrual cycle
_____ 3. ovaries
_____ 4. uterus
_____ 5. vagina
_____ 6. vulva
_____ 7. amniotic sac
_____ 8. amniotic fluid
_____ 9. placenta
_____ 10. umbilical cord

A. Carries oxygen and nutrients from the mother to the fetus

B. Structure that provides nutrition, excretion, and circulation to the fetus

C. Passageway for egg cells from the ovaries to the uterus

D. External structures of the female genitalia

E. Changes that occur in the ovaries and uterus between puberty and the end of child-bearing potential

F. Muscular tube extending from the uterus to the vulva

G. Two almond-shaped glands on either side of the pelvic cavity that produce and release eggs and secrete female hormones

H. Sac in which the fetus develops

I. Muscular structure in which the fetus develops

J. Double-membraned sac

K. Fluid that the fetus drinks and excretes

Multiple-Choice Items

Read each question carefully. For each item, select the answer that BEST completes the statement or answers the question, and place the letter of that answer in the space provided.

_a_ 1.   The neck of the uterus is called the:
    a.   cervix.
    b.   endometrium.
    c.   fundus.
    d.   vagina.

_b_ 2.   The innermost lining of the uterus is the:
    a.   cervix.
    b.   endometrium.
    c.   fundus.
    d.   vagina.

_d_ 3.   The _____ function(s) as a conduit for transport of the ova (egg cell) from the ovaries to the uterus.
    a.   cervix
    b.   corpus luteum
    c.   endometrium
    d.   fallopian tubes

_d_ 4.   The organ commonly referred to as the birth canal is the:
    a.   cervix.
    b.   corpus luteum.
    c.   fundus.
    d.   vagina.

_d_ 5.   The term used to refer to all of the female external genitalia is:
    a.   labia majora.
    b.   mons veneris.
    c.   vestibule.
    d.   vulva.

_c_ 6.   When fertilization does not occur, a portion of the lining of the uterus is expelled, causing a process known as:
    a.   gestation.
    b.   menopause.
    c.   menstruation.
    d.   nidation.

_d_ 7.   The placenta is an organ that provides:
    a.   nourishment for the endometrium.
    b.   oxygen to the fetus.
    c.   waste removal for the fetus.
    d.   b and c.

_b_ 8.   The umbilical cord is a pipeline between the placenta and the fetus and is about _____ inches in length.
    a.   15
    b.   21

c. 30

d. 42

_C_ 9. The umbilical cord contains:

a. one artery and one vein.

b. one artery and two veins.

c. two arteries and one vein.

d. two arteries and two veins.

_b_ 10. Typically, during pregnancy the pulse rate is _____ than the patient's usual nonpregnant pulse rate.

a. significantly higher

b. slightly higher

c. slightly lower

d. significantly lower

_C_ 11. Typically, during pregnancy the blood pressure is _____ than the patient's usual nonpregnant blood pressure.

a. significantly higher

b. slightly higher

c. slightly lower

d. significantly lower

_d_ 12. A woman in her last month of pregnancy is found lying on her back in bed. Her blood pressure is low, and she is complaining of dizziness. She does not have any vaginal bleeding. You should suspect:

a. eclampsia.

b. preeclampsia.

c. premature delivery.

d. supine hypotension syndrome.

STUDY GUIDE ASSIGNMENT 30-2

▪ Assessment of the Gynecologic and Obstetric Patient
▪ Gynecologic Emergencies
▪ Complications of Pregnancy

Reading Assignment: pages 696-704

Matching Items

Match each of the terms in the left column with the BEST definition in the right column by placing the letter of that definition in the space next to the term. Each definition may be used once or not at all.

_____ 1. abortion

_____ 2. abruptio placenta

_____ 3. eclampsia

_____ 4. ectopic pregnancy

_____ 5. placenta previa

A. Condition in which the placenta implants itself in a lower portion of the uterus than is normal

B. Hypertensive disorder specific to pregnancy

C. Termination of a pregnancy before the fetus is viable

_____ 6. preeclampsia

_____ 7. pelvic inflammatory disease

D. Premature separation of the placenta

E. Appearance of the presenting part of the fetus at the vaginal opening

F. Serious toxemic disorder, characterized by high blood pressure, albuminuria, oliguria, and convulsions; etiology is unknown

G. Occurs when a fertilized ovum implants itself outside the uterus

H. Infective process that leads to inflammation of the pelvic organs

Multiple-Choice Items

Read each question carefully. For each item, select the answer that BEST completes the statement or answers the question, and place the letter of that answer in the space provided.

b 1. In assessing the patient with vaginal bleeding, it may be useful to ask how many tampons or pads have been used. The average tampon or pad contains an average of _____ mL of blood when completely saturated.
   a. 10
   b. 25
   c. 50
   d. 75

c 2. Your patient, a 19-year-old sexually active female, is complaining of severe abdominal pain that is localized in the right lower quadrant. The pain radiates to her right shoulder. She gives a history of heavy vaginal discharge and an irregular menstrual cycle. Vital signs are within normal limits. The presumptive diagnosis is:
   a. amenorrhea.
   b. cholecystitis.
   c. pelvic inflammatory disease.
   d. placenta previa.

c 3. The most common cause of acute abdominal pain in young adult females is:
   a. appendicitis.
   b. ectopic pregnancy.
   c. pelvic inflammatory disease.
   d. ruptured ovarian cyst.

d 4. A 26-year-old patient has suffered trauma to her genital area and has been bleeding vaginally for 30 minutes. Vital signs are BP 82/52, pulse 124, and respiration 24. Treatment should include oxygen, placement in shock position, and:
   a. ice packs to the vulva and femoral area.
   b. insertion of tampon, 20 gauge needle with IV normal saline or lactated Ringer's, and massage of lower abdomen.
   c. 16 gauge needle with IV D_5W, and 20 units oxytocin.
   d. 16 gauge needle with IV normal saline or lactated Ringer's, and pneumatic anti-shock garment.

_a_ 5. Your medic unit responds to a call to find a 22-year-old rape survivor. Which of the following questions should you ask in your history taking?
   a. Are you hurt anywhere?
   b. Did your attacker penetrate you?
   c. How did the rape occur?
   d. Were you a virgin?

_b_ 6. Vaginal bleeding in pregnancy is usually classified as early (first trimester) or as late (third trimester). The most common "early bleeds" are:
   a. abortion and abruptio placenta.
   b. abortion and ectopic pregnancy.
   c. placenta previa and abruptio placenta.
   d. placenta previa and ectopic pregnancy.

_b_ 7. A 20-year-old female provides a history of having missed two periods. She complains of pain in the lower left abdomen and slight vaginal bleeding. She is hypotensive. The presumptive diagnosis is:
   a. acute appendicitis.
   b. ectopic pregnancy.
   c. placenta previa.
   d. ruptured ovarian cyst.

_d_ 8. The type of abortion characterized by a closed cervix and vaginal bleeding that may subside is called a(an) _____ abortion.
   a. incomplete
   b. inevitable
   c. missed
   d. threatened

_b_ 9. The type of abortion characterized by cervical dilation and copious vaginal bleeding, to the point where termination of pregnancy cannot be prevented, is called a(an) _____ abortion.
   a. incomplete
   b. inevitable
   c. missed
   d. threatened

_c_ 10. The type of abortion characterized by fetal death within the uterus and delayed expulsion of the fetus is called a(an) _____ abortion.
   a. incomplete
   b. inevitable
   c. missed
   d. threatened

_a_ 11. The type of abortion characterized by pain, vaginal bleeding, and cervical dilation, with part of the products of conception expelled and part retained, is called a(an) _____ abortion.
   a. incomplete
   b. inevitable
   c. missed
   d. threatened

_a_ 12. The termination of pregnancy before viability is called:
    a. abortion.
    b. abruptio placenta.
    c. placenta previa.
    d. uterine rupture.

_d_ 13. Treatment for abortion, with hypotension, includes:
    a. IV D$_5$W, diazepam, and transport.
    b. IV lactated Ringer's, oxytocin, pneumatic anti-shock garment, and transport.
    c. oxygen, IV D$_5$W, and transport.
    d. oxygen, IV normal saline or lactated Ringer's, pneumatic anti-shock garment, and transport.

_d_ 14. The condition during late pregnancy that is characterized by malaise, headache, edema, and hypertension is called:
    a. ectopic pregnancy.
    b. hydatiform mole.
    c. peripheral neuritis.
    d. preeclampsia.

_a_ 15. When the pregnant female has a convulsion, especially in her third trimester, the most probable cause is:
    a. eclampsia.
    b. epilepsy.
    c. preeclampsia.
    d. supine hypotension syndrome.

_a_ 16. Eclampsia is a life-threatening condition. In transporting patients with preeclampsia, one should place _____ on standby.
    a. diazepam and magnesium sulfate.
    b. diazepam and methylergonovine.
    c. oxytocin and diphenhydramine.
    d. oxytocin and methylergonovine.

_c_ 17. The most common "late bleeds" (third trimester vaginal bleeding) are:
    a. abortion and abruptio placenta.
    b. abortion and ectopic pregnancy.
    c. placenta previa and abruptio placenta.
    d. placenta previa and ectopic pregnancy.

_c_ 18. In managing the eclamptic patient, the paramedic should:
    a. expedite transport with lights and sirens.
    b. keep the patient compartment well-lighted for observation.
    c. maintain an open airway.
    d. position the patient on her right side.

<u>C</u> 19. A 29-year-old female who is 9 months pregnant awakened during the night in a pool of blood. She complains of dizziness and of being frightened but otherwise feels fine. The patient exam reveals a slightly low blood pressure, but otherwise normal vital signs and a soft uterus. The presumptive diagnosis is:

    a.   abruptio placenta.
    b.   ectopic pregnancy.
    c.   placenta previa.
    d.   preeclampsia.

<u>a</u> 20. Your patient is a 31-year-old female who is 8 months pregnant. She has experienced a sudden onset of dizziness and weakness associated with severe, constant abdominal pain. Her uterus is rigid to palpation. Vital signs are BP 88/60, pulse 132, and respirations 22. The presumptive diagnosis is:

    a.   abruptio placenta.
    b.   Braxton-Hicks contractions.
    c.   placenta previa.
    d.   uterine rupture.

STUDY GUIDE ASSIGNMENT 30-3

- Labor and Delivery
- Care of the Newborn

Reading Assignment: pages 704-717

Matching Items

Match each of the terms in the left column with the BEST definition in the right column by placing the letter of that definition in the space next to the term. Each definition may be used once or not at all.

_____ 1. breech
_____ 2. complete breech
_____ 3. crowning
_____ 4. footling breech
_____ 5. frank breech
_____ 6. labor
_____ 7. prolapsed umbilical cord
_____ 8. shoulder lie

A. Presentation of the buttocks or lower extremity during childbirth

B. A transverse lie during delivery in which the shoulder may become wedged in the pelvic canal

C. Presentation during delivery when one or both feet of the baby are folded under the buttocks

D. Premature expulsion or compression of the umbilical cord

E. Process of expelling the fetus and placenta from the uterus and vagina

F. Appearance of the presenting part of the fetus at the vaginal opening

G. Occurs when a fertilized ovum implants itself outside the uterus

H. Legs are flexed at the hips, knees are extended, and the feet and head are close together

I. Fetal delivery in which the legs are flexed at the hips, but one or both knees are also flexed

Multiple-Choice Items

Read each question carefully. For each item, select the answer that BEST completes the statement or answers the question, and place the letter of that answer in the space provided.

___C___ 1. "Show" is defined as the:
- a. gush of blood following delivery of the placenta.
- b. delivered placenta.
- c. discharge composed of mucus with traces of blood.
- d. domed appearance of the pregnant abdomen.

___C___ 2. Cervical effacement is the _____ of the cervix.
- a. dilation and thickening
- b. elongation and thinning
- c. shortening and thinning
- d. shortening and thickening

___b___ 3. Cervical dilation is said to be complete when the cervical os (opening) has widened to _____ centimeters.
- a. 4-5
- b. 10
- c. 16
- d. 20

___C___ 4. The first stage of labor begins with:
- a. cervical dilation.
- b. crowning.
- c. uterine contractions.
- d. vaginal show.

___C___ 5. The second stage of labor concludes with:
- a. cervical dilation.
- b. crowning.
- c. infant delivery.
- d. placental delivery.

___C___ 6. Delivery of the placenta is considered to end the _____ stage of labor.
- a. first
- b. second
- c. third
- d. fourth

___C___ 7. The average length of first labor is _____ hours.
- a. 4
- b. 8
- c. 14
- d. 20

_a_ 8. A 27-year-old woman is pregnant with her third child. Contractions are 2 minutes apart and visual inspection reveals a bulging perineum. You should:
   a. prepare the patient for home delivery.
   b. request police escort during transport.
   c. transport and deliver the infant en route if necessary.
   d. transport the patient to the nearest hospital.

_d_ 9. The IV fluid of choice for home delivery is:
   a. D₅W.
   b. lactated Ringer's.
   c. normal saline.
   d. b or c.

_b_ 10. Once your IV is started for home delivery, you should set your IV to run at _____ mL/hour.
   a. 20-30
   b. 100
   c. 150
   d. 200

_a_ 11. To prevent explosive delivery of the infant's head, you should support the infant's head by:
   a. applying gentle pressure with the palm of the hand on the crowning head.
   b. maintaining finger pressure against the center of the head.
   c. placing the palm of the hand firmly against the head.
   d. using the thumb and index fingers to hold traction on the labia majora.

_d_ 12. Once the head is delivered, the first thing you should do is:
   a. assist delivery of the anterior shoulder.
   b. check for a nuchal cord.
   c. check for spontaneous respirations.
   d. suction the mouth and nose.

_b_ 13. Once the head is delivered, the second thing you should do is:
   a. assist delivery of the anterior shoulder.
   b. check for a nuchal cord.
   c. check for spontaneous respirations.
   d. suction the mouth and nose.

_a_ 14. You can assist the birth of the anterior shoulder by:
   a. gently guiding the infant's head downward.
   b. gently guiding the infant's head upward.
   c. rotating the infant's head and body 45 degrees.
   d. rotating the infant's head and body 180 degrees.

_c_ 15. Following the birth of the infant and cessation of umbilical cord pulsation, the cord may be cut at _____ inches from the infant's umbilicus.
   a. 6-9
   b. 6-12
   c. 8-10
   d. 10-20

d 16. What should the paramedic do with the placenta after it is delivered and placed in a plastic bag?
   a. Give it to the father or next of kin.
   b. Take it to the pathology laboratory.
   c. Throw it away at the hospital in a "human waste" container.
   d. Transport it with the mother to the hospital.

b 17. Delivery of the placenta is normally associated with _____ mL of blood loss.
   a. 100-200
   b. 300-500
   c. 600-800
   d. 800-1000

c 18. The technical term for "difficult labor" is:
   a. caput.
   b. dyspareunia.
   c. dystocia.
   d. vernix caseosa.

c 19. The most common type of breech presentation is one in which the buttocks present with the hips flexed and the legs extended against the chest and abdomen. This type of breech is called a(an) _____ breech.
   a. complete
   b. footling
   c. frank
   d. incomplete

d 20. An 18-year-old female is in active labor. Inspection of the vaginal opening reveals a single arm presentation. The paramedic should:
   a. do nothing, because the delivery will be normal.
   b. reach into the vagina and turn the infant.
   c. reinsert the infant's arm into the vagina and gently push the infant back up the birth canal.
   d. transport immediately; this is a true emergency.

c 21. Upon examining a 20-year-old woman, you discover that the umbilical cord is protruding from her vagina. All care for this patient is aimed at:
   a. cutting the cord.
   b. preventing the delivery.
   c. relieving pressure on the cord.
   d. replacing the cord.

b 22. When one is caring for a mother with a prolapsed cord, which of the following is the best position in which to place the patient?
   a. Fowlers
   b. Knee-Chest
   c. Lithotomy
   d. Sims

_d_ 23. Postpartum bleeding may be caused by:
   a. laceration of the birth canal.
   b. retained fragments of the placenta.
   c. uterine atony.
   d. all of the above.

_a_ 24. Oxytocin is the drug of choice to firm the uterus and reduce postpartum bleeding. After mixing 10-20 units of oxytocin in 1000 mL of normal saline or lactated Ringer's solution, you should run the oxytocin drip at:
   a. 1-4 mL/min.
   b. 50 mL/min.
   c. 100 mL/hr.
   d. 1000 mL/3 hr.

_a_ 25. The paramedic's primary responsibility to the newborn is to:
   a. clear the airway and provide warmth.
   b. cut and clamp the cord.
   c. record the time of delivery.
   d. show the baby to the mother.

_b_ 26. A newborn with a 1-minute Apgar score of 4 is:
   a. healthy and active.
   b. in a guarded condition.
   c. in need of resuscitation.
   d. moribund.

_b_ 27. Any infant born before the 38th week of gestation, or weighing less than _____ pounds, is said to be premature.
   a. 4.5
   b. 5.5
   c. 7.0
   d. 8.0

CHAPTER 31

Behavioral and Psychiatric Emergencies

STUDY GUIDE ASSIGNMENT 31-1

- Misconceptions
- Forms of Emotional Disorders
- Characteristics of Emotional Disorders
- Assessment of Behavioral Emergencies

Reading Assignment: pages 720-726

Multiple-Choice Items

Read each question carefully. For each item, select the answer that BEST completes the statement or answers the question, and place the letter of that answer in the space provided.

b 1. Toxicity, infections, and brain injury are examples of causes associated with the _____ category of emotional disorders.
   - a. innate
   - b. organic
   - c. functional
   - d. psychotic

d 2. General symptoms of emotional disorders triggered by functional causes include:
   - I. changes in level of consciousness.
   - II. depression.
   - III. hallucinations.
   - IV. anxiety.
       - a. I, II, and III
       - b. II, III, and IV
       - c. I, III, and IV
       - d. II, III, and IV

c 3. A transient emotional disorder is defined as:
   - a. a disruption of one or two main areas of life.
   - b. a severe mental derangement with significant impairment.
   - c. a temporary mental derangement usually as a result of severe stress.
   - d. a disturbance in motor function with delusions and illusions.

_a_ 4. Common causes of anxiety states include:
   I. previous emotional trauma.
   II. drugs.
   III. genetic factors.
   IV. severe stress.
   V. biochemical abnormalities.
      a. I and IV
      b. I, II, and III
      c. II, III, and IV
      d. I, II, III, IV, and V

_d_ 5. Emotional disturbance(s) described as long-term or lifelong include:
   a. psychosis.
   b. transient disorders.
   c. anxiety states.
   d. a and c.

_a_ 6. A psychiatric emergency is any situation in which:
   a. the patient's moods, thoughts, or actions are disordered to the point of posing a risk of harm to self or others.
   b. a disordering of the patient moods, thoughts, or actions occurs but is viewed as not being harmful.
   c. the patient loses consciousness as a result of ingestion of excessive amounts of drugs or alcohol.
   d. b and c.

_b_ 7. Examples of true behavioral emergencies include:
   I. suicidal behavior.
   II. violent behavior.
   III. acute agitation.
   IV. severe depression.
   V. grief after loss.
      a. I, II, and III
      b. I, II, and IV
      c. II, III and IV
      d. III, IV, and V

_d_ 8. The first step in assessing a patient in a behavioral emergency is to:
   a. contact the local police.
   b. determine past history.
   c. assess vital signs.
   d. determine the problem.

C 9. The function of the mental status examination is to:
   a. attempt to divert the patient's attention from his or her current situation and focus on other information.
   b. keep the paramedic and patient from getting bored while on the scene or en route to the hospital.
   c. assist in gathering information about the patient's behavioral, psychological, and intellectual functions.
   d. a and b.

C 10. The components of the mental status examination include:
   I. thought.
   II. speech.
   III. appearance.
   IV. mood.
   V. psychosis.
       a. I, II, and III
       b. I, III, and V
       c. I, II, III, and IV
       d. I, II, III, IV, and V

a 11. Hallucinations, illusions, and delusions are the most common distortions in:
   a. perception.
   b. depression.
   c. emotions.
   d. suicide.

STUDY GUIDE ASSIGNMENT 31-2

▪ Other Factors Associated with Behavioral Emergencies
▪ Principles of Crisis Intervention
Reading Assignment: pages 726-732

Multiple-Choice Items

Read each question carefully. For each item, select the answer that BEST completes the statement or answers the question, and place the letter of that answer in the space provided.

d 1. Factors affecting reactions to chemical substances may include the:
   a. size and weight of the user.
   b. mental attitude and motivation of the user.
   c. personality of the user.
   d. all of the above.

c 2. The first step when one is involved in a potential elder abuse situation is to:
   a. reduce stress in the environment.
   b. confront the family for details of the incident.
   c. calmly but effectively protect the person who may have been abused.
   d. contact local law enforcement immediately.

_a_ 3. The victim of a sexual assault should be treated with:
  a. respect, dignity, and reassurance.
  b. objectivity and skepticism.
  c. a police officer present at all times.
  d. b and c.

_c_ 4. Which of the following patients would be considered at high risk for a suicide attempt?
  I. A 32-year-old female whose husband abuses her.
  II. A 6-year-old male about to face major surgery.
  III. A 40-year-old male who has just lost his job.
  IV. A 75-year-old female who has just lost her spouse.
  V. A 50-year-old socialite who has lost a tennis match.
    a. I, II, and V
    b. I, III, and IV
    c. III and IV
    d. I, II, III, IV, and V

_d_ 5. During the initial contact, the paramedic may institute procedures that will reduce the potential for suicidal behavior. These procedures include:
  a. pointing out the patient's options.
  b. taking all suicidal threats seriously.
  c. developing the patient's trust.
  d. all of the above.

_b_ 6. _____ is a set of action-oriented, but temporary, strategies designed to reduce the negative impact of a distressing event on a person or group and to restore normality.
  a. Chronic emotional stability
  b. Crisis intervention
  c. Emotional reactivity
  d. Mental distress coping

_a_ 7. The main objectives the paramedic should consider when working with a patient in the midst of a crisis include:
  a. protection from further stress.
  b. maintenance of a state of dysfunction.
  c. non-restraint of unacceptable behavior.
  d. all of the above.

_c_ 8. When involved in crisis intervention, it is helpful for the paramedic to work within a framework of elements. This framework includes:
  I. helping to set long-term goals.
  II. non-support of decisions made by the person in crisis.
  III. focus on the immediate situation.
  IV. encouraging self-reliance.
  V. closing out the intervention.
    a. I, II, and III
    b. II, III, and IV
    c. III, IV, and V
    d. I, II, III, IV, and V

_a_ 9. Inappropriate behavior for a paramedic assisting an individual through a crisis includes:
   a. withholding the truth.
   b. talking directly to the person in crisis.
   c. allowing the people in crisis to express themselves.
   d. a and c.

_b_ 10. When dealing with a severely disturbed patient, the paramedic should:
   I. threaten or challenge the patient when necessary.
   II. respect the patient and maintain dignity.
   III. communicate with the patient and build trust.
   IV. ignore the questions of an irrational patient.
   V. not encourage thought distortions.
      a. I, II, and IV
      b. II, III, and V
      c. II, IV, and V
      d. I, III, and V

_d_ 11. Occasionally, when involved in a case of severe mental disturbance, the paramedic may find it necessary to restrain the patient. Patient restraint:
   a. should be used only as a last resort.
   b. should be used as a threat early in the situation.
   c. should not be attempted without adequate personnel.
   d. a and c.

_c_ 12. While transporting the potentially violent patient, the paramedic who is administering patient care should assume a position:
   a. close to the driver's compartment for possible paramedic escape.
   b. at the head of the cot in order to be able to restrain the patient's head if necessary.
   c. between the patient and the doors to prevent the patient's exit from a moving vehicle.
   d. a and b

_d_ 13. To determine the legal implications of applying restraint and dealing with disturbed patients, the paramedic should:
   a. consult any EMS textbook.
   b. study appropriate state and local laws.
   c. be familiar with medical protocols.
   d. b and c.

Answer Key

All of the questions in this guide can be answered by referring to the text *Advanced Emergency Care for Paramedic Practice*. The page number(s) in parentheses following each multiple-choice answer indicate(s) on which page the correct answer can be found. Refer to the glossary to help you review the answers to the matching items.

Chapter 1
ASSIGNMENT 1-1

Matching

1. C
2. F
3. B
4. A
5. E

Multiple Choice

1. c. The performance of the health professional cannot be affected in any way by personal dislike of the patient or distain for the actions of the patient. The drunk driver may be legally and morally to blame, but the paramedic cannot allow personal judgment or anger interfere with the patient's medical treatment. (pg. 4)

2. c. The role of the professional is complex; it involves serving the medical interests and needs of patients in a society of multiple values and customs. (pg. 4)

3. b. Remember that integrity and diligence are assumed in the fulfillment of professional responsibilities. (pg. 4)

4. d. Today, with extensive training, testing, and physician direction, the tasks performed by the paramedic are many and multifaceted. Patient care is only one aspect in the role of the paramedic. (pg. 6)

5. d. The patient run report is an integral part of the patient's medical history and management and also serves as a legal document. (pg. 6-7)

ASSIGNMENT 1-2

Matching

1. B
2. A
3. D
4. E

Chapter 2

ASSIGNMENT 2-1

Matching

1. D	3. B	5. A
2. F	4. E	6. G

Multiple Choice

1. a. Medical control or medical direction refers to the physicians' roles and responsibilities in supervising and monitoring all medical aspects of the EMS system. (pg. 10)

2. d. Standing orders are authorizations for specific protocols to be initiated before or without direct voice contact with the medical control physician. (pg. 11)

3. b. Off-line medical control refers to the administrative components of medical control, including protocols and standing orders. (pg. 11)

4. a. On-line medical control refers to the supervision of patient care provided by the paramedic at the scene and en route to the hospital via voice communication between the paramedic and emergency physician. (pg. 11)

5. a. On-line medical control refers to the supervision of patient care provided by the paramedic at the scene and en route to the hospital via voice communication between the paramedic and emergency physician. (pg. 11)

6. c. These are the four operational units that make up the emergency medical services delivery system. (pg. 12)

7. c. The required design characteristics of ambulances are outlined in state EMS rules and regulations. (pg. 13)

ASSIGNMENT 2-2

Matching

1. D	3. A	5. E
2. C	4. F	

Multiple Choice

1. c. Time of day is not a factor. Helicopters can fly either in the day or at night. (pg. 14)

2. b. Hazards arise from the two helicopter rotors, the main rotor and the tail rotor. (pg. 15)

3. d. In most states, the EMT-P is trained in advanced management of trauma and cardiac care. (pg. 16)

4. b. Speedy access through the development of 911 as a nationally recognized emergency telephone number has heightened the capabilities of EMS to respond to an emergency. (pg. 16)

5. a. Communications operators are a critical link in the system. (pg. 16)

6. a. This system uses a single channel that allows communication between two points in only one direction at a time. (pg. 17)

Chapter 3
ASSIGNMENT 3-1

Matching

1. C	4. H	7. J
2. A	5. B	8. E
3. F	6. G	9. I

Multiple Choice

1. a. Civil law refers to private law, as it applies to agreements between any two recognizable parties, which may be individuals, corporations, or other entities. (pg. 20)

2. b. Administrative law pertains to the government's authority to enforce the rules, regulations, and pertinent statutes of governmental agencies. (pg. 20-21)

3. d. Upon being convicted of committing a crime, the defendant is punished by the state through imprisonment, fines, or both. (pg. 20)

4. b. Such statutes identify the aspects of medical practice that may be delegated by a physician to a paramedic. (pg. 21)

5. d. Civil law includes actions based on a contract or tort. (pg. 21)

6. b. As with other laws, this one varies from state to state. (pg. 21)

7. d. The use of lights and sirens is not a defense to liability and is only one factor considered in the determination of fault. (pg. 21)

ASSIGNMENT 3-2

Matching

1. A	5. H	9. B
2. D	6. L	10. I
3. G	7. K	11. E
4. C	8. M	12. J

ASSIGNMENT 3-3

Matching

1. B	4. G	7. C
2. D	5. I	8. A
3. H	6. E	

Chapter 4
ASSIGNMENT 4-1

Matching

1. E	4. A	7. G
2. I	5. H	8. D
3. B	6. C	

ASSIGNMENT 4-2

Matching

1. C	3. A	5. F
2. E	4. D	

Chapter 5
ASSIGNMENT 5-1

Matching

1. B	4. E	6. G
2. F	5. C	7. D
3. H		

Chapter 6
ASSIGNMENT 6-1

Matching

1. D	4. F	6. C
2. E	5. H	7. A
3. B		

Chapter 7
ASSIGNMENT 7-1

Matching

1. A	3. B	5. G
2. F	4. C	6. D

ASSIGNMENT 7-2

Matching

1. I	5. G	9. D
2. A	6. C	10. L
3. J	7. E	11. F
4. B	8. K	

Chapter 8
ASSIGNMENT 8-1

Matching

1. C	3. A	5. E
2. D	4. F	

Multiple Choice

1. b. (pg. 79)
2. a. (pg. 79)
3. d. (pg. 79)
4. b. (pg. 79)
5. c. (pg. 79)

6. a. (pg. 79)
7. d. (pg. 79)
8. d. (pg. 80)
9. c. (pg. 80)

10. b. (pg. 80)
11. b. (pg. 80)
12. a. (pg. 81)
13. c. (pg. 81)

ASSIGNMENT 8-2

Matching

1. B
2. I
3. D
4. K
5. H
6. U
7. N

8. V
9. E
10. T
11. S
12. F
13. R
14. A

15. Q
16. M
17. O
18. C
19. P
20. G
21. L

Labeling

1. A. sagittal
   B. midsagittal
   C. frontal
   D. transverse

2. A. dorsal
   B. cranial
   C. spinal
   D. abdominal
   E. pelvic
   F. thoracic
   G. abdominopelvic
   H. ventral

Chapter 9
ASSIGNMENT 9-1

Matching

1. F
2. I
3. E

4. H
5. G
6. C

7. A
8. B

ASSIGNMENT 9-2

Matching

1. P
2. O
3. A
4. J
5. Q
6. E
7. I

8. F
9. H
10. S
11. G
12. R
13. M
14. L

15. T
16. B
17. U
18. C
19. D
20. N

Multiple Choice

1. c. The degree of thoroughness and the evaluation method are dependent on the acuteness and specific circumstances of each patient situation. (pg. 103)

2. a. The direct method allows the patient to focus on a single detail, but it can lead the paramedic into a "tunnel vision" approach to patient care. (pg. 105)

3. d. All of these components are part of a complete patient evaluation. (pg. 106-107)

4. d. Medications and allergies are separate sections of a patient history. (pg. 106-107)

5. c. The purpose of the medical history is to identify any of the patient's past medical health problems that may affect the current illness or injury. (pg. 107)

6. b. Auscultation can provide important information about the patient, particularly concerning the respiratory system. (pg. 107)

7. d. A thorough neurologic assessment is obtained as information is gathered throughout the secondary survey. (pg. 109)

8. a. Interpretation of a single term can vary from one practitioner to another. (pg. 109)

9. c. Normal breathing has a regular pattern; medium depth (about 500 mL tidal volume) is effortless and almost silent. (pg. 110)

10. d. The secondary survey allows the paramedic to quantify and evaluate the patient's pulse. (pg. 110-111)

11. d. Bradycardia can occur abnormally or normally. (pg. 111)

12. d. Reassessment of the blood pressure is often necessary to interpret findings and to keep track of dynamic physiologic functions. (pg. 111)

13. b. False high and false low blood pressure readings can distort the perception of the actual condition of the patient. (pg. 112)

14. c. The ability to hear blood pressure sounds is hampered frequently in the prehospital environment. (pg. 112-113)

15. d. Any infant or child involved in trauma and all children beyond the age of 3 or 4 years should have their blood pressure measured. (pg. 114)

16. c. Cardiac tamponade and heart failure may cause a narrowed pulse pressure. (pg. 114)

17. b. Insignificant alterations indicate a negative tilt test. (pg. 114-115)

18. a. Rectal, rather than oral, temperatures should be taken on infants and children up to age 6. (pg. 115)

19. d. Bilateral dilated and fixed pupils can also result from hypoxia or severely increased intracranial pressure. (pg. 117)

20. a. Subcutaneous emphysema occurs when air escapes into the tissues. (pg. 118)

21. b. Rales can be simulated by rolling hair between the thumb and forefinger close to one's ear. (pg. 117)

22. c. Extra sounds may be normal and benign for some individuals. (pg. 118)

23. b. Abnormal postures are primitive responses that indicate severe intracranial pressure. (pg. 119)

ASSIGNMENT 9-3

Multiple Choice

1. d. The numerical values are added to the Adult Glasgow Coma Scale to give a total trauma score. (pg. 119)

2. c. Eye opening - 2, verbal response - 2, and motor response - 4. (pg. 121)

Chapter 10
ASSIGNMENT 10-1

Matching

1. A
2. I
3. K
4. F

5. G
6. M
7. C
8. B

9. L
10. H
11. E
12. J

Labeling

1. A. nasal cavity
    B. oral cavity
    C. larynx
    D. trachea
    E. esophagus
    F. nasopharynx
    G. oropharynx
    H. laryngopharynx

2. A. epiglottis
    B. vallecula
    C. vestibular fold
    D. vocal folds
    E. arytenoid cartilage

Multiple Choice

1. d. By definition, the upper airway ends at the cricoid cartilage. The cricoid cartilage is the dividing point between the upper airway and the lower airway. (pg. 126)

2. c. The amount of water required for humidification increases with the respiratory rate. This explains the dehydration that results from hyperventilation. (pg. 126-127)

3. b. The mucous layer contains bactericidals that engulf and kill bacteria that enter through the nose, thus preventing infection, and also provides heat and humidification. (pg. 127)

4. d. Because these patients have lost the function of the nose to warm and humidify air, a priority is to supply warm and humidified air. (pg. 127)

5. a. The eustachian tube allows for equalization of pressure between the middle ear and the pharynx. This is important for the functioning of the tympanic membrane. (pg.128)

6. d. The larynx protects the lower airway by using the epiglottis and the cough reflex. (pg. 128)

7. c. Because the larynx has been bypassed, the cough reflex is diminished, making the lower airway more vulnerable to foreign matter and mucus buildup. (pg. 128)

8. c. Frequently foreign objects lodge in the larynx at the vocal cords because the adult airway is narrowest at this point. (pg. 129)

9. c. Laryngeal spasm can be induced by manipulation such as tracheal suctioning or tracheal intubation. The depth and duration of suctioning can be controlled by the paramedic so as not to induce spasm. (pg. 129)

10. d. Laryngeal edema can be caused by both medical and traumatic conditions, such as blunt trauma to the larynx, tracheal intubation, epiglottitis, and anaphylaxis. (pg. 129)

ASSIGNMENT 10-2

Matching

1. E	4. I	7. G
2. D	5. B	8. H
3. J	6. F	9. A

Multiple Choice

1. b. Injuries that involve striking a fixed object such as a fence should increase the index of suspicion of laryngeal trauma. (pg. 129)

2. c. The jaw-thrust method is the safest method of opening the airway and should always be used on a patient suspected of having cervical spine injury. (pg. 130)

3. b. The history of the current episode enables the paramedic to determine how long the particular problem has been present. This allows the paramedic to differentiate between acute and chronic problems. (pg. 130)

4. d. Restlessness, combativeness, or drowsiness often indicates profound hypoxemia or hypercarbia. Slurred speech is most indicative of central nervous system interruption from stroke, drugs, head injury, or hypoglycemia. (pg. 131)

5. a. Central cyanosis is indicative of hypoxemia. Peripheral cyanosis in the extremities may indicate hypoxemia, although it may also be caused by poor circulation, hypothermia, or orthopedic disorders. (pg. 131)

6. a. This condition is termed "pulsus paradoxus" and is caused by significantly increased intrathoracic pressures created by breathing against obstruction. (pg. 131)

ASSIGNMENT 10-3

Matching

1. C	5. K	9. A
2. H	6. L	10. F
3. B	7. G	11. D
4. E	8. J	

Multiple Choice

1. b. Endotracheal intubation is the definitive technique for protecting the lower airway. An endotracheal tube allows for direct access to the lower airway. All the other devices listed allow for indirect access to the lower airway. (pg. 132)

2. b. Increasing the fraction of inspired oxygen above that present in room air increases the amount of oxygen in the alveoli. Because movement of oxygen into the pulmonary capillary bed is governed by simple diffusion, increasing the amount of oxygen in the alveoli improves oxygen concentration in the blood unless a severe diffusion disorder is present. (pg. 132)

3. c. Dead air space in the nasopharynx acts as a reservoir for oxygen. The patient does not need to breathe through the nose; oxygen is entrained through the device even with mouth breathing. (pg. 133)

4. a. Because of their simplicity and because few complications arise from their use, oropharyngeal and nasopharyngeal airway devices are ideal for use in a patient whose airway requires maintenance for only a short period of time. (pg. 135)

5. c. If the patient accepts an oropharyngeal airway without gagging, placement of an endotracheal tube should be considered. Patients whose gag reflex is not intact cannot protect their airways. (pg. 136)

6. a. Selection of the correct size is done by nostril size. (pg. 136)

7. a. Suctioning should not be done for more than 5 seconds; it removes air from the lungs as well as fluid from the airway. (pg. 137)

8. d. Complications associated with pressure-regulated devices include pneumothorax and gastric rupture. These complications contraindicate the use of these ventilators in children. (pg. 138)

9. b. Regardless of which device is used, the limiting factor until the patient is intubated is the seal of the mask. (pg. 138)

10. a. The first function of the laryngoscope blade is to align the structures of the upper and lower airways to enable the endotracheal tube to pass through them into the trachea. Its second function is to provide direct visualization of the larynx and vocal cords, through which the endotracheal tube is passed. (pg. 141)

11. c. Intubation, EGTA, and EOA are not first-line airway-control techniques. If respirations are absent or inadequate, ventilation with supplemental oxygen and a less sophisticated airway device should be initiated. (pg. 139 and 142)

Chapter 11
ASSIGNMENT 11-1

Matching

1. B	13. A	24. J
2. A	14. D	25. E
3. J	15. B	26. D
4. C	16. H	27. D
5. D	17. E	28. F
6. I	18. I	29. E
7. K	19. A	30. H
8. F	20. C	31. G
9. G	21. B	32. I
10. E	22. G	33. C
11. F	23. H	34. A
12. G		

ASSIGNMENT 11-2

Multiple Choice

1. a. The mitochondria are organelles (small organs) within the tissue cells and are responsible for the production of energy. They do require and use oxygen, but the delivery of oxygen to the mitochondria is through the process of diffusion. Answers *b*, *c*, and *d* are all components of the Fick principle. (pg. 176)

2. b. Active transport involves the use of energy to move molecules. Menhidrosis is vicarious menstruation through the sweat glands, or literally "sweating blood." Osmosis is the movement of water from areas of lower concentration to areas of higher concentration. (pg. 181)

3. d. Menidrosis is an alternative spelling of menhidrosis. (pg. 181)

4. a. Because this movement is against the natural flow, energy must be present to transport molecules through the membrane. Proteins in the membrane also act as carriers to assist in this process. (pg. 181)

5. a. Examples of hypertonic solutions include $D_5 0.9\%$ NaCl, $D_5 0.45\%$ NaCl, $D_{10}W$, and D_5LR. (pg. 182)

6. b. Half-normal saline is an example of a hypotonic solution. (pg. 182)

7. c. In the adult, total body water represents 50-60% of total body weight. (pg. 182)

8. c. Electrolytes are substances that separate into ions when in solution and conduct a weak electrical current. (pg. 183)

9. d. Positively charged ions are called cations. Sodium is the most important cation in the fluid outside the cell. (pg. 184)

10. c. Potassium is the most important cation inside the cell. (pg. 184)

11. c. Barometric pressure is atmospheric pressure, or the weight of the atmosphere on the surface of the earth. Osmotic pressure is the pressure that develops in a solution as a result of the net osmosis into that solution. (pg. 184)

12. b. Blood accounts for about 8% of total body weight. (pg. 184)

13. b. The formed elements (red blood cells, white blood cells, and platelets) are suspended in the plasma. (pg. 185)

14. a. The red blood cell carries oxygen and carbon dioxide. (pg. 185)

15. b. A hematocrit of 45 means that 45% of whole blood is composed of red blood cells. The average adult male has a hematocrit of 45 + or - 7; the average female has a hematocrit of 42 + or - 5. (pg. 186)

16. b. The leukocytes, or white blood cells, are outnumbered by red cells 700 to 1 and tend to be colorless. Several types of leukocytes are found in the body. One type engulfs and destroys invaders. Another type, called the lymphocyte, is largely responsible for providing immunity to infectious disease. (pg. 186)

17. d. Platelets are the smallest formed elements in the blood and are actually not cells in themselves, but fragments of cells. When blood is put in contact with tissue other than the inside of the blood vessels, as in an injury, the platelets stick together and form a plug that seals the wound. (pg. 186)

18. d. An acid is defined by its ability to donate hydrogen ions. (pg. 187)

19. c. A base is defined by its ability to accept hydrogen ions. (pg. 187)

20. c. Blood plasma is slightly alkaline and has a normal range from 7.35 to 7.45; any value within this range is considered a neutral state for blood. (pg. 187)

21. a. A blood pH of 7.30 equals acidosis, and a blood pH of 7.50 equals alkalosis. The lower limit at which a person can live more than a few hours is about 6.8, and the upper limit is about 8.0. (pg. 187)

22. a. The buffer system involves weak acids and weak bases within the body that combine with stronger bases and stronger acids to form weaker compounds. The three major buffer systems in body fluids are bicarbonate buffer, phosphate buffer, and protein buffer. Protein is actually part of the buffer system but is less important than bicarbonate and phosphate in its buffering potential. The renal system and the respiratory system both work to regulate acid-base balance, but they do so less quickly than the buffer system does. (pg. 188)

23. c. Ventilation is controlled by the brain stem, which is sensitive to pH changes. Respiration is increased to "blow off" carbon dioxide in acidotic states and is decreased to retain carbon dioxide in alkalotic states. (pg. 188)

24. c. The use of narcotics in drug overdose promotes respiratory depression. Decreased ventilation results in carbon dioxide retention and a plunge in pH. (pg. 189)

25. d. When a patient hyperventilates, excessive elimination of carbon dioxide results and pH rises. (pg. 190)

26. a. The normal PCO_2 level rules out respiratory acidosis and alkalosis. Diabetics in ketoacidosis produce large amounts of ketones, which are acidic and lower blood pH. The Kussmaul breathing is actually a compensatory process designed to "blow off" carbon dioxide and adjust pH upward. (pg. 190)

27. b. The normal PCO_2 level rules out respiratory acidosis and alkalosis. Peptic ulcer patients can ingest sufficient quantities of bases (sodium bicarbonate in baking soda and calcium carbonate in antacid tablets) to elevate their blood pH. (pg. 191)

ASSIGNMENT 11-3

Multiple Choice

1. d. Vagal activity (parasympathetic action) is decreased in shock, during which sympathetic activity dominates. Increased peripheral vascular resistance is achieved through peripheral vasoconstriction. (pg. 191)

2. d. High-flow, high-concentration oxygen is desirable in shock patients so that red blood cells, which may be reduced in number from hemorrhage, are maximally loaded with oxygen molecules for delivery to ischemic tissues. (pg. 195)

3. c. When air is heated it expands. The cold air trapped in the garment will expand when exposed to a warmer environment, and the garment will become tighter. Although there are safety features to prevent the garment from becoming too tight (pop-off valves and slipping of the Velcro), the patient should be examined for the presence of distal pulses and his or her blood pressure should be evaluated. (pg. 195)

4. c. Thoracic trauma with associated hemorrhage and the presence of pulmonary edema are contraindications for the use of the pneumatic anti-shock garment. (pg. 196)

5. d. Either normal saline or lactated Ringer's solutions is an acceptable volume expander for the shock patient. D_5W is not considered an adequate volume expander because it leaves the vascular space so rapidly. (pg. 203)

Chapter 12
ASSIGNMENT 12-1

Matching

1. A	6. G	10. B
2. E	7. N	11. F
3. J	8. C	12. M
4. I	9. K	13. D
5. H		

Multiple Choice

1. b. Many different parts of animals have been used as drug sources. (pg. 207)

2. a. This act provided added protection against untested drugs. (pg. 207)

3. d. The Drug Enforcement Agency is the enforcer of all drug legislation. (pg. 208)

ASSIGNMENT 12-2

Matching

1. C	9. L	17. K
2. A	10. O	18. E
3. D	11. J	19. I
4. F	12. M	20. F
5. G	13. P	21. B
6. B	14. N	22. Q
7. H	15. D	23. A
8. G	16. H	

ASSIGNMENT 12-3

Multiple Choice

1. d. Aqueous solutions need to be shaken prior to use. (pg. 210)

2. d. The oral route is used for absorption of drugs through the lining of the gastrointestinal system. (pg. 212)

3. b. Intravenous drug therapy leaves no margin for error, because the drug bypasses absorption barriers and is injected directly into the bloodstream. (pg. 213)

4. d. Drugs given through the tracheal route are rapidly absorbed and delivered to the heart for distribution. (pg. 214)

5. b. The combined effects of drugs are greater than if each were given individually. (pg. 214)

6. a. In general, most drugs pass into the brain more slowly than into other tissues. (pg. 214)

7. a. As a drug begins to act, the free components are metabolized into substances for elimination. (pg. 215)

8. d. An antagonist occupies a receptor site but causes no physiologic response. (pg. 215)

9. b. These responses prepare the body for fight or flight from a dangerous situation. (pg. 216-217)

10. d. They also cause slight vasodilation in skeletal muscle. (pg. 217)

11. a. Isuprel (isoproterenol) is generally used in cases of symptomatic bradycardia and heart blocks. (pg. 217-218)

12. d. This condition is counteracted by using atropine as an antagonist. (pg. 218)

ASSIGNMENT 12-4

Multiple Choice

1. c. (pg. 219)

1 tablespoon = 3 teaspoons
1 tablespoon = 30 mL

2. c. (pg. 219)

```
          97.72   or rounded off to 98 kg
2.2. )215.0.0
       198
       170
       154
       160
       154
        60
        44
        16 (remainder)
```

3. d. (pg. 220)

```
   5.1          5.100
   8.25         8.250
 + 3.006   or + 3.006
               16.356
```

4. c. (pg. 220)

```
                4 11 16 1
   52.7         52.70
 - 23.81   or - 23.81
                28.89
```

5. b. (pg. 220)

```
     7.5
  x  125
    375
    150
    75
    9375    add decimal point   937.5
```

275

6. c. (pg. 220)

$$0.25\overline{)7.80.0}$$

$$\begin{array}{r} 31.2 \\ \hline 7\ 5 \\ 30 \\ 25 \\ 50 \\ 50 \\ \hline 00 \end{array}$$

7. a. (pg. 221)

$$\text{Volume} = \frac{2.5 \text{ mg} \times 2 \text{ mL}}{10 \text{ mg}} = \frac{5}{10} = 0.5 \text{ mL}$$

8. c. (pg. 221)

$$\text{Volume} = \frac{50 \text{ mg} \times 10 \text{ mL}}{100 \text{ mg}} = \frac{500}{100} = 5 \text{ mL}$$

9. c. (pg. 221)

$$\text{Volume} = \frac{4 \text{ mg} \times 500 \text{ mL}}{2000 \text{ mg} = 2 \text{ g}} = \frac{2000}{2000} = 1 \text{ mL}$$

Using microdrip tubing:

$$\text{gtt/min} = \frac{1 \text{ mL}}{1 \text{ min}} \times \frac{60 \text{ microgtt}}{1 \text{ mL}} = 60 \text{ microgtt/min}$$

10. d. Intramuscular injections are absorbed quicker than subcutaneous injections. (pg. 227)
11. b. The maximum volume deliverable via the subcutaneous route is 2.0 mL. (pg. 227)
12. d. The direct and rapid access to the peripheral circulation through an intraosseous route allows the administration of virtually any fluid or medication that can be given through a peripheral IV site. (pg. 247 and 251)

Chapter 13
ASSIGNMENT 13-1

Matching

1. C
2. F
3. G
4. A
5. D
6. K

7. H
8. J
9. E
10. B
11. D

12. G
13. C
14. A
15. F
16. E

ASSIGNMENT 13-2

Matching

1. F
2. B
3. G

4. H
5. D
6. I

7. C
8. A

Multiple Choice

1. b. The extent of tissue damage depends on these three factors. (pg. 269)
2. b. A bullet that breaks into many small fragments on impact or one that fragments as it leaves the gun, such as a shotgun bullet, increases the frontal area significantly. (pg. 269)
3. a. A handgun is an example of a medium-energy weapon. (pg. 270)
4. d. Valuable time is saved when the initial consideration of the paramedic is to determine the mechanism of injury. (pg. 271)
5. c. In addition to the car being crashed, the occupants and their internal organs are also damaged. (pg. 271)
6. a. In order of frequency of occurrence, the most common sites of injury in automobile trauma without restraints are the head, thorax, abdomen, and long bones. (pg. 273)
7. c. Depending on the type of collision, the structural damage to the car is similar to the damage sustained by the patient, in both location and amount of energy exchange. Therefore, by assessing the location and extent of car damage, the paramedic can anticipate the injuries the patient may have sustained. (pg. 273)
8. a. In the down-and-under pathway, the unrestrained occupant's body travels down into and slides over the edge of the car seat. In the up-and-over pathway, the head of the unrestrained occupant is the lead point of the human missile. (pg. 274)
9. c. If the head rest is improperly positioned, the cervical spine is the recipient of the initial energy exchange, with backward extension over the top of the seat. Severe cervical strains, commonly called whiplash, can result. (pg. 275-276)
10. c. Pedestrian-car collisions occur in three stages: the car-body impact, the body-to-car hood thrust, and the body-to-ground fall. (pg. 277)
11. c. Whereas the adult attempts to escape from the impact, a young child looks to see what is happening. This action may result in frontal injury rather than the lateral or posterior injury that is more common in the adult. (pg. 279)
12. b. To make accurate assessments and provide information to emergency department personnel, the paramedic must be familiar with the pattern of injury and the kinematics of trauma. (pg. 279)

13. a. The types of neck injuries include cervical compression and vertebral fractures due to hyperextension, hyperflexion, or lateral flexion. The most common vertebral fractures are at C-1, C-2, C-5, and C-6. (pg. 280)

14. c. The arch of the aorta and the heart are fairly movable. When rapid deceleration occurs, whether from lateral or frontal impact, the stationary thoracic aorta remains with the chest wall, and the heart and aortic arch swing like a pendulum. (pg. 280)

15. d. Attached only to the diaphragm, the liver descends into the abdominal cavity and is stopped by the ligamentum teres in the perineal area. The capsule can split like cutting cheese. The result is a midpoint laceration of the liver. (pg. 281)

16. a. The astute paramedic at the scene of a blast accident is alert to the three blast forces that cause injury and assesses the victim for eye, lung, ear, extremity, and thermal injuries. (pg. 281)

17. c. A blast is an explosive force. Blast injuries can occur several feet or many yards away from the incident. (pg. 281)

Chapter 14
ASSIGNMENT 14-1

Matching

1. D	4. J	7. I
2. A	5. B	8. G
3. F	6. H	9. C

Multiple Choice

1. a. Soft-tissue injuries involve the skin and underlying musculature. An injury to these tissues is commonly referred to as a wound. (pg. 287-288)

2. d. A contusion is a bruise; a blood clot that forms at the injury site is called a hematoma; crush injuries are usually caused by extreme external forces that crush both tissue and bone. (pg. 288)

3. b. As blood accumulates in the area, a characteristic black and blue mark is seen. (pg. 288)

4. d. Before managing any patient with open wounds, the paramedic should put on a pair of latex gloves for personal protection against the transmission of blood-borne diseases. (pg. 288)

5. c. In an abrasion, usually only the epidermis and part of the dermis is lost. A little bleeding may result, but rarely do more than a few drops ooze from injured capillaries. (pg. 288)

6. a. As the bacteria grow, they produce a toxin that provokes serious muscle spasms and interferes with breathing. Puncture wounds are fertile ground for the tetanus organism, which flourishes in an oxygen-poor environment. (pg. 289)

7. c. If the avulsed skin is still attached by a flap of skin and the skin is folded back, circulation to the flap can be severely compromised. (pg. 290)

8. c. In complete amputations the body part is completely severed. Partial amputations have more than 50% of the body part severed. In degloving amputations the skin and adipose tissue are torn away, but underlying tissue is left intact. (pg. 290)

9. d. Because blood vessels are elastic, they tend to have spasms and to retract into surrounding tissue in cases of complete amputations. (pg. 290)

10. c. Once the part has been cleaned, wrapped, and placed in plastic bags, it should be put in a container of ice or ice water. Never use dry ice or the tissue will become frozen. (pg. 291)

11. a. If the object is impaled in the cheek, bleeding into the mouth and throat can impair breathing. If the object is removed it may be necessary to pack the inside of the cheek, between the cheek wall and the teeth, with sterile gauze to help control bleeding and, thus, decrease the risk of aspiration. (pg. 291-292)

ASSIGNMENT 14-2

Matching

1. C
2. B
3. G

4. F
5. D

6. E
7. A

Multiple Choice

1. b. Thermal burns are caused by hot liquids, solids, super-heated gases, and flames. Electrical burns are caused by low- or high-voltage current and lightning. Chemical burns are caused by wet or dry corrosive substances, and radiation burns are caused by ultraviolet light and atomic explosions. (pg. 292)

2. d. Superficial burns are confined to the epidermal layers of the skin. Partial-thickness burns involve the entire epidermis and may extend deep into the dermis. Full-thickness burns cause destruction of both the epidermis and dermis. Severe full-thickness burns may even involve damage to the subcutaneous tissue, muscle, and bone. (pg. 293)

3. a. This method gives a rough estimate and should be used only to calculate surface area that is minimally burned. (pg. 295)

4. d. Associated injuries can also complicate the care of the burn-injured patient. Fractures or internal injuries that may be suffered from explosions, motor vehicle accidents associated with fire, or falls when the patient has jumped from a burning building can alter the eventual outcome of the burn-injured patient. (pg. 296)

5. c. These age groups are not able to handle stress very well, and the thickness of the dermal layer of the skin is thinner in the very young and old. The same injuries that cause a partial-thickness burn in a young adult could result in a full-thickness burn in the thinner skin of a very young or old person. The people who respond best to therapy are those between 5 and 34 years of age. (pg. 296)

6. c. Carbon monoxide is a colorless, odorless, and tasteless gas. It passes through the lungs and combines with hemoglobin to produce carboxyhemoglobin. The hypoxia that results from carbon monoxide poisoning is caused by a decrease in circulating oxygen. (pg. 297)

7. b. Moderate levels in the blood produce confusion, lethargy, and depressed ST segments as well as all the early signs. Eventually, coma and death ensue if intervention does not occur. (pg. 297)

8. b. Labored breathing is a symptom, hoarseness; cough, singed nasal hair, and blisters around the mouth are signs. (pg. 298)

9. a. In burn emergencies, the number-one priority is the safety of the rescuers. (pg. 298)

10. d. The primary survey is always the first step once the paramedic is at the patient's side. (pg. 298)

11. c. This can be remembered by using the acronym "AMPLE." (pg. 299)

12. d. The proper steps are to stop the burning process, secure the airway and breathing, and administer 100% oxygen by mask. (pg. 299)

13. a. Large amounts of intravenous fluids are used to flush the kidneys of myoglobin, a by-product of the breakdown of muscle tissue. (pg. 300)

14. c. Flushing should begin immediately with copious amounts of water. Do not use neutralizing agents because they may cause an additional reaction. (pg. 300)

15. d. A more moderate loss occurs over the next 12 to 16 hours. (pg. 301)

16. c. In addition, the level of consciousness should be normal, and urine output should be kept at 30 mL/hour. (pg. 301)

Chapter 15
ASSIGNMENT 15-1

Matching

1. D	11. B	20. N
2. L	12. E	21. B
3. K	13. J	22. G
4. G	14. R	23. K
5. H	15. D	24. A
6. I	16. I	25. L
7. F	17. P	26. O
8. A	18. C	27. F
9. C	19. Q	28. H
10. E		

Labeling

1. A. auricle
    B. tympanic membrane
    C. malleus
    D. incus
    E. stapes
    F. eustachian tube

2. A. cornea
    B. vitreous body
    C. optic nerve
    D. pupil
    E. lens
    F. iris
    G. conjunctiva
    H. retina
    I. sclera

ASSIGNMENT 15-2

Multiple Choice

1. d. A break in the skull can result in the loss of cerebrospinal fluid into the nearby cavities and eventually out through the ears or nose or both. (pg. 305)

2. c. Direct pressure to stop the fluid leak should be avoided because this action can, in turn, increase the intracranial pressure. Sterile dressings gently packed in and around the ear will help prevent infection and will allow fluid to escape, therefore decreasing the pressure within the skull. (pg. 306)

3. d. Particles lodged under the lower lid may be removed by pulling down the lower lid, exposing the inner surface. The corner of a piece of sterile gauze can be used to remove the foreign object. (pg. 308)

4. b. A hole should be cut in the center of a bulky dressing. The dressing should be moistened, and the injured globe should protrude through the hole. A protective cup should be secured over

the pad. The uninjured eye should also be bandaged to prevent sympathetic eye movement. (pg. 308)

5. c. A fracture of the skull allows blood to seep from the cranium into the sinus cavities and then out the nostrils. Facial injuries that result from blunt trauma usually cause a nosebleed. Infections within the nose, bleeding disorders, sinusitis, and high blood pressure can all cause a nosebleed. (pg. 310)

6. d. All of these techniques should control the bleeding. Application of cold also helps to stop a nosebleed because cold constricts blood vessels. (pg. 310)

7. a. The difference between mean arterial pressure and the intracranial pressure is normally sufficient to maintain adequate cerebral perfusion. If the intracranial pressure is increased through cerebral edema or hemorrhage, cerebral perfusion pressure is decreased and blood flow to the brain is decreased. If the intracranial pressure becomes equal to or exceeds the mean arterial pressure, blood flow to the brain effectively ceases. (pg. 311)

8. c. Cushing's triad is a clear but late sign of increasing intracranial pressure. (pg. 312)

9. a. Differing signs and symptoms occur in these three areas as pressure intensifies and lower areas of the brain stem are affected. (pg. 312)

10. d. Decorticate posturing occurs when the stage of cerebral herniation usually is reversible with prompt surgical intervention to remove the compressing force. (pg. 312)

11. b. When a painful stimulus is applied, the patient may exhibit decerebrate posturing. Few patients who reach this stage ever function again. (pg. 312)

12. c. A cerebral concussion has classically been defined as a transient episode of neuronal dysfunction after a violent jar or shock to the brain, with a rapid return to normal neurologic activity. (pg. 313)

13. d. Short-term memory loss produces repetition of questions. A major cause of this type of behavior is frontal lobe injury, and some of these patients may be combative. (pg. 313)

14. a. Depending on the area of the brain involved, a neurologic deficit may or may not be evident. (pg. 314)

15. d. Blood travels into the periorbital subcutaneous tissue, producing the typical racoon's eyes appearance. (pg. 315)

16. b. Epidural bleeds represent 2% of head injuries that result in hospitalization. About 15% to 20% of these patients die. (pg. 315)

17. c. Typically, the hemorrhage is caused by a congenital arterial aneurysm that ruptures spontaneously, often during exertion. (pg. 316)

18. d. In each of these categories the paramedic determines the best response the patient can make to a set of standardized stimuli. (pg. 317)

19. a. The more depressed the level of consciousness, the more likely it is that a one-sided fixed and dilated pupil represents herniation of brain structures secondary to increased intracranial pressure. (pg. 317)

20. d. Any trauma above the clavicle suggests cervical spine injury. (pg. 317)

21. b. Prehospital treatment of any patient with head injury focuses on maintaining adequate oxygenation and cerebral blood flow. Hyperoxygenation is effective in providing oxygen to hypoperfused cells. (pg. 317)

22. b. An IV line of lactated Ringer's or normal saline at a to-keep-open (TKO) rate should be started in case signs of shock appear. (pg. 317)

23. c. The method that can be used to decrease intracranial pressure and prevent brain stem herniation is hyperventilation with 100% oxygen, which causes cerebral vasoconstriction and subsequently decreases intracranial pressure. (pg. 317)

ASSIGNMENT 15-3

Multiple Choice

1. d. The integrity of the larynx, mandible, and other bony structures of the face and neck should be carefully evaluated. (pg. 318)

2. a. Plastic wrap is well suited for this purpose. The wrap should be sealed on all sides to make the seal airtight. Direct pressure should be applied over the occlusive dressing to control bleeding. (pg. 319)

3. d. Axial loading can occur in several ways. Most commonly, this compression of the spine occurs when the head strikes an object and the weight of the still-moving body bears against the stopped head. (pg. 319)

4. c. Shock secondary to spinal cord injury is called spinal shock. (pg. 320)

5. d. Note, however, that the absence of these signs does not rule out bony spine injury. (pg. 321)

6. b. These methods can cause movement of both the cervical and lower spine. (pg. 321)

7. c. This is because the posterior musculature is not well developed. (pg. 323)

Chapter 16
ASSIGNMENT 16-1

Matching

1. I	5. J	8. F
2. B	6. G	9. D
3. C	7. K	10. E
4. H		

Multiple Choice

1. b. Vital signs are part of the secondary survey. (pg. 326)

2. a. This quick listen identifies only the presence of breath sounds in each of the lung fields and their absence in the stomach. (pg. 327)

3. b. These diminished breath sounds can be extremely difficult to distinguish from the breath sounds on the other side or from tracheal sounds. (pg. 327)

4. c. These can be injuries to the chest wall, diaphragm, lungs, or heart or injuries to the thoracic vascular system. (pg. 327)

5. a. Such associated injuries might include a pneumothorax or pulmonary contusion. (pg. 328)

6. c. This combination of fractures creates a "flail" segment of the chest wall, which is made up of the segments of the fractured ribs between the fractures that no longer have a firm bony attachment to the rest of the rib cage. (pg. 328)

7. d. The decreased oxygenation associated with a pulmonary contusion requires the primary focus to be patient care. (pg. 328)

8. b. When a flail segment is present, the negative pressure in the chest during inspiration causes the flail segment of the chest to be pulled inward instead of expanding outward with the rest of the chest wall. Similarly, during expiration, the higher pressure in the chest causes the flail segment to move outward instead of relaxing inward with the rest of the chest wall. (pg,. 328)

9. d. Treatment of a patient with a flail chest should be focused on providing supplemental oxygen to overcome the hypoxemia that may accompany the reduced ventilatory capacity and

aggressive treatment of any associated injuries. If a large flail segment is present, endotracheal intubation and positive pressure ventilation may be necessary to provide adequate ventilation. (pg. 328)

10. c. Because pulmonary contusion frequently is accompanied by other ventilation-compromising injuries, the cumulative effect of all the injuries on the patient's ability to breathe may be profound. The pulmonary contusion is the major pathologic process that effects the morbidity and mortality associated with a flail chest. (pg. 329)

11. a. This condition is one of the few that require the pneumatic anti-shock garment to be deflated in the field. (pg. 330)

12. d. In a normal, otherwise healthy patient, a small simple pneumothorax may be tolerated rather well, because the normal lung usually has a good deal of reserve capacity. In a patient with multiple injuries, respiratory compromise may be serious, because positive-pressure ventilation increases the size of a pneumothorax or even converts it to a tension pneumothorax. (pg. 331)

13. c. A mediastinal shift creates a profound compromise of ventilation and reduces cardiac output because it reduces blood flow to the left atrium by kinking the vena cava and increasing pulmonary vascular resistance. (pg. 331)

14. c. The purpose of the field thoracentesis is to convert the tension pneumothorax into an open pneumothorax by allowing escape for the air that is accumulating in the pleural space. (pg. 332)

15. c. Another complication is inducing a pneumothorax unnecessarily if performed when a tension pneumothorax is not actually present. (pg. 332)

16. b. Such an open wound may be the result of a variety of penetrating trauma forces such as gunshot or stab wounds. (pg. 335)

17. d. It is important to appreciate, however, that the patient with an open pneumothorax may easily develop a tension pneumothorax because of either the nature of the external wound or the treatment applied in the field. (pg. 335-336)

18. c. Notably, however, the blood accumulation in a hemothorax most often moves to the lower lung fields, producing reduced breath sounds much lower than those found in a pneumothorax. (pg. 336)

19. c. A bundle-branch block, usually caused by a right muscular contusion, produces ST-segment elevation and enzyme changes. (pg. 336)

20. a. This rapid and profound decrease in cardiac output and increase in preload give rise to the signs and symptoms of cardiac tamponade, which include hypotension out of proportion to apparent blood loss, distended neck veins, narrowing pulse pressure, muffled heart sounds, and paradoxical pressure and pulse. (pg. 339)

21. c. Without aggressive treatment, cardiac tamponade can be rapidly fatal. The only effective emergency treatment for life-threatening cardiac tamponade is pericardiocentesis, a procedure that involves the insertion of a needle into the pericardial sac and aspiration of the accumulating blood. (pg. 339)

22. d. A significant difficulty with any intrathoracic bleeding is that the presence of even major hemorrhage may not be evident on the exterior of the body. (pg. 340)

23. b. The first step in this process is red blood cell oxygenation in the lungs. (pg. 340)

24. d. All three steps are important to provide adequate oxygenation of the red blood cells. (pg. 340)

25. b. The paramedic should try to understand what is happening to the patient, but diagnosing the problem should not be done in the field. (pg. 340)

ASSIGNMENT 17-1

Matching

1. A	3. F	5. E
2. D	4. C	

Multiple Choice

1. d. Traumatic abdominal injury may result in hemorrhage, inflammation, infection, or loss of organ function. The particular complication that predominates often depends on the type of abdominal structure that has been injured. That is why it is convenient to classify abdominal groups. (pg. 342)

2. c. The stomach is a hollow organ. (pg. 343)

3. d. Both of these structures carry large volumes of blood between the heart and body tissues. As a result, injury to either of these structures may produce major bleeding and hypovolemic shock. (pg. 343)

4. a. The spleen is in close anatomical relation to the left lower thorax. For this reason, patients who have sustained trauma to the chest wall should be carefully evaluated for rib fractures. (pg. 343)

5. d. The large blood supply and soft consistency of the spleen make it particularly vulnerable to hemorrhage. Hypovolemic shock is a serious and frequent complication of splenic fracture and has associated tachycardia, not bradycardia. (pg. 343)

6. b. Because the liver is so large, it is frequently subject to injury; in fact, in cases of both blunt and penetrating abdominal trauma, it ranks as one of the most frequently injured abdominal structures. (pg. 343)

7. d. Because blood loss can be severe, hypertension is not a factor in injury to the liver. (pg. 343)

8. d. If, as is commonly the case, injury to other organs is found, then uncontrolled hemorrhage and its associated clinical signs may be present. (pg. 344)

9. b. General signs of peritonitis include tenderness, guarding, and rebound. (pg. 344)

10. c. The clinical manifestations, for the most part, are nonspecific; they are the result of the release of highly acidic and irritative contents from the stomach, which invariably occurs after perforation. (pg. 344)

11. a. Percussion of the abdomen is frequently difficult in the prehospital setting and, for the most part, may be omitted also. (pg. 345)

12. c. Because intra-abdominal hemorrhage is a major complication of abdominal trauma, its presence should be actively sought and treated. If clinical signs of hypovolemia are present, the measures of establishing intravenous access with volume replacement and applying the pneumatic anti-shock garment should be considered. (pg. 346)

13. b. This helps preserve sterility and prevents excessive loss of moisture. (pg. 346)

14. c. Volume replacement should be with normal saline or lactated Ringer's solution. (pg. 346)

15. a. Transport should be initiated as soon as feasible. (pg. 346)

Chapter 18
ASSIGNMENT 18-1

Matching

1. B
2. G
3. C
4. J

5. L
6. F
7. H
8. K

9. E
10. M
11. I
12. A

Labeling

1. A. cervical
    B. thoracic
    C. lumbar
    D. sacral
    E. coccygeal

2. A. clavicle
    B. lateral humeral condyle
    C. humerus
    D. medial humeral condyle
    E. ulna
    F. radius
    G. carpals
    H. metacarpals
    I. phalanges
    J. scapula

3. A. greater trochanter
    B. patella
    C. neck of femur
    D. lesser trochanter
    E. femur
    F. fibula
    G. tibia
    H. medial malleolus
    I. tarsals
    J. metatarsals
    K. phalanges
    L. head of femur
    M. calcaneus

Multiple Choice

1. d. Though movement is the most familiar function of muscles, they also play a significant role in the production of body heat, and they aid in the maintenance of posture. (pg. 350)

2. a. Smooth muscle is innervated by nerve fibers of the autonomic nervous system. (pg. 352 and 355)

3. c. Most voluntary muscles end in tough, whitish cords (tendons, also called leaders), by which they are attached to the bones that they move. (pg. 352)

4. b. The fascia is a tough fibrous tissue that also covers the muscle. (pg. 352)

5. d. Cardiac muscle is a special type of muscle found only in the heart. (pg. 355)

6. c. Because skeletal muscle cells are both highly active and numerous, they produce a major portion of the body heat. Skeletal muscle contractions, therefore, constitute one of the most important parts of the mechanism that maintains a balance of temperature. (pg. 355)

7. a. Because of its resiliency, articular cartilage acts as a cushion against jars or blows. (pg. 356)

8. d. Between each two vertebrae is a fluid-filled pad of tough cartilage, called the intervertebral disc, which acts as a shock absorber. These discs are extremely susceptible to injury from twisting, grinding, or improper lifting of heavy objects. (pg. 357)

9. d. The cervical and lumbar areas are the least protected of the spinal column. (pg. 357)

10. c. These ribs are not connected directly to the sternum. (pg. 359)

11. c. This is the most freely movable joint in the body and is easily dislocated. (pg. 359)

12. b. The pelvic girdle is actually composed of three separate bones that, during developmental periods, fuse together to form a single irregular bone. The strongest and lowermost bone is the ischium; the anteriormost, the pubis. (pg. 361)

13. c. The femur is also called the thigh bone. (pg. 362)

14. a. The knee joint is a strong hinge joint that, like the elbow, allows angular movement only. The tibia's broad upper surface receives condyles of the femur to form the knee joint. (pg. 362)

15. b. Bones of the skull form fibrous joints. (pg. 363-364)

16. d. Provides motion like a door on a hinge; permits flexion and extension. Examples are the fingers, elbows, and knees. (pg. 364)

17. c. Flexion decreases the angle between bones, such as bending. Extension increases the angle between bones, such as straightening. Adduction moves a bone toward the midline. (pg. 365)

18. a. Pronation turns the forearm so that the palm of the hand faces posterior or inferior. Gliding slides one surface back and forth over the other. Circumduction moves a bone so that its distal end describes a circle and the rest of the bone describes a cone. (pg. 365)

ASSIGNMENT 18-2

Matching

1. D	4. A	7. B
2. C	5. E	8. H
3. G	6. I	

Multiple Choice

1. b. A strain is characterized by pain on active movement. The muscle fibers involved may be stretched or partially torn. Most strain injuries occur in the back. (pg. 365)

2. c. A sprain is usually precipitated by the sudden twisting of a joint beyond its normal range of motion. Sprains most commonly affect the knees and ankles and are characterized by pain, tenderness, swelling, and discoloration over the joint. (pg. 365)

3. d. This care helps ease the pain and swelling often associated with sprains. It also facilitates healing of the injury by preventing any further aggravation of the involved tissues. (pg. 366)

4. b. Diseases of the bone weaken it until only slight stress can cause it to fracture. (pg. 366 and 368)

5. c. This type of fracture is most common among children, whose bones are more elastic than those of adults. (pg. 368)

6. a. The pain is usually localized to the fracture site. (pg. 370)

7. d. All life-threatening injuries should be treated prior to treating fractures. (pg. 370)

8. c. The shoulder, elbow, fingers, hips, and ankles are the joints most frequently affected. (pg. 370)

Chapter 19
ASSIGNMENT 19-1

Matching

1. J	6. C	10. L
2. D	7. G	11. M
3. H	8. N	12. I
4. B	9. E	13. A
5. K		

Labeling

1. A. right bronchus
   B. bronchiole
   C. visceral pleura
   D. parietal pleura
   E. trachea
   F. diaphragm
   G. esophagus
   H. terminal bronchiole
   I. respiratory bronchiole
   J. alveoli

Multiple Choice

1. b. Foreign particles are caught in the mucus and moved up the ciliary escalator by the rhythmic movement of the cilia. (pg. 379)

2. a. Surfactant prevents the alveoli from collapsing by lowering the fluid surface tension along the alveolar walls. (pg. 381)

3. d. The tissues most affected by hypoxia are the brain, lungs, heart, and liver. (pg. 381)

4. c. With normal lungs, the PaO_2 can be increased to values as high as 120 mm Hg. (pg. 381)

5. b. Use of the accessary muscles is a clinical sign of respiratory decompensation. (pg. 383)

6. c. A sigh hyperinflates the lungs and may serve to re-expand atelectatic areas. (pg. 383)

7. c. The intercostal muscles are innervated by the spinal nerves that exit the spinal column successively from the first to the twelfth thoracic vertebrae. Therefore, cervical cord injuries that are below the C-3, C-4, or C-5 level affect rib expansion and its function in ventilation. (pg. 384)

8. d. Overall control of respiration is influenced by several factors. Most prominent among these factors, the pH of the cerebrospinal fluid, coupled with the $PaCO_2$, provides about 80% of the control of respiration. (pg. 384)

9. a. The patient's respiratory rate and depth respond to PaO_2 levels below 60 mm Hg. Because of the low levels of PaO_2 required to maintain respiration, the patient is said to operate on a hypoxic drive. (pg. 385)

ASSIGNMENT 19-2

Matching

1. B	5. F	9. J
2. L	6. D	10. H
3. A	7. G	11. I
4. K	8. C	

Multiple Choice

1. b. Patients who describe dyspnea that begins only with exertion and whose dyspnea goes away immediately after exertion may be describing dyspnea of cardiac origin. (pg. 385)

2. d. The impedance to flow from the right heart to the left also is responsible for creating pulsus paradoxus. Unlike the loss of elastic recoil and the formation of blebs, the cardiac effects of

hyperinflation are generally reversible with proper treatment. (pg. 394-395)

3. b. Holding the lungs inflated for several seconds after injection may enhance drug distribution to the terminal airways. (pg. 397)

4. a. Singed facial and nasal hairs and facial burns are suggestive of airway burns. Visible swelling and blistering of the pharynx confirms the presence of airway burns. An explosion causes traumatic injury. (pg. 400-401)

5. c. A tentative diagnosis of hyperventilation syndrome can be made only after the possibility of more serious conditions has been eliminated. (pg. 402)

6. a. The presence of signs of infection is the final cardinal sign assessed during the chief complaint and may be useful in clarifying the cause of dyspnea. (pg. 386)

7. b. In chronic respiratory disease, the patient's subjective report is the most accurate indicator of acuity available on the scene. (pg. 386)

8. c. Corticosteroids are anti-inflammatory, anti-allergic drugs. Because of their anti-inflammatory action, toxicity is not a problem on an acute basis. (pg. 387)

9. d. A history of cardiac, seizure, or diabetic problems is especially important, because medications the paramedic may give are potentially cardiotoxic, lower the seizure threshold, and occasion the release of sugar into the blood, causing hyperglycemia. (pg. 387)

10. c. In the presence of respiratory distress, confusion, agitation, or combativeness frequently indicates hypoxemia or hypercapnia. (pg. 389)

11. a. Retractions and the use of accessory muscles are caused by breathing against an obstruction. (pg. 389)

12. d. Nasal flaring and tracheal tugging, along with retractions (intercostal, sternal, or clavicular), are all indicators of airway obstruction. (pg. 389)

13. b. Especially significant in the patient with respiratory distress is tachycardia, which often indicates hypoxia. (pg. 389)

14. c. Breath sounds heard posteriorly tend to be clearer and louder; one can hear the lower lobes only when listening from the back or sides. Sounds heard from the sides do not, however, tend to be clearer and louder. (pg. 390)

15. b. Because the airways naturally narrow somewhat during expiration, wheezes frequently start during expiration. (pg. 391)

16. a. As the patient's condition deteriorates, wheezes may also become evident during inspiration. (pg. 391)

17. d. Stridor is caused by the narrowing of the upper airway rather than by that of the bronchi and bronchioles. (pg. 391)

18. b. The easiest way to distinguish between rales and rhonchi is to determine whether the sound is continuous or is made up of a series of short, discrete sounds. Rhonchi are continuous sounds and rales are discontinuous. (pg. 391)

19. d. The term "obstructive lung disease" refers to several diseases that have obstruction of the lower airway in common. Included in this group are asthma, emphysema, and chronic bronchitis. (pg. 393)

20. a. Air trapping is a feature shared by all obstructive lung diseases. (pg. 394)

21. c. Theophylline's effect is that of bronchodilation, diuresis, tachycardia, palpitations, hypertension, and muscle tremors. (pg. 398)

22. d. Collapse of the alveoli, known as atelectasis, is a common result of pneumonia. Another condition found with pneumonia is pleuritis, which is an inflammation of the pleura. Pneumonia is the most common cause of sepsis. (pg. 399)

23. a. Entrapment in a closed space indicates a heavy exposure to both heat and smoke. Coughing sooty sputum is suggestive of smoke inhalation. Oxygen at 100% is required and decreases the half-life of carbon monoxide from 5 hours to 30 minutes. IV access must be established, and because of the presence of bronchospasm (wheezing), bronchodilators are also appropriate. (pg. 401)

Chapter 20
ASSIGNMENT 20-1

Matching

1. H	8. A	15. D
2. L	9. F	16. F
3. I	10. C	17. H
4. G	11. E	18. C
5. J	12. B	19. K
6. D	13. E	20. I
7. K	14. G	21. A

Labeling

1.
   A. brachiocephalic artery
   B. superior vena cava
   C. right pulmonary artery
   D. right pulmonary veins
   E. right atrium
   F. right ventricle
   G. inferior vena cava
   H. left common carotid artery
   I. left subclavian artery
   J. left pulmonary artery
   K. left pulmonary veins
   L. left atrium
   M. left ventricle
   N. descending thoracic aorta

2.
   A. sinus node
   B. AV node
   C. bundle of His
   D. right bundle branch
   E. left bundle branch
   F. purkinje fibers

Multiple Choice

1. a. Arteries carry blood to the body, whereas veins carry blood to the heart. Blood passes through the heart chambers and valves as a result of pressure changes and valvular openings and closings. (pg. 407)

2. c. The intima is composed of epithelial tissue and is the innermost arterial wall. The media is composed of muscle tissue and is the middle lining. The adventitia, also known as the externa, is composed of connective tissue and is the outermost arterial wall. (pg. 407)

3. b. The mediastinum is the "middle space" between the lungs and above the diaphragm, in which the heart sits. Endometrium is the innermost lining of the uterus. Periosteum is the membrane covering bone. Platypodia is the medical term meaning flat-footed. (pg. 410)

4. c. The pericardium is a double-walled sac covering the heart. The endocardium is the innermost wall of the heart. The myocardium is the muscular middle wall of the heart. The

subendocardium is the myocardial area beneath the endocardium. (pg. 411)

5. b. The pulmonic valve is the exit valve for the right ventricle to the pulmonary artery. The aortic valve is the exit valve for the left ventricle to the aorta. The tricuspid and bicuspid (mitral) valves are atrioventricular valves. (pg. 412)

6. c. Diastole is the relaxation phase of the cardiac cycle. Milieu is a term meaning environment. Tocus is a medical term meaning childbirth or parturition. (pg. 413)

7. a. The ventricles fill with blood during diastole. This phase lasts much longer than systole (0.52 second vs. 0.28 second at a heart rate of 75 beats per minute). An increase in heart rate more significantly reduces the length of diastole than of systole. The duration of the diastolic phase is important; this is when about 70% of coronary artery flow occurs and complete filling of the ventricles takes place. (pg. 413)

8. a. This volume is about 60 to 100 mL, although a healthy adult heart has a great capacity to increase this amount. (pg. 413)

9. d. Sympathetic stimulation occurs with the release of norepinephrine, which binds with beta receptor sites in the heart, causing increased heart rate, enhanced conduction, and contractility. (pg. 414)

10. a. *B* describes the electrical property of excitability. *C* describes the electrical property of conductivity. *D* describes the mechanical property of contractility. (pg. 415)

11. d. The AV node is a secondary or "backup" pacemaker for the heart, whereas the Purkinje system serves as the pacemaker of "last resort." (pg. 415)

12. b. The inherent rate of the SA node is 60-100, and the ventricular inherent rate is 20-40. (pg. 416)

ASSIGNMENT 20-2

Matching

1. C	5. H	9. D
2. A	6. L	10. K
3. E	7. B	11. I
4. J	8. G	

Multiple Choice

1. a. Chest or epigastric pain is the most common presenting complaint. (pg. 417)

2. c. The intima is composed of epithelial tissue and is the layer that is abnormally thickened and hardened, resulting in a loss of elasticity. (pg. 418)

3. d. Because the heart has such a high demand for oxygen, it must have a continuous reliable supply of oxygenated blood. Any event that reduces the supply, and any event that increases the demand without an increase in supply, places the heart in jeopardy of ischemia. (pg. 419)

4. c. Cardiomegaly is general enlargement of the heart. Myocardial infarction is the death of heart muscle tissue. Ventricular hypertrophy is the enlargement of the ventricular wall. (pg. 419)

5. d. Catecholamines such as epinephrine and norepinephrine may contribute to angina by increasing the heart's work load, but they are responsive factors rather than initiating factors. Decreased hemoglobin in the blood (anemia) can place a patient at higher risk for angina but is not the direct cause. Poor oxygen saturation of the blood can contribute to the "supply" side problem, but is not the entire cause of angina. Angina is due to a discrepancy between the oxygen needed by the heart given a particular myocardial workload (demand) and the blood supplied to the heart through the coronary arteries (supply). (pg. 419)

6. d. Angina is distinguished from acute myocardial infarction in that there is no death of heart muscle tissue in angina. (pg. 419)

7. b. Chest pain usually dissipates within 3-5 minutes after the patient comes to rest or takes nitroglycerine. (pg. 420)

8. a. The term myocardial infarction means heart muscle death. There is always some cellular death in some portion of heart muscle tissue in myocardial infarction. (pg. 420)

9. a. Pump failure (heart failure) is the second most common cause of death, and cardiogenic shock, the most severe form of pump failure, carries a 80-90% mortality rate. Cardiac tamponade is seen with ventricular rupture, dissecting aortic aneurysm, and penetrating trauma to the chest. Cardiac tamponade is commonly lethal and presents as a form of pump failure with eventual cardiac arrest. (pg. 420)

10. a. Although complaints of shortness of breath (dyspnea) and odd heart sensations (palpitations) are seen in a heart attack, they are not so common as chest pain, which is said to affect about 90% of patients. Radiation of chest pain to the left shoulder is said to occur in about 25% of patients. (pg. 420)

11. c. Other arrhythmias, although not immediately life-threatening, may be warning arrhythmias or forerunners of more serious disturbances and require early prehospital intervention. (pg. 421)

12. c. Each of the procedures may be deemed appropriate in local medical protocols. (pg. 421)

13. b. The ineffective forward pumping action of the left ventricle causes a pressure of blood to be backed up into the pulmonary circulation, ultimately resulting in a condition called pulmonary edema. (pg. 422)

14. d. Enlarged and tender liver (hepatomegaly) and jugular vein distention are seen in right heart failure. Hemoptysis literally translates as "spitting up blood" but in this case refers to the pink, frothy sputum that results from red blood cells mixing with plasma in the alveoli. Orthopnea means that the patient must sit up to breathe. Paroxysmal nocturnal dyspnea (PND) is a cardinal sign of left pump failure. PND occurs about 2-3 hours after the patient retires to sleep. The supine position in sleep results in increased venous return from the extremities, which in turn causes pump overload and signs of left failure. Rales, rhonchi, and wheezes are all seen in left pump failure. (pg. 422)

15. b. D₅W is preferred over normal saline in pump failure because the salt in saline could add to the patient's fluid load. The patient should be positioned sitting with legs dangling. The supine position increases blood return to the already overloaded heart. (pg. 423)

16. d. *A*, *b*, and *c* can all directly cause right pump failure, in the absence of left pump failure. An obstruction of the left anterior descending coronary artery will result in a left ventricular infarction, which may directly cause left pump failure but will only indirectly cause right pump failure. (pg. 423)

17. c. Although cardiogenic shock is the most severe form of pump failure, the patient should be positioned supine to insure adequate cerebral perfusion. (pg. 424)

18. a. Sudden death accounts for 60% of all deaths from atherosclerotic heart disease and, in a significant number of patients, is the first manifestation of cardiac disease. (pg. 424)

19. c. Ventricular fibrillation may be a primary arrhythmia caused by myocardial ischemia, or it may be a secondary arrhythmia caused by other conditions, such as hypothermia, drug toxicity, or drowning. (pg. 424)

20. b. Chronic obstructive pulmonary disease is not associated with electromechanical dissociation. Electromechanical dissociation describes the circumstance in which the heart appears to be functioning electrophysiologically (hence a potentially life-sustainable rhythm is seen on the monitor) but is not functioning mechanically (the heart is either not contracting or is contracting insufficiently, and hence there is no pulse). In cardiac tamponade, as the

pericardium distends with blood, the chambers are compressed so that blood flow through the heart is impeded. In hypovolemia, the blood volume may be so inadequate that although the heart is pumping, the stroke volume is so low that no pulse is created. In tension pneumothorax, the heart may be laterally displaced so that the aorta is coarctated (pinched) with resulting impediment to stroke volume and cardiac output. (pg. 426)

21. b. Hypertension and wide pulse pressures are not seen in cardiac tamponade. (pg. 427)

22. a. Pulsus paradoxus is thought to occur as a result of inspiration trapping more blood in the lungs so as to decrease blood return to the left heart, thus decreasing stroke volume. Pulsus paradoxus may be seen in normal individuals but is most pronounced in cardiac tamponade. (pg. 427)

ASSIGNMENT 20-3

Matching

1. B	4. F	7. H
2. G	5. A	8. J
3. I	6. E	9. D

Multiple Choice

1. c. Oxygen is the most potent antiarrhythmic agent known to medical science. Answers *a*, *b*, and *d* are potential second-line agents. Furosemide can be used if the patient displays signs of pump failure. Morphine is useful in terms of analgesia and reduction of preload. Procainamide is useful for ventricular ectopy but is second-line to lidocaine for premature ventricular complexes. (pg. 430)

2. c. This scenario is more consistent with a probable presumptive diagnosis of angina. Morphine and nitrous oxide are potential second-line agents for treatment of myocardial infarction. Nifedipine has potential uses in hypertensive crisis. (pg. 431)

3. c. Morphine is both an analgesic and a peripheral vasodilator, which abates pain and reduces pulmonary edema. Atropine is useful in the treatment of symptomatic bradycardia and would not be indicated for a patient with a heart rate of 132. Lidocaine should not be used on non-monitored patients and should be used only for certain presentations of premature ventricular complexes. Theophylline ethylenediamine is a bronchodilator, but it has cardiac side effects and should be used cautiously in a patient presenting with cardiac symptoms. (pg. 431)

4. b. Dopamine is the agent of choice because it increases blood pressure without damaging the kidneys or intestines. (pg. 432)

5. c. Epinephrine is the first drug given in ventricular asystole. (pg. 433)

6. d. Sodium bicarbonate may be useful in some cases, but it carries a number of potentially deleterious side effects. As a consequence it is reserved as a late-line drug. (pg. 433)

ASSIGNMENT 20-4

Matching

1. F	4. B	7. C
2. D	5. I	8. E
3. G	6. H	

Multiple Choice

1. a. The rate is 94 and regular. P waves are present and normal, and PR and QRS are within normal limits. Therefore, this is normal sinus rhythm. (pg. 440)
2. d. Normal sinus rhythm does not produce any signs or symptoms by itself. (pg. 440)
3. c. Though other management interventions may be necessary for this patient, no specific arrhythmia management is indicated. (pg. 440)

ASSIGNMENT 20-5

Matching

1. C
2. A
3. G
4. B

5. E
6. H
7. L
8. K

9. J
10. I
11. F

Multiple Choice

1. d. The rate is 65 and irregular. P waves are present, with the seventh P wave premature and different in shape from the sinus P waves. PR and QRS durations are within normal limits: sinus rhythm with one premature atrial complex. (pg. 449)
2. c. The type of chest pain the patient complains of, combined with the associated complaints, is suggestive of hyperventilation syndrome. Jaw pain, congestion, and syncope are not usually seen in hyperventilation. Hyperventilation patients complain of "sticky-stabby" kinds of chest pain, but they rarely describe their pain as crushing. Palpitations due to the premature atrial complexes are the only logical additional complaints this patient is likely to offer. (pg. 449)
3. c. Although other management interventions may be necessary for this patient, no specific arrhythmia management is indicated. (pg. 449)
4. D. The rate is 125 and regular. P waves are present, and PR and QRS are within normal limits: sinus tachycardia. (pg. 444)
5. c. Sinus tachycardia is usually a "secondary" arrhythmia; that is, it is most commonly caused by some other factor or influence. In this case, the tachycardia is probably caused by the patient's fever. It is estimated that heart rate increases about 4 beats per minute for each degree of elevated body temperature. This sinus tachycardia is best treated by reducing the patient's fever, thus removing the cause. (pg. 444)
6. d. The rate is 140 and irregular. P waves are absent, with fibrillatory "f" waves present. The PR cannot be calculated. QRS is normal in duration: uncontrolled atrial fibrillation. (pg. 457)
7. c. Fast heart rates are associated with a decline in cardiac output due to inadequate ventricular filling time, especially in the diseased heart. (pg. 457)
8. d. Atropine is clearly not indicated for this patient because it would increase rate. There is no indication for the use of lidocaine in the absence of ventricular ectopy. Verapamil can be useful for reducing heart rate in atrial flutter and fibrillation, but it should be withheld if the patient is hypotensive. In addition, the patient should be questioned concerning any known history of Wolff-Parkinson-White (WPW) syndrome, because verapamil may actually speed the rate of atrial fibrillation in patients with WPW syndrome. (pg. 457)
9. a. The rate is 214 and regular. P waves are not discernible, and the QRS is within normal limits: paroxysmal supraventricular tachycardia (PSVT). (pg. 452)
10. c. This patient is considered to be a "stable" PSVT patient because there is no chest pain, dyspnea, hypotension, or signs of ischemia or pump failure. First-line therapy according to

the stable ACLS algorithm is vagal stimulation. (pg. 452)

11. d. After vagal maneuvers have failed to convert the PSVT, verapamil may be tried. Another drug that is being used by some EMS systems prior to verapamil is adenosine. Adenosine is not yet a part of the ACLS PSVT algorithm. (pg. 452)

12. b. The rate is 60 and regular. P waves are absent, with flutter "F" waves present. The QRS is within normal limits: atrial flutter. (pg. 455)

13. a. Atrial flutter arises from a single irritable ectopic focus in the atrial conduction system. The "F" waves achieve their characteristic "sawtoothed" appearance through "circus" or circular movement in the atria, with the wave form upsweeping as it moves toward the monitoring positive electrode and downsweeping as the impulse circles back upward in atrium. (pg. 455)

ASSIGNMENT 20-6

Matching

1. C	5. E	9. D
2. H	6. K	10. I
3. B	7. F	11. G
4. L	8. J	

Multiple Choice

1. d. The rate is 150 and regular. P waves and PR intervals are absent, and the QRSs are wide and bizarre. Therefore, this is ventricular tachycardia. Torsade is a form of ventricular tachycardia that appears to be coiled about the baseline. (pg. 476)

2. b. The patient is considered "stable" because the patient is conscious with a pulse and has no signs of chest pain, dyspnea, pulmonary edema, or hypotension. Lidocaine is the first-line therapy for stable ventricular tachycardia. A precordial thump may be used prior to cardioversion and is a later-line intervention given this scenario and the ACLS protocol. (pg. 476)

3. b. Repeat lidocaine at half dose. (pg. 476)

4. d. The rate is 31 and regular. P waves are absent, and the QRS is wide and bizarre: ventricular escape rhythm. (pg. 468)

5. b. The patient should be treated according to the electromechanical dissociation algorithm, because evidence of electrical activity is not matched by a perfusing pulse. (pg. 468)

6. d. IV epinephrine is the next appropriate therapy in the electromechanical dissociation algorithm. (pg. 468)

7. d. The rate is 107 and irregular. P waves are present before sinus complexes but are absent prior to the two paired ectopics. PR is normal prior to sinus complexes. Sinus QRS durations are normal, and ectopic QRS is 0.12: sinus tachycardia with couplet PVCs. (pg. 471)

8. c. Lidocaine is indicated for couplet or paired PVCs. In addition, the PVCs are uncomfortably close to the preceding T wave, which is a second indication for lidocaine. (pg. 471)

9. d. The rate is 0 and the non-perfusing waveforms are chaotically irregular. P, PR, and QRS are absent: ventricular fibrillation. (pg. 480)

10. c. Epinephrine stimulates electrical activity through its beta properties and makes ventricular fibrillation more convertible. (pg. 480)

11. a. The rate is 60 and regular. P waves are absent. The QRS is within normal limits: junctional escape rhythm. (pg. 462)

12. d. Because the rate is 60, vital signs are within normal limits and there is no ventricular ectopy; no immediate pharmacologic intervention is indicated. Obviously, because junctional escape rhythm is an abnormal rhythm, this patient should be transported to a medical facility for further evaluation. (pg. 462)

13. b. The rate is 0 with no regular QRS complexes. P waves are present at a rate of 30: ventricular asystole. (pg. 481)

14. a. The initial treatment for asystole is CPR, with epinephrine being the first-line drug. It might be noted that asystole carries a poor prognosis, especially in light of the scenario described. (pg. 481)

ASSIGNMENT 20-7

Matching

1. A
2. E
3. B
4. F
5. D

Multiple Choice

1. b. The rate is 68 and regular. P waves are absent, and pacing spikes appear prior to wide QRSs. Therefore, this is an artificial pacemaker rhythm. (pg. 495)

2. d. The artificial pacemaker is functioning properly with capture. A functioning artificial pacemaker should not produce any cardiac signs or symptoms. (pg. 495)

3. c. Although other management interventions may be necessary for this patient, no specific arrhythmia management is indicated. (pg. 495)

4. c. The rate is 36 and regular. P waves are present at a rate of 58; PR varies. QRS is wide at 0.12 second: third degree AV block. (pg. 488)

5. c. *A, b* and *d* are all present with some form of chest pain. Silent myocardial infarction describes the condition in which heart attack presents without chest pain. This condition is principally seen in the elderly and in diabetics and is thought to result from decline of or damage to the sensory nervous system. (pg. 488)

6. c. Uncorrected third degree AV block may progress to asystole. (pg. 488)

7. c. The rate is 33 and regular. P waves are present at a 2:1 ratio with the QRSs. PR is considered constant at 0.22-0.24 (note that total PR variation of less than 0.04 is considered "constant"). QRS duration is within normal limits: type II second degree AV block. (pg. 487)

8. a. The treatment of choice for symptomatic bradycardia is atropine. (pg. 487)

9. c. The rate is 94 and regular. P waves are present. The PR is prolonged at 0.26-0.28 second. The QRS is within normal limits: sinus rhythm with first degree AV block. (pg. 483)

10. d. Although other management interventions may be necessary for this patient, no specific arrhythmia management is indicated. (pg. 483)

ASSIGNMENT 20-8

Matching

1. E
2. K
3. D
4. J
5. C
6. H
7. B
8. I
9. A
10. F

ASSIGNMENT 20-9

Strip 1
Rate: 107/min
Rhythm: Regular
P wave: Sinus P waves present
PR interval: 0.16 sec
QRS complex: 0.12 sec
Rhythm interpretation: Sinus tachycardia with bundle branch block

Strip 2
Rate: Atrial, 400/min or greater; ventricular, 90/min
Rhythm: Irregular
P wave: Fibrillation waves present
PR interval: Not discernible
QRS complex: 0.06-0.08 sec
Rhythm interpretation: Atrial fibrillation

Strip 3
Rate: 80/min
Rhythm: Irregular
P wave: Sinus P waves present
PR interval: 0.12 sec
QRS complex: 0.08-0.10 sec
Rhythm interpretation: Normal sinus rhythm with premature junctional complexes

Strip 4
Rate: 188/min
Rhythm: Regular
P wave: Not discernible
PR interval: Not discernible
QRS complex: 0.08 sec
Rhythm interpretation: Atrial tachycardia

Strip 5
Automatic interval rate: 72/min
Analysis: The first two complexes are paced complexes, followed by a patient complex, three paced complexes, a patient complex, and two paced complexes
Rhythm interpretation: Normal pacemaker function

Strip 6
Rate: 45/min, dropping to 25/min
Rhythm: Irregular
P wave: Sinus P waves present
PR interval: 0.26-0.28 sec
QRS complex: 0.06 sec
Rhythm interpretation: Sinus rhythm with sinus arrest, a junctional escape beat, and first degree AV block

Strip 7
Rate: 188/min
Rhythm: Regular

296

P wave: Not discernible
PR interval: Not discernible
QRS complex: 0.16 sec
Rhythm interpretation: Ventricular tachycardia

Strip 8
Rate: Atrial, 62/min; ventricular, 35/min
Rhythm: Regular
P wave: Sinus P waves not relating to the QRS complexes
PR interval: Varying greatly
QRS complex: 0.12 sec
Rhythm interpretation: Normal sinus rhythm; complete AV block with pacemaker origin from the ventricles

Strip 9
Rate: 83/min
Rhythm: Irregular
P wave: Sinus P waves present
PR interval: 0.20 sec
QRS complex: 0.06 sec (sinus complexes); 0.12 sec (premature complexes)
Rhythm interpretation: Normal sinus rhythm with multifocal, multiform premature ventricular complexes

Strip 10
Rate: Atrial, 300/min; ventricular, 150/min
Rhythm: Regular
P wave: Two flutter waves to each QRS complex
PR interval: Not discernible
QRS complex: 0.04-0.06 sec; 0.12 sec (premature beat)
Rhythm interpretation: Atrial flutter with 2:1 AV conduction and one premature ventricular complex

Strip 11
Rate: 60/min
Rhythm: Regular
P wave: Sinus P waves present
PR interval: 0.24 sec
QRS complex: 0.08 sec
Rhythm interpretation: Normal sinus rhythm with first degree AV block

Strip 12
Rate: 100/min
Rhythm: Regular
P wave: Sinus P waves present
PR interval: 0.12 sec
QRS complex: 0.06-0.08 sec
Rhythm interpretation: Normal sinus rhythm

Strip 13
Rate: 72/min
Rhythm: Regular
P wave: Absent

PR interval: Unmeasurable
QRS complex: 0.08-0.10 sec
Rhythm interpretation: Accelerated junctional rhythm

Strip 14
Rate: 115/min
Rhythm: Regular
P wave: Sinus P waves present
PR interval: 0.16 sec
QRS complex: 0.04-0.06 sec
Rhythm interpretation: Sinus tachycardia

Strip 15
Rate: 40/min
Rhythm: Irregular
P wave: Sinus P waves present
PR interval: 0.18-0.20 sec
QRS complex: 0.08-0.10 sec
Rhythm interpretation: Sinus bradycardia and sinus arrhythmia

Strip 16
Rate: 79/min
Rhythm: Irregular
P wave: Sinus P waves present; two inverted P waves with premature complexes present
PR interval: 0.12 sec (sinus complexes); 0.08 sec (premature complexes)
QRS complex: 0.04-0.06 sec
Rhythm interpretation: Normal sinus rhythm with two premature junctional complexes

Strip 17
Rate: 0/min
Rhythm: Irregular and chaotic
P wave: Not discernible
PR interval: Unmeasurable
QRS complex: Absent
Rhythm interpretation: Ventricular fibrillation

Strip 18
Rate: 38/min
Rhythm: Regular
P wave: Sinus P waves present
PR interval: 0.16 sec
QRS complex: 0.08-0.10 sec
Rhythm interpretation: Sinus bradycardia

Strip 19
Rate: 188/min
Rhythm: Regular
P wave: Not discernible
PR interval: Unmeasurable
QRS complex: 0.16 sec
Rhythm interpretation: Ventricular tachycardia

Strip 20

Rate: Atrial, 75/min; ventricular, 60/min
Rhythm: Irregular
P wave: Sinus P waves present
PR interval: 0.24 sec, progressing to 0.32 sec
QRS complex: 0.12 sec
Rhythm interpretation: Normal sinus rhythm with second degree AV block, type I, and bundle branch block

Strip 21

Automatic interval rate: 94/min
Analysis: The first complex is a patient complex, followed by a sensing malfunction, a paced complex, loss of capture, a patient complex, loss of capture, a patient complex, a sensing malfunction, a paced complex, loss of capture, a patient complex, loss of capture, a patient complex, and a sensing malfunction
Rhythm interpretation: Loss of capture and sensing malfunction in the presence of sinus bradycardia with first degree AV block and bundle branch block

Strip 22

Rate: Atrial, over 200/min; ventricular, 115/min
Rhythm: Irregular
P wave: Pointed atrial P waves present
PR interval: Varies
QRS complex: 0.12 sec; 0.16 sec (premature complex)
Rhythm interpretation: Atrial tachycardia with variable AV block, bundle branch block, and a premature ventricular complex

Strip 23

Rate: 107/min
Rhythm: Regular
P wave: Inverted
PR interval: 0.08-0.10 sec
QRS complex: 0.04-0.06 sec
Rhythm interpretation: Junctional tachycardia

Strip 24

Rate: Atrial, 400/min or greater; ventricular, 100/min
Rhythm: Irregular
P wave: Fibrillation waves present
PR interval: Unmeasurable
QRS complex: 0.06 sec; 0.16 sec (premature complexes)
Rhythm interpretation: Atrial fibrillation with three premature ventricular complexes

Strip 25

Rate: 75/min
Rhythm: Regular
P wave: Sinus P waves present
PR interval: 0.12 sec
QRS complex: 0.08 sec
Rhythm interpretation: Normal sinus rhythm; pacemaker spikes are noted in complexes 4 and 5

Strip 26
Rate: 83/min
Rhythm: Irregular
P wave: Sinus P waves present; one premature, abnormal P wave present
PR interval: 0.16 sec
QRS complex: 0.12 sec
Rhythm interpretation: Normal sinus rhythm with bundle branch block and one premature atrial complex

Strip 27
Rate: 58/min
Rhythm: Irregular
P wave: Varying in size and shape
PR interval: 0.16-0.18 sec
QRS complex: 0.08-0.10 sec
Rhythm interpretation: Wandering atrial pacemaker

Strip 28
Rate: Atrial, 40/min; ventricular, 10/min
Rhythm: Irregular
P wave: Sinus P waves present
PR interval: Unmeasurable
QRS complex: 0.12-0.14 sec
Rhythm interpretation: Ventricular standstill

Strip 29
Rate: 48/min
Rhythm: Irregular
P wave: Sinus P waves present
PR interval: 0.20 sec
QRS complex: 0.04-0.06; 0.18-0.20 sec (premature complexes)
Rhythm interpretation: Sinus bradycardia with premature ventricular complexes in a bigeminal pattern

Strip 30
Rate: 100/min
Rhythm: Irregular
P wave: Sinus P waves present; one P wave missing
PR interval: 0.18-0.20 sec
QRS complex: 0.08 sec
Rhythm interpretation: Sinus tachycardia with sinoatrial block

Strip 31
Rate: 270/min
Rhythm: Regular
P wave: Not discernible
PR interval: Unmeasurable
QRS complex: 0.06-0.08 sec
Rhythm interpretation: Atrial tachycardia

Strip 32

Rate: Atrial, 94/min; ventricular, 60/min

Rhythm: Irregular

P wave: Sinus P waves present

PR interval: 0.24 sec, progressing to 0.28 sec

QRS complex: 0.06-0.08 sec

Rhythm interpretation: Normal sinus rhythm with second degree AV block, type I

Strip 33

Rate: Atrial, 88/min; ventricular, 80/min

Rhythm: Irregular

P wave: Sinus P waves present

PR interval: 0.20 sec, progressing to 0.30 sec

QRS complex: 0.12 sec

Rhythm interpretation: Normal sinus rhythm with second degree AV block, type I, and bundle branch block

Strip 34

Rate: Atrial, 76/min; ventricular, 38/min

Rhythm: Regular

P wave: Two sinus P waves to each QRS complex

PR interval: 0.24 sec with constant relationship to the QRS complexes

QRS complex: 0.12 sec

Rhythm interpretation: Sinus rhythm with 2:1 second degree AV block, type II; clinical correlation is suggested to diagnose type II when 2:1 conduction is present

Strip 35

Rate: 20/min

Rhythm: Irregular

P wave: Absent

PR interval: Unmeasurable

QRS complex: 0.12-0.14 sec

Rhythm interpretation: Ventricular standstill

Strip 36

Rate: 72/min

Rhythm: Regular

P wave: Inverted

PR interval: 0.08-0.10 sec

QRS complex: 0.06-0.08 sec

Rhythm interpretation: Accelerated junctional rhythm

Strip 37

Rate: 50/min

Rhythm: Regular

P wave: Absent

PR interval: Unmeasurable

QRS complex: 0.08 sec

Rhythm interpretation: Junctional rhythm

Strip 38

Rate: 75/min
Rhythm: Regular
P wave: Varying in size and shape
PR interval: 0.10-0.12 sec
QRS complex: 0.10 sec
Rhythm interpretation: Wandering atrial pacemaker

Strip 39

Rate: 68/min
Rhythm: Regular
P wave: Sinus P waves present
PR interval: 0.36-0.38 sec
QRS complex: 0.06 sec
Rhythm interpretation: Normal sinus rhythm with first degree AV block

Strip 40

Rate: Atrial, 300/min; ventricular, 150/min
Rhythm: Irregular
P wave: Two flutter waves before each QRS complex
PR interval: Varies
QRS complex: 0.04-0.06 sec; 0.12 sec (premature complex)
Rhythm interpretation: Atrial flutter with 2:1 AV block and one premature ventricular complex

Strip 41

Rate: 115/min
Rhythm: Irregular
P wave: Inverted
PR interval: 0.08-0.10 sec
QRS complex: 0.04 sec; 0.12 sec (premature complex)
Rhythm interpretation: Junctional tachycardia with one premature ventricular complex

Chapter 21
ASSIGNMENT 21-1

Matching

1.	I	8.	F	15.	E
2.	B	9.	M	16.	G
3.	J	10.	K	17.	F
4.	A	11.	C	18.	D
5.	N	12.	D	19.	C
6.	O	13.	H	20.	A
7.	L	14.	G		

Multiple Choice

1. c. Hormones belong to different chemical classes, including amines, polypeptides, glycoproteins, and steroids. (pg. 522)

2. d. Tropic hormones have minimal direct biologic effects themselves and are primarily regulatory hormones that stimulate or inhibit release of hormones from the various endocrine glands. (pg. 523)

3. b. Effector hormones are released by the target endocrine glands and are responsible for producing biologic effects in the organism. (pg. 523)

4. a. Endocrine glands are distinguished from other glands by the fact that they do not possess ducts but, instead, secrete their products directly into the systemic circulation. (pg. 523)

5. b. The pituitary gland is located at the base of the brain in a small depression in the sphenoid bone known as the sella turcica. (pg. 524)

6. a. Because of the pituitary's role as a link between the central nervous system and the body's endocrine system and its regulatory control over the major endocrine glands, it is often referred to as the body's "master endocrine" gland. (pg. 524)

7. c. The posterior pituitary secretes two polypeptide hormones, antidiuretic hormone and oxytocin. Both hormones are actually synthesized in the hypothalamus and transported down along nerve axons to the posterior pituitary, where they are stored until needed. (pg. 525)

8. b. The extensive blood supply to the thyroid gland and its close proximity to the cricoid cartilage make a complete understanding of its anatomy critical to cases in which emergency airway management calls for a cricothyroidotomy, so that the serious complications of hemorrhage and damage to the gland can be avoided. (pg. 526)

9. b. In hypoparathyroidism, biochemical abnormalities result in convulsions, and the QT interval on the EKG is prolonged, without associated U waves. (pg. 527)

10. c. The adrenal glands are located retroperitoneally and lie in close association with the upper part of each kidney. (pg. 527)

11. c. The adrenal medulla secretes as its primary hormones the catecholamines epinephrine and norepinephrine. (pg. 528)

12. d. Release of adrenal catecholamines results in the typical "fight or flight" response, with increased heart rate, cardiac output, and systemic blood pressure. (pg. 528)

13. a. Adrenocortical insufficiency manifests itself with multiple system effects. The patient may be extremely ill and be in a state of hypovolemic shock when first encountered. (pg. 528)

14. d. The pancreas is located retroperitoneally in the upper portion of the abdomen behind the stomach and in close proximity to the duodenum and spleen. (pg. 528)

15. b. The overall effects of glucagon tend to be opposite those of insulin; its most important action is to increase blood glucose levels. (pg. 528)

16. c. The most important stimulator of insulin release is the concentration of blood glucose. When blood glucose levels are high, such as after a meal, the pancreas increases its release of insulin. (pg. 528)

17. b. Insulin promotes the uptake of blood glucose into body tissues, of amino acids into muscle tissue, and of triglycerides into fat tissue. The clinical results are lowered blood glucose, increased muscle protein synthesis, and increased fat deposition. (pg. 529)

18. b. Type I is distinguished by its onset during childhood or early adulthood, by minimal to no pancreatic production of insulin, and by a tendency toward development of ketosis. (pg. 529)

19. c. In secondary diabetes, the underlying cause for the persistent elevation in blood sugar is a preexisting condition. (pg. 529)

ASSIGNMENT 21-2

Matching

1. B
2. A
3. C

Multiple Choice

1. a. The major clinical findings of diabetic ketoacidosis can be traced to hyperglycemia and hyperketonemia. Hyperglycemia leads to polyuria and dehydration, which may present as hypotension. Hyperketonemia may cause Kussmaul's breathing. Weight loss is due to the body's breakdown of fat and muscle. This causes hyperketonemia and is not a result of it. (pg. 530)

2. b. The presence of infection is a major physiologic stress that acts to increase the body's insulin requirements and cause severe diabetic ketoacidosis. (pg. 531)

3. d. Diabetic ketoacidosis often presents with tachycardia; deep, rapid, labored respirations; and warm, flushed, and dry skin; abdominal pain may be present and the abdomen tender to palpation. (pg. 531)

4. b. In the field, it is frequently difficult to distinguish among hypoglycemia, diabetic ketoacidosis, and hyperosmolar hyperglycemic nonketotic coma. Hypoglycemia can produce a serious and potentially life-threatening condition. (pg. 532)

5. c. Hyperosmolar hyperglycemic nonketotic coma occurs more frequently in older people who have some precipitating cause, such as cerebrovascular accident, infection, or trauma. (pg. 532)

6. d. The pulse is rapid, and respirations are normal or shallow. The skin is often cool, pale, and diaphoretic. (pg. 533)

Chapter 22
ASSIGNMENT 22-1

Matching

1. H
2. M
3. B
4. G
5. N
6. D
7. R

8. O
9. P
10. A
11. Q
12. S
13. C

14. T
15. J
16. L
17. K
18. F
19. E

Labeling

1. A. epidural space
   B. subarachnoid space
   C. dura mater
   D. subdural space
   E. arachnoid mater
   F. pia mater

2. A. cerebrum
   B. diencephalon
   C. midbrain
   D. pons
   E. medulla oblongata
   F. cerebellum

Multiple Choice

1. a. The central nervous system is composed of the brain and spinal cord. (pg. 536)

2. d. The basic unit of the nervous system is the individual nerve cell, which is called the neuron. (pg. 536)

3. d. Damage to the nerves in the brain and spinal cord usually is permanent, because they do not possess this outer covering (myelin sheath and neurilemma) and, therefore, are unable to regenerate. (pg. 538)

4. a. The space between the dura mater and the periosteum of the skull is referred to as the epidural space. The prefix epi- means "on top of" and "dura" refers to the dura mater. Thus, "epidural space" means a space that is located on top of the dura. (pg. 538)

5. b. The area between the dura mater and the arachnoid membrane is known as the subdural space. The prefix sub- means "under, beneath, or below" and dura refers to the dura mater. Thus the term "subdural space" refers to a space beneath or under the dura mater. (pg. 538)

6. d. The subarachnoid space is that area below the arachnoid membrane but above the pia mater. The prefix sub- means "under, beneath, or below" and "arachnoid" refers to the arachnoid membrane. Thus the term "subarachnoid space" refers to a space beneath the arachnoid membrane. (pg. 539)

7. d. The two vertebral arteries and the internal carotid arteries provide the majority of the blood supply to the brain. (pg. 539)

8. b. The circle of Willis allows one of the other vessels to supply the blocked area of the brain if one of the main vessels becomes occluded. (pg. 540)

9. a. The cerebrum controls sensory and motor functions and also houses the centers for memory, speech, emotions, and thought processes. (pg. 540)

10. d. The hypothalamus serves as a bridge between two separate communication systems, the nervous system and the endocrine system. (pg. 542)

11. c. The hypothalamus also plays a crucial role in the mechanism that maintains normal body temperature. (pg. 542)

12. d. The cerebellum functions in the synergistic control of skeletal muscle movements. That is, it governs coordinated movement. (pg. 542)

13. c. The brain stem houses the medulla, pons, and midbrain. The pons accommodates the pneumotaxic centers, the midbrain contains reflex centers that coordinate pupillary reflexes, and the medulla contains reflex centers such as the cardiac, vasomotor, and respiratory centers. (pg. 543)

14. b. The second function of the spinal cord is that of a reflex center. Reflexes are natural protective measures for the body. (pg. 543)

15. c. The cervical vertebrae include the top seven bones. (pg. 543)

16. b. Loss of sensation that begins at the nipple line indicates damage at T-4. (pg. 545)

17. c. Loss of sensation at the umbilicus level results from damage at T-10. (pg. 545)

18. c. Many signs and symptoms detected in patients in the field are, in essence, the effects of the autonomic nervous system. (pg. 546)

19. b. The sympathetic division functions as the body's "emergency" system, often referred to as the "fight or flight syndrome." (pg. 547)

20. c. The vagal nerve controls certain actions of the heart, stomach, and GI tract. (pg. 548)

ASSIGNMENT 22-2

Matching

1. E
2. G
3. D
4. I

5. K
6. A
7. H

8. J
9. B
10. C

Multiple Choice

1. d. In the primary survey of the neurologic patient, the patient's responsiveness and respiratory status are the most serious concerns. (pg. 548)

2. d. The respiratory system is often affected by neurologic impediments. Respiratory patterns may be normal or may fall under one of several variations, such as Cheyne-Stokes respiration, central neurogenic hyperventilation, ataxic breathing, or apneustic breathing. Shallow tachypnea is a result of compensatory mechanisms rather than a result of neurologic impediments. (pg. 549)

3. b. It is common to see cardiac arrhythmias in the later stages of increasing intracranial pressure. Management should be aimed at reducing the intracranial pressure by aggressive hyperventilation rather than treating the arrhythmias. (pg. 549)

4. c. In addition to evaluation of the state of consciousness in the neurologic exam, patient assessment also includes the position in which the patient was found, speech patterns, movement of extremities, pupillary size and reaction, extraocular motions, and posturing. Pulse regularity is more a function of irritability or compensatory mechanisms of the heart itself than an effect of the neurological system. (pg. 549)

5. a. For coma to occur, either both right and left cerebral cortexes have to be affected or the reticular activating system has to be damaged. (pg. 551)

6. c. Metabolic coma is usually preceded by fever and is of slower onset, and the secondary exam is often symmetrical. (pg. 551)

7. b. Structural lesions include head trauma, tumors, and intracranial hemorrhage. (pg. 551)

8. b. Common medications administered to comatose patients, depending on the underlying cause, include 50% dextrose, naloxone, thiamine, and sodium bicarbonate. (pg. 552)

9. c. A seizure is a massive electrical discharge of one or more groups of neurons in the brain. A seizure is not a disease but a manifestation or symptom of an underlying disorder. Recurrent seizures constitute the definition of epilepsy. Epilepsy is the disease and is irreversible. A seizure is not a disease and is considered reversible. (pg. 552)

10. c. When patients suffer a partial complex seizure, they tend to repeat certain words or phrases and also to display local, nonpurposeful movements, such as "lip smacking" and rolling their fingers as if moving a marble between them. Though these patients may be unable to communicate, they remain conscious. (pg. 553)

11. d. Associated complications of status epilepticus include aspiration of blood and vomit, brain damage from the resulting hypoxia, long bone and spine fractures, and severe dehydration. (pg. 553)

12. d. One of the most common causes of status epilepticus is failure to take prescribed medications by people who have a history of seizure disorders. (pg. 554)

13. d. The universal medication used to treat seizures is diazepam. If the person is already taking seizure medication such as phenytoin, the physician may order this drug to be given IV. Another medication to consider is 50% dextrose. The patient may become hypoglycemic, or

hypoglycemia may be the cause of the seizures. (pg. 554)

14. c. Thrombosis and emboli both obstruct cerebrovasculature. Cerebrovascular hemorrhage is a bleed within the brain that is due to one of several causes. (pg. 555)

Chapter 23
ASSIGNMENT 23-1

Matching

1. B
2. D
3. A

4. J
5. F
6. I

7. C
8. H
9. G

Multiple Choice

1. c. Together, these three portions measure about 7 meters in length. (pg. 558)

2. b. Chemicals needed for the digestion of lipids (fats) and proteins are contained in other parts of the digestive system. (pg. 560)

3. c. The pancreas lies behind the parietal peritoneum and extends from the C-shaped curve of the duodenum to the spleen. (pg. 560)

4. a. The gallbladder is a pear-shaped organ that stores, concentrates, and releases bile to the small intestine to aid in digestion. (pg. 560)

5. a. The parietal peritoneum lines the abdominal wall, whereas the visceral peritoneum covers each abdominal organ. (pg. 561)

6. c. The solid organs of the abdominal cavity include the liver, spleen, pancreas, and kidneys. (pg. 561)

7. d. Other parts of the urinary system are the kidneys, ureters, and urethra. (pg. 561)

8. b. The kidneys' primary function is to maintain a normal composition and volume of body fluids. (pg. 561)

9. d. Sperm cells remain in the epididymis for 18 hours to 10 days until they are capable of fertilizing an egg. (pg. 562)

10. c. The prostate is a doughnut-shaped gland that surrounds the beginning of the urethra below the urinary bladder. (pg. 562)

11. d. The ovaries are walnut-sized organs attached to the pelvic cavity by ligaments. (pg. 563)

12. c. Injury to a solid organ may result in hemorrhage, whereas infection and inflammation may occur after injury to a hollow organ. When gas or intestinal contents do not pass normally through the intestinal tract, obstruction results. (pg. 563)

13. b. Diverticulitis occurs in the diverticula, sacs located in the intestinal wall. Cholecystitis is an inflammation of the gallbladder, usually due to gallstones. Pleuritis is an inflammation of the pleura covering the lungs. (pg. 563)

14. c. Pain can be caused by a variety of medical conditions, including intestinal obstruction, ulcers, inflammation of the gallbladder, inflammation of the intestine, appendicitis, or an abdominal aortic aneurysm. (pg. 563)

15. a. Although abdominal distention is associated with intestinal obstruction, it is a sign, not a symptom. (pg. 563)

16. d. The pain is usually described as "gnawing" or "burning." (pg. 563)

17. c. After a meal that contains fried, greasy, spicy, or fatty foods, the patient develops an acute onset of crampy pain in the right upper quadrant. (pg. 563)

18. c. This patient should be transported to an appropriate medical facility immediately. (pg. 564)

19. d. The patient may complain of a "tearing" pain in the lumbar region of the back. Hypotension may be present, and the patient may have weak or absent femoral and pedal pulses. (pg. 564)

20. c. Dark-red or bright-red bloody stool may occur as a result of bleeding in the lower gastrointestinal tract. (pg. 564)

21. d. If shock is present or suspected, a second IV line should also be started. If indicated, the pneumatic anti-shock garment should be applied. The patient should be transported rapidly but gently to an appropriate medical facility. (pg. 566)

22. b. The patient in chronic renal failure who is not treated with dialysis is likely to develop pericarditis, pericardial tamponade, hyperkalemia, fluid overload, and pulmonary edema. (pg. 566)

23. a. Eventually, these deposits will dislodge and travel down the ureters. When this occurs, the patient will experience intense pain that develops in the flanks and may radiate to the groin. (pg. 566)

24. c. When a urinary obstruction is present, anuria may also occur.

25. b. The patient with an open shunt may suffer fatal hemorrhage if a damaged shunt tube is not rapidly occluded. The paramedic should never attempt to obtain a blood pressure or start an IV on an extremity containing a dialysis shunt or fistula. (pg. 567)

26. c. More aggressive management should be instituted if traumatic injury has occurred to the testes or penis. (pg. 568)

27. b. If the condition progresses and the tube ruptures, the patient will hemorrhage and shock will occur. Vaginal bleeding may not be present. (pg. 568)

28. d. If the patient appears shocky, the IV fluid should be lactated Ringer's or normal saline infused with a large-bore catheter. (pg. 569)

Labeling

1. A. pharynx
    B. esophagus
    C. liver
    D. gallbladder
    E. duodenum
    F. ascending colon
    G. appendix
    H. stomach
    I. pancreas
    J. transverse colon
    K. jejunum
    L. descending colon
    M. ileum
    N. rectum

2. A. ureter
    B. bladder
    C. scrotum
    D. epididymis
    E. testis
    F. seminal vesicle
    G. rectum
    H. prostate

Chapter 24

ASSIGNMENT 24-1

Matching

1. F	4. B	7. G
2. A	5. J	8. E
3. H	6. D	9. I

Multiple Choice

1. b. It is estimated that a person in the United States has a lifetime risk of 0.4% of suffering an anaphylactic reaction. Although the number of insect sting fatalities in the United States is low, the paramedic must always consider an anaphylactic reaction of this type to be potentially serious. (pg. 572)

2. d. The immune response is a positive adaptive response that mobilizes the body's protective cells to recognize, fight, and destroy intruders. (pg. 572)

3. c. Immunity is the body's natural protective state of being resistant to poisons and foreign substances. (pg. 572)

4. d. Antibodies are also sometimes referred to as immune bodies or immunoglobulins. Defending the body from foreign substances is their major function. (pg. 572)

5. a. An allergy is individualized. Only certain susceptible persons will have a reaction to a given substance. (pg. 573)

6. b. Anaphylaxis is derived from "ana," meaning without, and "phylaxis" meaning protection. The reaction is more severe than a simple allergic reaction. (pg. 573)

7. d. Inhalation is the least common route of exposure. (pg. 573)

8. c. Persons with allergies to penicillin may also be allergic to other similar antibiotics. (pg. 573)

9. d. Both the bumblebee and the yellow jacket are members of the order Hymenoptera. Honeybees and white-faced hornets also belong to this order. A sting from any of these insects may increase the allergic response to that of any of the others. (pg. 573-574)

10. a. This reaction triggers the release of histamine, serotonin, bradykinin, and other chemicals. (pg. 574)

11. b. Body systems generally affected include the skin, respiratory, gastrointestinal, and cardiovascular systems. The patient may also experience headache, dizziness, and a decreased level of consciousness. (pg. 574)

12. d. Although cardiovascular abnormalities, hypovolemia, and seizures are possible occurrences in the patient experiencing anaphylaxis, laryngeal edema is the primary event that may lead to death. The paramedic should observe the patient closely for signs and symptoms that may indicate the development of airway obstruction. (pg. 574)

13. d. Other important information includes medic alert tags and medications the patient takes regularly. The physical examination should be very thorough, with frequent reassessments of the primary survey. (pg. 575)

14. b. Frequent reassessment of circulatory function should also be an essential part of patient care in suspected anaphylaxis. (pg. 576)

15. b. If respiratory involvement ensues without shock, the epinephrine may be given subcutaneously. (pg. 576)

16. d. Dosage depends on whether the patient has had any theophylline products in the last 36 hours. (pg. 576)

17. a. Remember that epinephrine is capable of inducing cardiac arrhythmias. It is important to monitor the blood pressure carefully, because administration of this medication to a patient with hypertension is not recommended. (pg. 576)

18. d. Other gastrointestinal side effects may also occur. (pg. 576-577)

19. d. Further preventive action includes avoiding flower beds, clover fields, picnic grounds, and other locations frequented by the insects to which the individual is allergic. (pg. 577)

Chapter 25
ASSIGNMENT 25-1

Multiple Choice

1. c. The local effects include cutaneous burns, blisters, erythema, and contact dermatitis. (pg. 581)

2. d. Upper and lower airway signs and symptoms may precede systemic toxicity. (pg. 581)

3. a. Absorption must occur across gastrointestinal mucosa before toxic effects occur. (pg. 581)

4. c. Substances with a high volatility and low surface tension, such as some hydrocarbons, can be aspirated even without emesis. (pg. 582)

5. b. Naloxone reverses respiratory depression due to narcotics. (pg. 582)

6. c. Excess chemicals can generate heat upon exposure to water. (pg. 583)

7. c. Once the dose is administered, emesis usually occurs within 20 minutes. (pg. 583)

8. b. Dosage of 15 mL (3 teaspoons or 1 tablespoon) is given with 4 to 8 ounces of clear fluid. (pg. 583)

9. d. The complications of aspiration and additional injuries are possible with these situations. (pg. 583)

ASSIGNMENT 25-2

Multiple Choice

1. d. In the worst case, the immediate emergency may be airway management. (pg. 584)

2. d. If the product is gulped by the child, burns to the mouth may be minimal compared to those in the esophagus. (pg. 584)

3. a. Rust remover is a commercial product that often creates acid burns. (pg. 584)

4. c. Therapy that utilizes a beta-2 stimulating drug is the best way to treat bronchospasm. (pg. 585)

5. a. Ethylene glycol is metabolized more rapidly than methanol and may have a more rapid onset of symptoms. (pg. 585)

6. c. Fire-retardant fabrics and building materials resist combustion but promote pyrolysis, which generates toxic gases. (pg. 585)

7. c. Amyl nitrate produces methemoglobin, which binds cyanide. (pg. 586)

8. d. The simple mixing of household bleach with an acid can release chlorine and cause a household exposure to toxic fumes. (pg. 587)

9. d. These insecticides are well absorbed by all routes of exposure. (pg. 587)

10. b. Organophosphates inhibit the enzyme acetylcholinesterase, which is involved in modulating nerve impulse transmission in the neuromuscular junction. (pg. 587)

11. d. The initial dose of atropine is 2 mg for an adult repeated in 15 minutes if no effect is seen. (pg. 587-588)

12. c. Syncope and weakness may be the chief complaints, and hypotension and electrolyte imbalance may be the immediate problems that require treatment. (pg. 588)

13. c. The neurotoxic venom can cause muscle spasm, rigidity, and paralysis initially in the anatomical region of the bite. (pg. 590)

14. d. Ice and cold packs may result in severe necrosis of the skin and deep frostbite injury at the bite. (pg. 590)

15. a. Narcotic overdoses classically present in coma with respiratory depression and constricted pupils. (pg. 591)

16. d. The paramedic should be prepared to restrain or withdraw from a patient given naloxone. (pg. 591)

17. a. Barbiturates can produce numerous reactions, such as excitation, sedation, hypnosis, anesthesia, and deep coma. (pg. 591)

18. d. Overdoses with these drugs can cause serious metabolic derangements, liver failure, and death. (pg. 592)

19. c. Tricyclic antidepressants also cause sedation and have central and peripheral anticholinergic effects. (pg. 592)

20. d. A narcotic addict given naloxone can experience withdrawal symptoms within 1 hour of administration. (pg. 596)

21. b. The psychotic response can be highly variable. The patient can sustain and inflict considerable trauma. (pg. 596)

22. c. Thiamine should be given to prevent the onset of Wernicke's encephalopathy. Wernicke's encephalopathy presents as mental confusion, vertical and horizontal nystagmus, disconjugate gaze, and ataxia (gait disturbances). (pg. 598)

23. c. Within 6 to 8 hours after abstinence begins, symptoms appear and a tremor develops. (pg. 599)

Chapter 26
ASSIGNMENT 26-1

Matching

1. I	4. G	7. F
2. D	5. H	8. B
3. J	6. C	9. E

Multiple Choice

1. c. The lymphatic system is a system of vessels that serves to convey excess tissue fluid back to the blood circulation system. (pg. 602)

2. c. The lymph nodes do not produce antigens. Antigens are substances that are foreign to the body. (pg. 602)

3. a. Cellular immunity defends the body against viruses, fungi, and some bacteria. (pg. 602)

4. b. Foveation means pitted, like the skin following smallpox. Piloerection is the medical term for "goosebumps," which occurs when the piloerector muscle contracts, pulling each hair follicle straight. Sicchasia is another term meaning nausea. (pg. 603)

5. d. Viral meningitis is not readily communicable. (pg. 603)

6. c. Ingestion must take place into the body. (pg. 603)

ASSIGNMENT 26-2

Matching

1. F	7. C	13. R
2. H	8. Q	14. L
3. A	9. D	15. S
4. J	10. P	16. E
5. N	11. O	17. G
6. M	12. I	18. B

Multiple Choice

1. c. Rashes and seizures are not commonly associated with tuberculosis. Hemoptysis is the presence of blood in the sputum. (pg. 603)

2. d. Because tuberculosis is spread by airborne droplets, face masks on the patient and paramedic offer maximum protection. Showering and changing clothing are not routinely recommended. (pg. 603)

3. b. The most common type of communicable hepatitis is hepatitis A, caused by the hepatitis A virus. This disease is most common in children but does occur in adults. Alcoholic hepatitis is not a form of viral hepatitis. (pg. 604)

4. c. Cheyne-Stokes respirations and yellow vision are not commonly associated with hepatitis. (pg. 604)

5. d. Wearing a face mask is not routinely recommended in caring for patients with hepatitis A, which is spread primarily through fecal-oral routes. (pg. 604)

6. d. Wearing a face mask is not routinely recommended in caring for patients with hepatitis B, which is primarily a blood-borne disease. (pg. 604)

7. a. Hepatitis C is a blood-borne disease that is the most common cause of post-transfusion hepatitis. (pg. 604)

8. d. Dark urine and dysphagia (difficulty in swallowing) are not associated with meningitis. (pg. 605)

9. a. Bacterial meningitis is easily transmissible; viral meningitis is not. (pg. 605)

10. b. Use of a gown or apron is not routinely recommended for meningitis, which is spread through contact with respiratory secretions. (pg. 605)

11. d. Once the herpesvirus has invaded the body, it takes up residence in the ganglia of nerve and resides there until triggered to be active. (pg. 605)

12. b. Fever blisters or cold sores are usually herpes simplex 1 eruptions, although they are infrequently due to herpes simplex 2 virus. (pg. 605)

13. d. Herpes simplex is not thought to be spread through contact with fomites (personal articles such as sheets or bedding). (pg. 605-606)

14. b. Cytomegalovirus is a latent viral infection in most immune-compromised individuals. Psoriasis is a chronic inflammatory skin disease unrelated to herpesvirus. Rosacea is a chronic skin disease that produces a flushed appearance of the affected area but is unrelated to the herpesviruses. (pg. 606)

15. a. Diclofenac is a non-steroidal anti-inflammatory drug (NSAID). Sucralfate is an antiulcer medication. Zidovudine is the generic name for AZT (azidothymidine), which is an anti-retroviral agent used in treating AIDS patients. (pg. 606)

16. c. Photophobia, or sensitivity to light, is seen in measles infections but not in varicella. Oral

candidiasis, or thrush, is a fungal infection producing white patches on the tongue and is seen in AIDS patients but not in varicella. (pg. 606)

17. d. Varicella Zoster Immune Globulin (VZIG) is recommended for chickenpox prophylaxis rather than gamma globulin. (pg. 606)

18. d. Herpes zoster does not precipitate the other herpes viral infections. (pg. 606-607)

19. a. Being of Mediterranean descent is a risk factor for Kaposi's sarcoma, a cancer also seen in AIDS patients, but it is unrelated to cytomegalovirus infection. Being either very old or young is not associated with cytomegalovirus infection. (pg. 607)

20. d. Dark urine production is seen in hepatitis but is not associated with gonorrhea. Nausea and vomiting are not common symptoms and signs of gonorrhea. (pg. 607)

21. d. Face masks and protective eye wear are not recommended precautions for dealing with patients with scabies or lice. (pg. 608)

22. b. Malaria is a protozoal disease affecting the red blood cells, but it is not prevented by the MMR. Malta fever is a zoonosis (disease transmitted from animals to humans) caused by the Brucella bacteria. It produces swelling of the joints and spleen but is not prevented by the MMR. Rheumatic fever is thought to be due to the streptococcus bacteria. It is a systemic, febrile disease often producing damage to the heart. It is not prevented by MMR. Meningitis, an inflammation of the meninges, is not prevented by the MMR. Rubeola is the red measles or the hard measles, and is prevented by the MMR. Moniliasis, also known as candidiasis, is a fungal infection affecting mucous membranes. It is not prevented by the MMR. Rabies is an almost uniformly fatal disease produced by a virus and affecting the central nervous system. The MMR does not protect against rabies. (pg. 608)

23. d. Use of protective eye wear is not routinely recommended in caring for patients with mumps. (pg. 608)

24. d. This disease is transmitted by direct contact with nasopharyngeal secretions from an infected person. It is also transmitted by droplets and by direct contact with articles contaminated with blood, urine, and stool. (pg. 608)

25. d. Congenital rubella syndrome is associated with both mental retardation and multiple birth defects. Commonly seen birth defects include cataracts, deafness, heart defects, and microcephaly. Cryptorchidism (undescended testicles in male infants), while classified as a birth defect, is not one commonly seen in congenital rubella syndrome. (pg. 608)

26. d. The purple-red skin lesions seen in AIDS patients are manifestations of Kaposi's sarcoma. The red lesions seen in rubeola patients are simply the German measles. The white blotches on the tongues and in the mouths of AIDS patients are due to the fungal infection thrush, or oral candidiasis. (pg. 609)

27. d. Coxsackievirus is a viral disease that affects multiple organs and may produce meningitis. Coxsackievirus is not seen in AIDS patients. Cytomegalovirus is seen in AIDS patients and is the principle cause of blindness in AIDS, but it does not cause the disease. Epstein-Barr virus is a herpesvirus that causes mononucleosis. Epstein-Barr may be seen in AIDS patients but does not cause the disease. (pg. 609)

28. d. Kissing, saliva contact, and sharing household articles have not been shown to cause AIDS transmission. (pg. 610)

29. a. The vast majority of cases in which health care providers have seroconverted as a result of an occupational exposure have been related to needle stick injury. Contaminated personal articles probably present a low risk of exposure if they are contaminated with blood. Respiratory secretions are thought to be low-risk, unless they are stained with visible blood. Saliva does contain the AIDS virus in low concentrations, but it has not been shown to be a method of transmission. (pg. 610)

30. d. The Centers for Disease Control has labeled the term "universal precautions." (pg. 611)

31. d. The Centers for Disease Control recommends that needles not be recapped after use. The recapping procedure often results in needle stick injuries. Needles should not be cut or bent for disposal. Instead, the needle and syringe should be disposed of, as one intact unit, into a puncture-resistant container right after their use. Needles and syringes need to be disposed of as infectious waste, rather than as regular trash. (pg. 612-613)

32. a. A 1-to-10 ratio of bleach to water yields a 10% solution. (pg. 614)

Chapter 27
ASSIGNMENT 27-1

Matching

1. B	5. C	8. E
2. D	6. K	9. G
3. J	7. H	10. A
4. I		

Multiple Choice

1. a. Temperature is one of the many variables to which the body adjusts in the process of maintaining homeostasis. (pg. 619)

2. c. The hypothalamus also detects the return to normal temperature when compensation efforts begin and shuts down the compensatory mechanisms accordingly. (pg. 619)

3. a. Radiation is felt when the sun shines; it is a form of electromagnetic wave. (pg. 619)

4. c. Fluid greatly enhances conduction and evaporation, which in turn promotes convective loss if a breeze is present. (pg. 619)

5. d. Voluntary and involuntary responses make heat production in muscle the most important defense against excessive heat loss in cold weather. (pg. 620-621)

6. d. Increased cardiac output acts to distribute heat throughout the body. (pg. 622)

7. c. Most often, heat cramps follow a period of physical exertion in a hot environment. (pg. 622)

8. a. Heat stroke patients can deteriorate quickly to coma. (pg. 623)

9. d. Salt tablets are not recommended, because they may precipitate nausea. (pg. 622)

10. c. Overcooling is dangerous because the hypothalamus is not functioning. (pg. 623)

11. b. The elderly tend to loose heat gradually. The thermal balancing mechanisms and other defense systems that would protect them from excessive heat lose sensitivity with age. Hypothermia in the elderly can develop over a period of days in indoor surroundings that feel comfortable to the young, healthy adult. (pg. 624)

12. c. In moderate hypothermia, the core temperature remains above 32°C (90°F). (pg. 624)

13. d. Changes in the patient's level of consciousness and cardiac rhythm signal not only temperature drop but also the need for rewarming measures. (pg. 624-625)

14. a. Basic management of hypothermia includes handling the patient gently, removing wet clothing, and covering the patient to prevent further cooling. (pg. 625)

15. b. The cold exposure causes an initial spasm in the small blood vessels and slows or blocks circulation. *A* and *c* occur after *b*. (pg. 626)

ASSIGNMENT 27-2

Matching

1. B
2. A
3. I

4. G
5. H
6. E

7. F
8. D

Multiple Choice

1. c. Because no water enters the tracheal airway, dry drowning responds readily to artificial ventilation, and victims of this type of drowning account for 90% of those successfully resuscitated. (pg. 628)

2. a. The high concentration of salt contained in the water that has collected in the lungs draws fluid from the bloodstream into the lungs to equalize the concentration of salt. (pg. 628)

3. d. As a result of acidosis, ventricular ectopy as well as hypoxemia may occur. Hyperventilation is the first-line method of treating acidosis. If oxygenation, hyperventilation, and possibly sodium bicarbonate injection do not suppress ventricular ectopy, a bolus of lidocaine can be used to suppress the ectopy. (pg. 629)

4. c. The pressure of a gas forces it into solution; in other words, a higher pressure means more dissolved gas. (pg. 630)

5. d. The threat is much more serious in the central nervous system, as the tissue's fragility makes it vulnerable to damage from bubble pressure. (pg. 630)

6. c. Management of decompression sickness focuses on fundamental resuscitative measures when necessary and on pain control in the severe cases. (pg. 631-632)

ASSIGNMENT 27-3

Matching

1. J
2. H
3. K
4. I

5. C
6. E
7. F

8. A
9. D
10. B

Multiple Choice

1. b. Their function is to contain the release from a safe distance, keep it from spreading, and prevent exposure. (pg. 633)

2. d. Proper recognition and identification of hazardous materials are accomplished by using all resources available to the emergency responders. (pg. 633-638)

3. a. The NFPA 704 system is not used on transportation vehicles. (pg. 635-636)

4. b. This number system was adopted by the U.S. Department of Transportation to allow first responders immediate access to hazard information. (pg. 636)

5. d. To become familiar with the needs of their communities, responders should plan and prepare for local needs. (pg. 639)

6. c. Emergency medical personnel should take and record the vital signs of hazardous materials entry personnel before they initially go into the hot zone. (pg. 640)

7. a. Internal organs are not at risk unless particles gain access by way of contaminated food, open wounds, or inhalation. (pg. 642)

9. d. Medically trained personnel are often tempted to begin treatment within the hazardous area. (pg. 644)

Chapter 28
ASSIGNMENT 28-1

Multiple Choice

1. d. The three leading causes of death in the elderly population are heart disease, cancer, and cerebrovascular accident. (pg. 650)

2. a. As a result of normal anatomical and physiologic changes in the respiratory system, elderly people can suffer significantly from inadequate ventilations and chronic states of hypoxia. (pg. 651)

3. b. Reduction in cardiac output is caused by a decrease in stroke volume, a decrease in heart rate, degeneration of the conduction system, and left ventricular hypertrophy. As a result, syncope, falls, and heart failure can occur while the system is trying to compensate for a sudden drop in cardiac output. (pg. 651)

4. a. Peripheral vascular resistance may increase because of arteriosclerosis and, thus, often results in systemic hypertension. Hypertension is of particular significance in the elderly trauma patient, because a systolic blood pressure of 100 mm Hg may not provide adequate tissue perfusion if the elderly patient is normally hypertensive. (pg. 652)

5. a. Nocturia is excessive urination at night. (pg. 652)

6. c. In the elderly, urine is produced at the same rate day and night. The bladder becomes distended with urine at night, and the elderly suffer from a condition called nocturia (excessive urination at night). (pg. 652)

7. c. Intelligence is not affected by aging, nor is the ability to verbalize. Long-term memory is intact but short-term memory may decrease. (pg. 653)

8. d. Decreased mobility may cause slowed movement and responses. A degree of loss of flexibility may affect the elderly's balance and range of motion in the neck and extremities. Even with a lack of mobility, elderly people can still adapt to their changing environment. (pg. 653)

9. b. The gastrointestinal tract is the most common site of chronic distress in the elderly. About 56% of complaints in this age group involve the gastrointestinal tract. (pg. 653)

10. d. Many elderly people experience heartburn after meals, which is due to the relaxation of the muscles in the walls of the esophagus. (pg. 653)

11. a. The elderly may be wearing many layers of clothing as a result of sensitivity to cold. Elderly patients may not be aware of necrotic toes or decubitus ulcers. Elderly patients may also have a high pain threshold and may minimize small discomforts. (pg. 654)

12. b. Hemoptysis of several hundred milliliters of blood is usually the result of chronic use of anticoagulants, heavy use of aspirin, or epistaxis. (pg. 655)

13. c. The symptoms of coughing, wheezing, and nocturnal episodes of asthma increase with age. The intensity of coughing and wheezing does not differ and the precipitating factors do not increase; however, sensitivity to the precipitating factors of asthma does increase. (pg. 655)

14. d. Advancing age is just one of the predisposing factors that contribute to the development of emboli. Patients with heart disease, particularly those with atrial fibrillation and congestive heart failure, are at higher risk of developing a pulmonary embolism. (pg. 655)

15. a. The safety, efficacy, and relative ease of administration of aerosolized bronchodilators such as metaproterenol and albuterol make them the drugs of choice. Epinephrine is not recommended

for elderly patients. The administration of a sedative is never appropriate. (pg. 656)

16. b. An acute myocardial infarction in an elderly person may present quite differently from the signs and symptoms the paramedic is accustomed to seeing. The pain may be mild. Shortness of breath may be significant. (pg. 657)

17. c. Orthopnea is best defined as difficulty breathing related to body position. (pg. 657)

18. d. In a myocardial infarction without pain, syncope is commonly the first sign. (pg. 657)

19. b. Hyperextension of the neck in patients with atherosclerotic carotid arteries can temporarily occlude arteries in the cervical spine. This state is thought to be the cause of syncope and falls when elderly people reach up to change a ceiling light bulb or reach for objects on high shelves. (pg. 657)

20. d. In the elderly, coma is frequently a result of a combination of disorders that affect the functioning of the central nervous system, as opposed to coma in the young patient, which usually is caused by only one factor. (pg. 658)

21. a. One of the most common causes of seizures in the elderly is a cerebrovascular accident. (pg. 658)

22. c. Dementia is demonstrated by knowledge and memory loss, such as manifests itself in impaired ability to recall numbers or solve simple mathematical problems. It is not unusual to forget where one has put things or, on occasion, a neighbor's name. However, it is unusual to forget how to use something or how to perform simple mathematical operations. (pg. 659)

23. c. Dextrose-containing solutions should not be administered to any patient with the potential for underlying acute cerebral ischemia, because dextrose may worsen cerebral intracellular acidosis. (pg. 659)

ASSIGNMENT 28-2

Multiple Choice

1. c. Padding of splints is important because of the decreased fat stores in elderly people. (pg. 660)

2. b. Peptic ulcer disease is the most common cause of upper gastrointestinal bleeding in nonalcoholic elderly patients. (pg. 661)

3. d. The bleeding source in diverticula are the arterioles in the mesenteric walls. Therefore, bright red blood is found in rectal bleeding. Bleeding may be massive without much complaint of pain or minimal with moderate abdominal pain on physical examination. (pg. 661)

4. b. The risk of pneumonia is so great after rib fractures in the elderly that these injuries should be considered significant. (pg. 662)

5. d. The presence of coronary atherosclerosis makes the heart susceptible to ischemia and infarction with hypotension from blood loss. (pg. 662)

6. a. Hypothermia may be observed in patients in the early stages of pneumonia. Many of the signs and symptoms of hypothermia can also be associated with stroke, a diabetic emergency, or a cardiac event. (pg. 664)

7. c. Abnormalities within the body that result from chronic disease and the use of medications, as well as fatigue, further predispose the elderly to hyperthermia. (pg. 664)

Multiple Choice

1. d. Both the parent and the child may be sources of useful information. Establishing a relationship with a parent while the child looks on identifies the paramedic as more an ally than a stranger. (pg. 668)

2. c. An attempt should always be made to develop an atmosphere of cooperation, trust, and confidence. However, this process may require more time than is available if a life-threatening condition is known or suspected. (pg. 669)

3. a. Separation anxiety may occur not only in the child but also in the parent or caretaker. However, the parent or caretaker may have to be cautioned to keep his or her anxiety in check to avoid disturbing the child. (pg. 669)

4. c. Normal vital signs for a child in this age range generally are as follows: BP 75-115 systolic, pulse 100, respirations 20-24. (pg. 670)

5. d. The respiratory pattern of a young infant is usually irregular. In order to obtain an accurate calculation of the respiratory rate, use a full 60-second count whenever possible. (pg. 670)

6. c. The fontanelles are also known as soft spots. The anterior fontanelle can be used effectively to determine intracranial pressure or dehydration in an infant. (pg. 670-671)

7. d. This indicator is similarly important in the adult patient. Determining the level of consciousness in a pediatric patient may be more challenging for the paramedic as a result of fear and the reluctance of the patient to communicate. (pg. 671)

8. b. Examples of infectious processes that may cause airway obstruction and produce stridor are croup and epiglottitis. (pg. 671)

9. c. Growth is an increase in body size. Development is an improvement or maturation in organs and systems as well as skills and functions. (pg. 671)

10. b. The child of this age group also fears pain and separation from his or her parents. Because communication skills are limited, the paramedic must attempt to determine the child's level of understanding and talk with the child on that level. (pg. 672)

11. d. Accidents may include vehicular and bicycle accidents, falls, sports injuries, toxic ingestion, and drowning. (pg. 672)

ASSIGNMENT 29-2

Matching

1. B	4. I	7. H
2. D	5. A	8. E
3. C	6. G	

Multiple Choice

1. b. Sudden infant death syndrome is the leading cause of death in infants between 1 week and 1 year of age. The peak incidence occurs between 2 and 4 months of age. (pg. 673)

2. d. Local protocol should be followed in cases of suspected sudden infant death syndrome. Support for the parents and other family members is crucial. The family should be instructed on how to contact local and national SIDS support agencies. The paramedic must remember

that he or she may also experience feelings of grief over the loss of a tiny patient and should take steps to deal with these feelings. (pg. 673)

3. a. The most common illnesses associated with febrile seizures are pharyngitis, tonsillitis, and otitis media. However, meningitis should also be considered a possibility. (pg. 674)

4. d. Other signs of dehydration include reduced skin turgor, hyperpnea, sunken eyeballs, tachycardia, and a depressed anterior fontanelle (in the infant). (pg. 675)

5. b. Minimal management should be instituted unless shock is suspected. The fluid should be given as a bolus over less than 20 minutes. The patient's condition should then be reassessed and the bolus repeated as necessary. Transport should not be delayed for IV line placement. (pg. 675)

6. d. Meningitis may be caused by a bacteria or a virus. Signs and symptoms may vary between young children and older children. Supportive therapy, including frequent reassessment of primary survey components and monitoring of vital signs, should be instituted. If bacterial meningitis is diagnosed in the child patient, the paramedic, as well as others who came in contact with the patient, must be treated for the condition. (pg. 675)

7. a. Signs and symptoms that may be present include vomiting, lethargy, fever, and shock. (pg. 675)

8. c. A diagnosis of Reye's syndrome cannot be made in the field. The paramedic must collect information that makes it possible to rule out other causes such as alcohol or drug ingestion. Because no definitive care is available to the prehospital care provider, supportive therapy should be instituted. (pg. 676)

9. d. Coughing, gagging, choking, and wheezing may occur. The goal of emergency management is to allow for adequate air exchange. Techniques aimed at achieving this goal should be instituted. Respiratory and cardiac arrest and cardiac arrhythmias may occur as complications of the foreign body obstruction. (pg. 676)

10. a. Management should also include oxygenation. Intubation should be attempted if the signs of airway obstruction are present. (pg. 677)

11. a. Laryngotracheobronchitis, or croup, is the result of a viral infection. Those affected are normally children between the ages of 3 months and 3 years. (pg. 677)

12. b. If total airway obstruction is present, intubation will be difficult to impossible. If intubation is not rapidly accomplished, one should transport the patient immediately to an appropriate medical facility, while assisting ventilations with a bag-valve-mask device. Translaryngeal jet ventilation may be indicated for this condition. (pg. 678)

13. c. The patient may also exhibit cough, tachypnea, expiratory wheezing, and prolonged expiration. Complications include dehydration, pneumonia, pneumothorax, and apnea. (pg. 678)

14. d. Theophylline ethylenediamine should be considered in the patient over 1 year of age who does not respond to standard epinephrine therapy. (pg. 679)

15. b. Cardiac disorders rarely cause cardiac arrest in children. Hypoxia and respiratory arrest are often precipitating factors. Airway management is essential in treatment of the pediatric patient. (pg. 679)

16. d. If use of an IV or the pneumatic anti-shock garment is warranted, that treatment should be instituted after oxygenation has been initiated. (pg. 680)

17. d. Blunt trauma to the abdomen of a pediatric patient may cause liver and spleen damage, which is potentially life-threatening. (pg. 681)

18. d. Injuries that are inconsistent with how the injury is alleged to have occurred should arouse suspicion in the paramedic. (pg. 682)

19. b. In order for the judicial system to work properly, the paramedic should contact the proper authorities and comply with their directions. The sooner the incident of child abuse is reported, the sooner the child and family will receive the attention and assistance that they need. (pg. 683)

20. b. If a "pop-off" or pressure-relief valve is included on the model of pediatric or infant resuscitation bag currently in use by the paramedic, the valve should be occluded. (pg. 684)

21. c. Endotracheal tubes used in children under the age of 8 years should be uncuffed. (pg. 685)

22. a. Although macrodrip or regular tubing may be used with older children, fluid overload may be a consequence of its use in younger children. (pg. 685)

23. b. Children who weigh more than 10 kg should have fluid infused at 40 mL per hour. (pg. 686)

Chapter 30
ASSIGNMENT 30-1

Matching

1. C	5. F	8. K
2. E	6. D	9. B
3. G	7. H	10. A
4. I		

Multiple Choice

1. a. The endometrium is the innermost lining of the uterus. The fundus in the superior portion of the uterus opposite to the internal cervical os (opening). The vagina is the birth canal. (pg. 692)

2. b. The endometrium is the mucous membrane. This membrane extends through the opening of the fallopian tubes into the peritoneum and extends within the uterus through the cervix into the vaginal opening. (pg. 692)

3. d. Each fallopian tube is 10 cm in length. The ampulla is where fertilization of the ovum usually takes place. The inside of the fallopian tube is lined with a mucous membrane (endometrium). (pg. 692)

4. d. The vagina is the passageway for sperm, the excretory duct for menstrual flow, and part of the birth canal. (pg. 692)

5. d. The labia majora are the larger longitudinal outer lips. The mons veneris, also known as mons pubis, is the rounded protuberance superior to the symphysis pubis. The vestibule is the space between the parted labia minora in which the urethral meatus (opening) and vaginal orifice lie. (pg. 692)

6. c. Gestation refers to the term of pregnancy. Menopause is the cessation of the menses (menstrual cycles). Nidation is the actual implantation of the fertilized ovum into the uterine wall. (pg. 694)

7. d. The placenta provides oxygen, nutrients, and waste removal for the fetus. It is the endometrium that nourishes the placenta, not vice versa. (pg. 694)

8. b. The umbilical cord is a vital structure. Blood flow is so rapid that twisting or kinking is prevented. The cord is not innervated, so cutting it after delivery does not cause pain to the infant. (pg. 694)

9. c. The cord has one vein that carries oxygen and nutrients from the mother through the placenta's villi to the fetus. The cord has two arteries. Both carry blood with waste products from the fetus back to the villi of the placenta. (pg. 694)

10. b. In pregnancy, blood volume, heart rate, stroke volume, and cardiac output increase. Heart rate may increase by 15 beats per minute. (pg. 695)

11. c. In pregnancy, the arterial blood pressure and vascular resistance decrease. (pg. 695)

12. d. Supine-induced hypotension occurs in the last weeks of pregnancy when the weight of the gravid (pregnant) uterus can press on the inferior vena cava when the woman is supine and reduce blood return to the heart (preload) and can decrease cardiac output. Preeclampsia is a third-trimester problem in pregnancy related to difficulty with high blood pressure. Eclampsia is a more serious form of preeclampsia in which grand mal convulsions are present. Premature delivery is delivery of the fetus prior to term. (pg. 695)

ASSIGNMENT 30-2

Matching

1. C
2. D
3. F

4. G
5. A

6. B
7. H

Multiple Choice

1. b. The average tampon or pad is completely saturated when it contains an average of 25 mL—that is, a range of 20-30 mL. (pg. 697)

2. c. Pelvic inflammatory disease produces lower abdominal and pelvic pain, which may also radiate to the shoulder as "shoulder strap" pain. Amenorrhea is the absence or suppression of menstrual periods. Cholecystitis is inflammation of the gall bladder. It is associated with upper right quadrant pain, which may radiate to the angle of the scapula. Placenta previa is a third trimester complication of pregnancy. (pg. 699)

3. c. All possible options are causes of acute abdominal pain; pelvic inflammatory disease is the most common. (pg. 699)

4. d. A large-bore IV with a volume expander is indicated. The pneumatic anti-shock garment is indicated with systolic blood pressures less than 90 mm Hg. Ice packs, tampons, and oxytocin are not indicated. (pg. 699)

5. a. You should avoid questions concerning the details of the sexual assault and avoid any questions about the survivor's sexual history. (pg. 699-700)

6. b. Placenta previa and abruptio placenta are "late bleeds." (pg. 702)

7. b. The principal presentations of ectopic pregnancy are lower abdominal pain and slight vaginal bleeding. Blood loss from the ectopic pregnancy may be more internal than external. A ruptured ovarian cyst may produce similar symptoms but is not usually associated with missed menstrual periods. (pg. 702)

8. d. The vaginal bleeding may subside in a threatened abortion and the pregnancy may continue. (pg. 702)

9. b. Uterine contractions and cervical dilatation accompany the vaginal bleeding, and the abortion is imminent. (pg. 902)

10. c. Death of the fetus occurs in utero without expulsion for more than 4 weeks. (pg. 902)

11. a. Expulsion of a portion of the conceptus, usually the fetus, occurs. This may cause significant bleeding, and the patient requires hospitalization for operative care. (pg. 902)

12. a. Viability is usually defined as 24 to 26 weeks gestation or a weight of 400 to 600 g. (pg. 902)

13. d. Oxygen, volume expansion, and transport are indicated. Normal saline or lactated Ringer's solutions are preferred over D_5W for volume expansion. Diazepam and oxytocin are not indicated. (pg. 703)

14. d. Preeclampsia is characterized by elevated BP, protein in urine, hyperreflexia, and edema. Other signs and symptoms may include severe continuous headaches, dizziness, blurring of vision, persistent vomiting, and epigastric pain. Hydatiform mole, or "molar pregnancy," is a rare cause of second-trimester bleeding, occurring from a failed pregnancy in which the placenta continues to grow. Peripheral neuritis is an inflammation of the peripheral nervous system. (pg. 703)

15. a. Epilepsy does of course cause convulsions, but epilepsy tends to improve with pregnancy so that even patients who are difficult to control often have fewer seizures during gestation. Preeclampsia describes the condition preceding eclampsia and is distinguished from eclampsia by the absence of convulsions. (pg. 703)

16. a. Magnesium sulfate may be used as a prophylactic agent to suppress the onset of convulsions. Diazepam (Valium) may be used to suppress convulsions once they present. Methylergonovine (Methergine) is a drug used to control postpartum bleeding. Diphenhydramine is Benadryl. (pg. 703)

17. c. Abortion and ectopic pregnancy are "early bleeds". (pg. 703)

18. c. Bright lights and loud noises are known to potentiate convulsions in preeclamptic patients. In eclamptic patients with convulsions, lights and noises may enhance the duration of the convulsion. The patient compartment should be dimmed and lights and sirens used sparingly. The patient should be positioned on her left side. (pg. 703)

19. c. The cardinal sign of placenta previa is a painless third-trimester bleed. (pg. 703)

20. a. Abruptio placenta may or may not present with vaginal bleeding, depending on whether the separation is concealed or revealed. The pain associated with abruption tends to be constant, unlike Braxton-Hicks contractions, which are episodic and irregular. Placenta previa usually presents as a painless vaginal bleed. Uterine rupture should be accompanied by some vaginal bleeding, although the internal bleed may exceed the external bleed. (pg. 704)

ASSIGNMENT 30-3

Matching

1. A	4. C	7. D
2. I	5. H	8. B
3. F	6. E	

Multiple Choice

1. c. The traces of blood present in the mucus plug are blood from the cervical capillaries that hemorrhage from the pressure of the presenting fetal part. (pg. 705)

2. c. The cervix shortens and thins with the progress of labor. (pg. 705)

3. b. The cervix has completed dilation at 10 centimeters. (pg. 705)

4. c. Crowning occurs later in labor when the fetal head remains visible in the vaginal opening between contractions. Vaginal show is a discharge composed of mucus with traces of blood. (pg. 705)

5. c. The second stage of labor begins with full cervical dilatation and concludes with delivery of the fetus. (pg. 705)

6. c. The third stage of labor begins with delivery of the fetus and concludes with delivery of the placenta. (pg. 705)

7. c. Wide variations occur in the duration of labor. However, the average length of first labor is 14 hours. Subsequent labors tend to be about 6 hours shorter than the first. (pg. 705)

8. a. Contractions 2 minutes apart with bulging perineum mean imminent delivery, especially in a woman having her third child. (pg. 706)

9. d. A volume expander such as lactated Ringer's solution or normal saline is used in anticipation of the blood loss associated with infant delivery. (pg. 706)

10. b. This should be sufficient to maintain blood volume. (pg. 706)

11. a. Finger pressure at the center of the head could injure the infant's fontanelles (soft spots on the infant's head). Firm or excessive pressure against the head is a source of potential injury. Traction on the labia majora is not recommended. (pg. 707)

12. d. Protection of the infant's airway is vital. Suction the mouth first and then the nose. (pg. 707)

13. b. A nuchal cord occurs when the umbilical cord is looped around the baby's neck. The nuchal cord must be removed, either by slipping the cord over the head or by clamping and cutting it, prior to the birth of the infant's body. (pg. 707)

14. a. Gentle pressure should be used with both hands on the infant's head to guide the head downward to facilitate birth of the anterior shoulder. (pg. 707)

15. c. The cord should be cut approximately midway between the infant and placenta. The location for cutting the cord is precautionary in the event that the cord should bleed after cutting. Should the cut cord end bleed, the paramedic can apply additional clamps or ties proximal to the bleeding cord end to control the hemorrhage. (pg. 707)

16. d. The placenta should be taken to the hospital where it may be inspected more thoroughly. (pg. 707)

17. b. This amount is considered normal. (pg. 710)

18. c. Caput, or caput succedaneum, is a condition in which the soft tissues of the scalp are swollen from prolonged pressure on the fetal head during a protracted first stage of labor. Dyspareunia is the presence of pain during sexual intercourse. Vernix caseosa is the cheesy lubricant that covers the infant's skin during birth. (pg. 710)

19. c. Breech presentation is more common in the premature infant and with multiple births. (pg. 710)

20. d. An arm presentation is associated with "transverse lie," which means that the infant is not positioned properly for birth. The mother should be transported lights and siren to the hospital for an emergency cesarean section. (pg. 711)

21. c. The presenting part will exert pressure on the cord, which could reduce blood flow between the placenta and the yet unborn infant. (pg. 713)

22. b. The knee-chest position is one in which the patient is "on all fours," face down, knees pressed toward the chest, with the buttocks high in the air. This odd looking position utilizes gravity to hold the unborn infant off the cord. The disadvantage of this position is that it is difficult to maintain in a moving ambulance. If the knee-chest position is not used, the next preferred placement is the Trendelenburg position. Fowlers position is semisitting. Lithotomy position is supine with the hips and knees flexed with the legs elevated. Sims position is lateral recumbent (patient lying on the side) with the upper leg flexed. (pg. 713)

23. d. Lack of uterine tone is probably the most common cause. It is caused by prolonged labor in which the uterus tires of contracting. (pg. 713)

24. a. Titrate to the severity of hemorrhage and uterine response. (pg. 713)

25. a. The initial threats to life are associated with airway obstruction and inadequate warming. The airway may be obstructed with fluids such as amniotic fluid or meconium (fetal fecal material). Heat loss can be rapid in the inadequately cared for newborn. Hypothermia places the infant at risk for respiratory depression and cardiac arrest. (pg. 714)

26. b. The purpose of the Apgar score is to identify those infants who require routine care and those who need further assistance. (pg. 715)

27. b. After premature birth, the newborn is at increased risk for hypothermia because of lack of subcutaneous fat, high surface-mass ratio, and insensible loss from respiratory distress. (pg. 716)

Chapter 31
ASSIGNMENT 31-1

Multiple Choice

1. b. Organic causes are always considered initially. If no organic cause is found, a non-physiologic cause is assumed. (pg. 721)

2. d. Other general symptoms include confusion, poor decision making, frustration, anger, fear, and phobias. (pg. 721)

3. c. Common causes of transient disorders include overwhelming stress, physical injury, and sudden loss. (pg. 722)

4. a. Drugs are a common cause of transient disorders, whereas genetic and biochemical abnormalities result in psychosis. (pg. 722)

5. d. Transient disorders are temporary. (pg. 722)

6. a. A very real threat to the patient or others exists, and the situation must be quickly brought under control. (pg. 722)

7. b. Acute agitation, grief, panic attacks, and bizarre behaviors are examples of urgent behavioral emergencies that are potentially less serious than true behavioral emergencies. (pg. 723)

8. d. In order to render the best possible care to the patient, the paramedic must first determine the presenting problem. Further questioning should reveal what has caused the problem, whether it has previously occurred, and what has led to the present circumstance. A plan of action should then be developed. (pg. 723)

9. c. The mental status examination is a short, organized format developed by psychiatrists for emergency interviewing. (pg. 724)

10. c. The examination of the thought component may lead the paramedic to discover key signs of psychosis. However, psychosis itself is not a separate component of the examination. (pg. 724)

11. a. Perception is a natural subdivision of the thought segment of the mental status examination. Consistently misinterpreting actual stimuli and perceiving things that do not exist are indicators of serious mental derangement and are key signs of psychosis. (pg. 725)

ASSIGNMENT 31-2

Multiple Choice

1. d. Other factors include type and dosage of the substance; the situation in which the substance is used; tolerance, based on the user's previous experience with the substance; and other chemicals or foreign substances the user is also taking. (pg. 726)

2. c. The patient should be protected, separated from any potentially dangerous situation, and treated for any injuries that were sustained. Confrontation of the family is not appropriate and may even be dangerous to the paramedic and the patient. Local law enforcement officers should be contacted, if they are not already on the scene. However, the patient must be the paramedic's primary responsibility unless imminent danger is sensed. (pg. 727)

3. a. The paramedic should actively listen to the victim and communicate the plan of action for treatment. Unnecessary touching should be avoided. The genitalia should not be examined unless severe wounds are present. The victim's privacy must be protected. All evidence should be carefully documented on the run form. (pg. 727)

4. c. Examples I, II, and V do contain a risk significant enough to place them in a high-risk group but do not follow the emergency assessment scheme for the suicide victim. (pg. 728)

5. d. Other important steps the paramedic may take include an immediate reduction of environmental stress, caring for family members and significant others if a successful suicide has occurred prior to the paramedic's arrival, offering continuous emotional support and understanding to the patient, and transporting the patient to an appropriate medical facility as soon as possible. (pg. 727-728)

6. b. Long-term goals are not the intention of crisis intervention. (pg. 728)

7. a. Other objectives include helping persons in distress to mobilize resources available to them and restoring as much function as possible. (pg. 728)

8. c. The patient should be encouraged to set only limited goals. Decisions made by the person in crisis should be supported. Also, the person should be encouraged to take immediate action to resolve the crisis. (pg. 728-729)

9. a. The person in crisis should always be able to rely on the honesty of the paramedic. The paramedic should also be calm and exhibit confidence. (pg. 729)

10. b. The paramedic should exhibit a sense of calm control of the situation and should be cooperative with the patient, answering all questions. However, the paramedic should take care not to worsen the situation by encouraging disturbed or distorted thoughts. (pg. 729)

11. d. Patient restraint equipment or weapons should not be shown to the patient experiencing a severe mental disturbance unless the paramedic has exhausted all other options and has sufficient assistance to restrain the patient. The patient should be restrained only to the point where safety for the patient and others is ensured. (pg. 729)

12. c. Even if the patient appears calm, a sudden change may take place, and the paramedic must guard against the patient's jumping from the vehicle. (pg. 731)

13. d. EMS textbooks offer only general guidelines regarding legal implications. Paramedics should be well versed in state and local legislation concerning all legal issues involving emergency medical services. (pg. 732)

Flashcards

- EKGs
- Drugs
- Advanced Cardiac Life Support Treatment Protocols

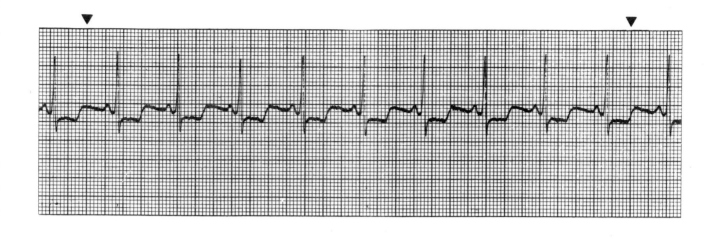

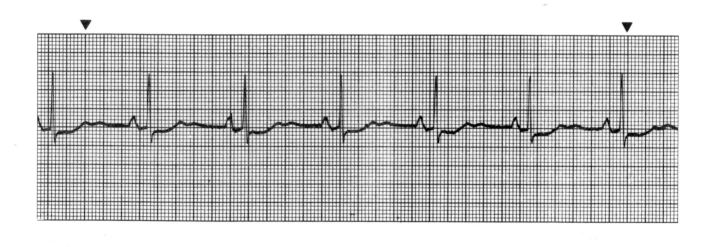

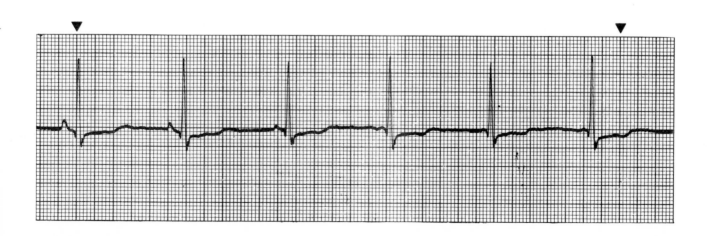

TREATMENT: ....
....
....
....
....
....
....
....
....
....
....
....
....

RATE: *88/min*
RHYTHM: *Regular*
P WAVE: *Sinus*
PR INTERVAL: *0.12 sec*
QRS COMPLEX: *0.06-0.08 sec*
RYTHYM INTERPRETATION: *Normal sinus rhythm*

TREATMENT: ....
....
....
....
....
....
....
....
....
....
....
....
....

RATE: *58/min*
RHYTHM: *Regular*
P WAVE: *Sinus*
PR INTERVAL: *0.18-0.20 sec*
QRS COMPLEX: *0.08 sec*
RYTHYM INTERPRETATION: *Sinus bradycardia*

TREATMENT: ....
....
....
....
....
....
....
....
....
....
....
....

RATE: *54/min*
RHYTHM: *Regular*
P WAVE: *Varying in size and shape*
PR INTERVAL: *0.12 sec*
QRS COMPLEX: *0.08-0.10 sec*
RYTHYM INTERPRETATION: *Wandering atrial pacemaker*

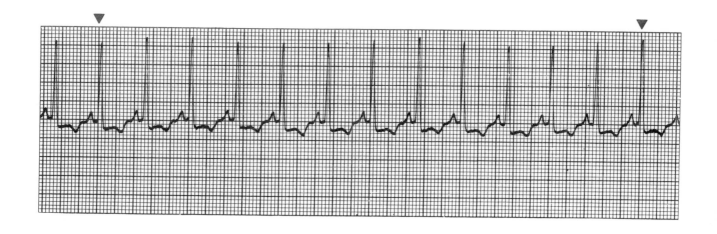

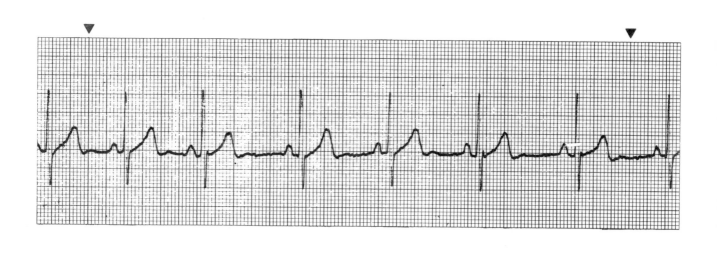

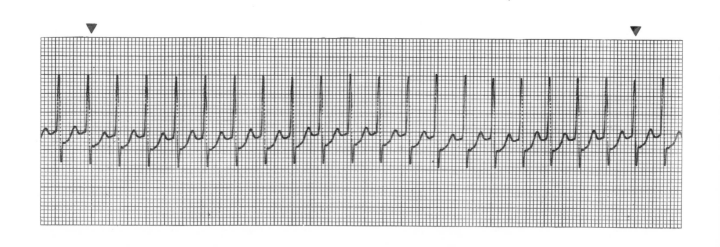

TREATMENT: ....
....
....
....
....
....
....
....
....
....
....
....
....
....

RATE: *125/min*
RHYTHM: *Regular*
P WAVE: *Sinus*
PR INTERVAL: *0.12 sec*
QRS COMPLEX: *0.06 sec*
RYTHYM INTERPRETATION: *Sinus tachycardia*

TREATMENT: ....
....
....
....
....
....
....
....
....
....
....
....
....
....

RATE: *63/min*
RHYTHM: *Irregular*
P WAVE: *Sinus*
PR INTERVAL: *0.14-0.16 sec*
QRS COMPLEX: *0.06-0.08 sec*
RYTHYM INTERPRETATION: *Sinus arrhythmia*

TREATMENT: ....
....
....
....
....
....
....
....
....
....
....
....
....
....

RATE: *188/min*
RHYTHM: *Regular*
P WAVE: *Not discernible*
PR INTERVAL: *Unmeasurable*
QRS COMPLEX: *0.06-0.08 sec*
RYTHYM INTERPRETATION: *Paroxysmal supraventricular tachycardia*

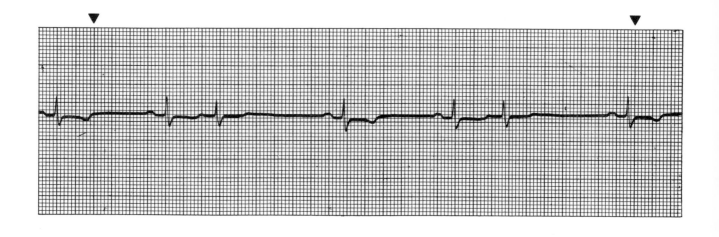

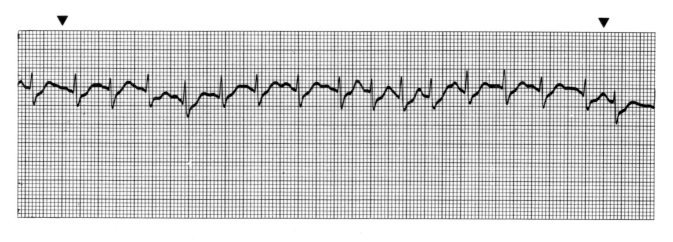

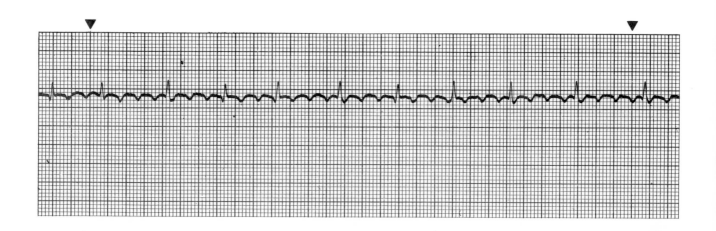

RATE: *Basic rate 50/min*
RHYTHM: *Irregular*
P WAVE: *Sinus P waves present; premature,
abnormal P waves with premature complexes*
PR INTERVAL: *0.20 sec*
QRS COMPLEX: *0.08 sec*
RYTHYM INTERPRETATION: *Sinus bradycardia with
two premature atrial complexes*

RATE: *Atrial, 400/min or more; ventricular,
150/min*
RHYTHM: *Irregular*
P WAVE: *Fibrillation waves*
PR INTERVAL: *Not discernible*
QRS COMPLEX: *0.08 sec*
RYTHYM INTERPRETATION: *Atrial fibrillation*

RATE: *Atrial, 300/min; ventricular, 90/min*
RHYTHM: *Irregular*
P WAVE: *Flutter waves*
PR INTERVAL: *Not discernible*
QRS COMPLEX: *0.06-0.08 sec*
RYTHYM INTERPRETATION: *Atrial flutter with
variable AV conduction*

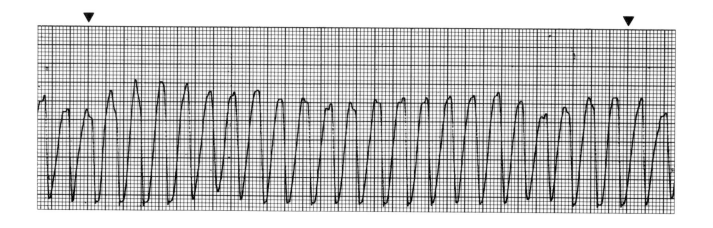

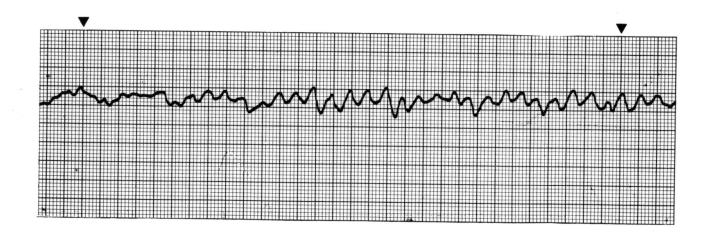

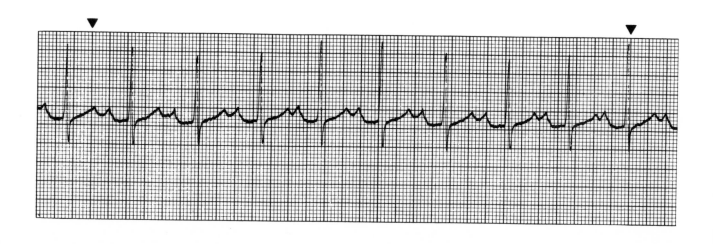

RATE: *230/min*
RHYTHM: *Regular*
P WAVE: *Not identified*
PR INTERVAL: *Not discernible*
QRS COMPLEX: *0.16-0.18 sec*
RYTHYM INTERPRETATION: *Ventricular tachycardia*

TREATMENT:

RATE: *0*
RHYTHM: *Chaotic*
P WAVE: *Absent; wave deflections are irregular and chaotic and vary in height, size, and shape.*
PR INTERVAL: *Not discernible*
QRS COMPLEX: *Absent*
RYTHYM INTERPRETATION: *Ventricular fibrillation*

TREATMENT:

RATE: *94/min*
RHYTHM: *Regular*
P WAVE: *Sinus P waves present*
PR INTERVAL: *0.28 sec*
QRS COMPLEX: *0.08 sec*
RYTHYM INTERPRETATION: *Sinus rhythm with first degree AV block*

TREATMENT:

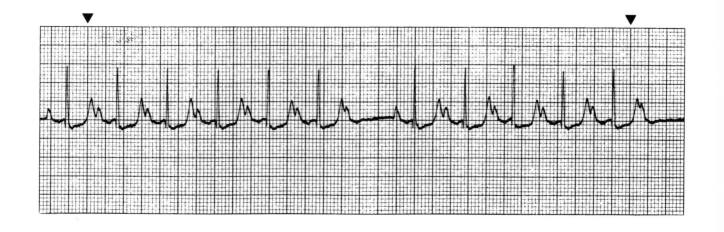

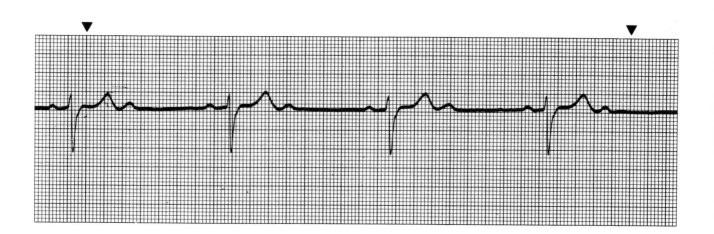

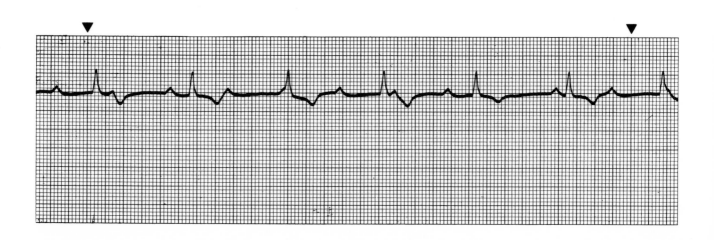

TREATMENT: ....

RATE: *Atrial, 107/min; ventricular, 100/min*
RHYTHM: *Irregular*
P WAVE: *Sinus P waves present*
PR INTERVAL: *0.20 sec, lengthening to 0.24 sec*
QRS COMPLEX: *0.04 sec*
RYTHYM INTERPRETATION: *Sinus tachycardia with second degree AV block, type I*

TREATMENT: ....

RATE: *Atrial, 70/min; ventricular, 35/min*
RHYTHM: *Regular*
P WAVE: *Two sinus P waves to each QRS complex*
PR INTERVAL: *0.22 sec and constant*
QRS COMPLEX: *0.10 sec*
RYTHYM INTERPRETATION: *Sinus rhythm with 2:1 second degree AV block, type II. Clinical correlation is suggested to diagnose type II when 2:1 conduction is present.*

TREATMENT: ....

RATE: *Atrial, 94/min; ventricular, 58/min*
RHYTHM: *Regular*
P WAVE: *Sinus P waves not relating to the QRS complexes*
PR INTERVAL: *Varies greatly*
QRS COMPLEX: *0.08 sec*
RYTHYM INTERPRETATION: *Sinus rhythm; complete heart block with pacemaker origin from the AV node*

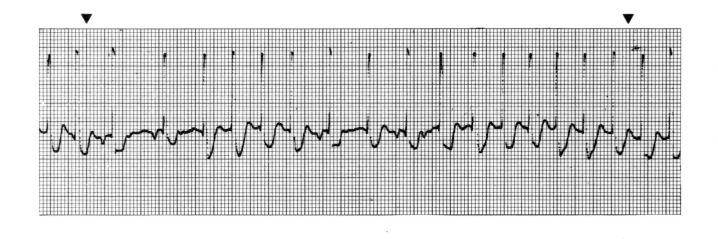

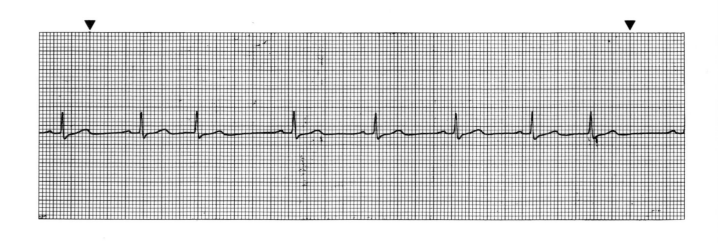

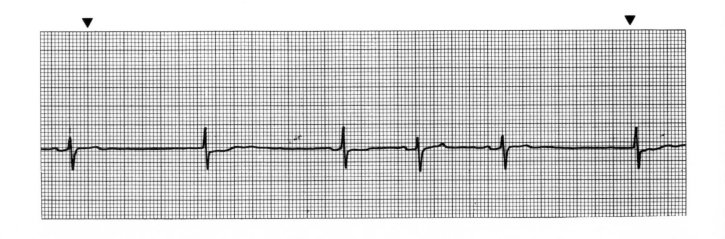

TREATMENT: ....
....
....
....
....
....
....
....
....
....
....
....
....

RATE: *Atrial, 400/min or greater; ventricular, 160/min*
RHYTHM: *Irregular*
P WAVE: *Fibrillation waves*
PR INTERVAL: *Not discernible*
QRS COMPLEX: *0.04-0.06 sec*
RYTHYM INTERPRETATION: *Atrial fibrillation*

TREATMENT: ....
....
....
....
....
....
....
....
....
....
....
....
....

RATE: *Basic rate 72/min*
RHYTHM: *Irregular*
P WAVE: *Sinus P waves present*
PR INTERVAL: *0.16 sec*
QRS COMPLEX: *0.08 sec*
RYTHYM INTERPRETATION: *Sinus rhythm with two premature junctional complexes*

TREATMENT: ....
....
....
....
....
....
....
....
....
....
....
....
....

RATE: *Basic rate 63/min*
RHYTHM: *Irregular*
P WAVE: *Sinus P waves present*
PR INTERVAL: *0.18 sec*
QRS COMPLEX: *0.06-0.08 sec*
RYTHYM INTERPRETATION: *Sinus rhythm with sinus arrest and two junctional escape complexes (complexes 2 and 6) and one atrial escape complex (complex 3)*

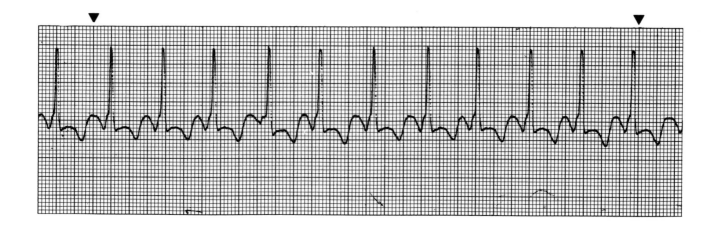

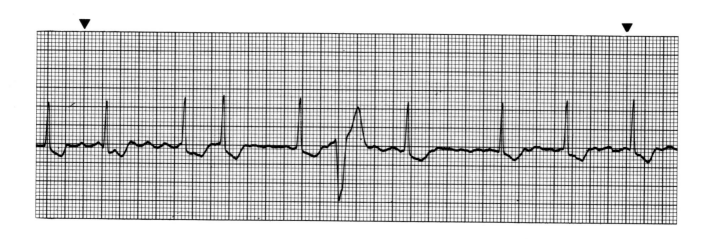

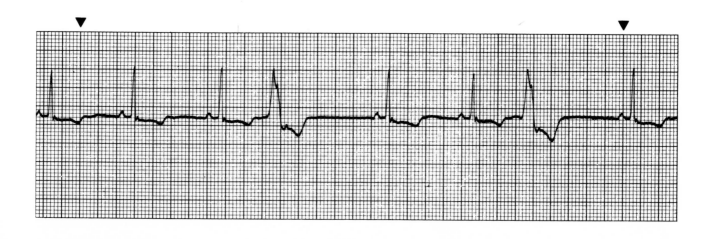

TREATMENT: ....
....
....
....
....
....
....
....
....
....
....
....
....

RATE: *107/min*
RHYTHM: *Regular*
P WAVE: *Inverted*
PR INTERVAL: *0.08 sec*
QRS COMPLEX: *0.06-0.08 sec*
RYTHYM INTERPRETATION: *Junctional tachycardia*

TREATMENT: ....
....
....
....
....
....
....
....
....
....
....
....
....

RATE: *Atrial, 400/min or more; ventricular, 80/min*
RHYTHM: *Irregular*
P WAVE: *Atrial fibrillation waves present*
PR INTERVAL: *Not discernible*
QRS COMPLEX: *0.06 sec (sinus complexes)*
            0.12 sec (premature complex)
RYTHYM INTERPRETATION: *Atrial fibrillation with a
premature ventricular complex*

TREATMENT: ....
....
....
....
....
....
....
....
....
....
....
....
....

RATE: *63/min*
RHYTHM: *Irregular*
P WAVE: *Sinus P waves present*
PR INTERVAL: *0.12-014 sec*
QRS COMPLEX: *0.04 sec*
            *0.12-0.14 sec (premature
            complexes)*
RYTHYM INTERPRETATION: *Sinus rhythm with two
premature ventricular complexes*

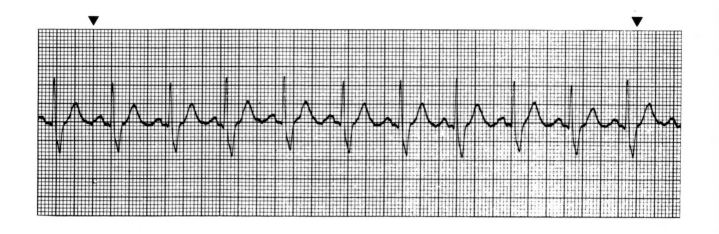

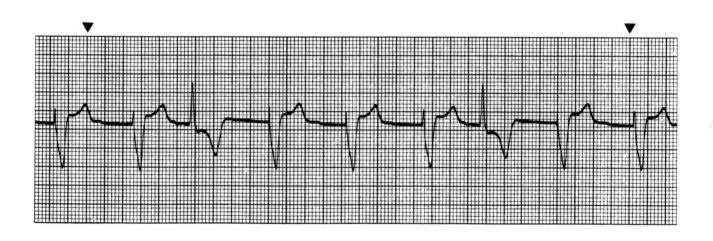

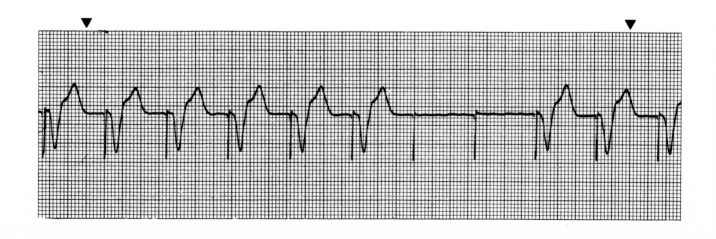

TREATMENT: ....
....
....
....
....
....
....
....
....
....
....
....
....

RATE: *94/min*
RHYTHM: *Regular*
P WAVE: *Sinus P waves present*
PR INTERVAL: *0.16 sec*
QRS COMPLEX: *0.12-0.14 sec*
RYTHYM INTERPRETATION: *Sinus rhythm with bundle branch block*

TREATMENT: ....
....
....
....
....
....
....
....
....
....
....
....
....

AUTOMATIC INTERVAL RATE: *72/min*
ANALYSIS: *The first two complexes are paced complexes, followed by a partient complex, three paced complexes, a patient complex, and two paced complexes.*
INTERPRETATION: *Normal pacemaker function*

TREATMENT: ....
....
....
....
....
....
....
....
....
....
....
....
....

AUTOMATIC INTERVAL RATE: *88/min*
ANALYSIS: *The first six complexes are paced complexes, followed by two pacemaker spikes with loss of capture and three paced complexes.*
INTERPRETATION: *Loss of capture*

Brand Name: Adenocard

Mechanism of Action:
Slows conduction through AV node; can interrupt re-entrant pathways through the AV node
Slows sinus rate
Has a direct effect upon supraventricular tissue

Indications and Field Use:
Conversion of supraventricular tachycardias, including those caused by Wolff-Parkinson-White syndrome
Not effective in conversion of atrial fibrillation or flutter or ventricular tachycardia

Adult Dosage:
6 mg IV bolus as rapidly as possible, followed by flushing the IV line, if rhythm does not convert within 2 minutes, repeat using 12 mg bolus

Pediatric Dosage:
Not used

Brand Name: None

Mechanism of Action:
Competitive inhibitor of acetylcholine in smooth muscle and glands, blocking parasympathetic response and allowing sympathetic response to take over

Indications and Field Use:
Sinus bradycardia with significant hypotension or ventricular ectopy
AV block
Asystole
Organophosphate insecticide poisoning
Counteracts physostigmine (Antilirium), neostigmine, edrophonium (Tensilon)

Adult Dosage:
Bradycardia: 0.5-1.0 mg rapid IV push or ET
Asystole: 1.0 mg rapid IV push or ET
(For either) - may be repeated at 5 minute intervals; maximum of 2 mg except in insecticide poisoning

Pediatric Dosage:
0.01 mg/kg (minimum of 0.2 mg) rapid IV push

Brand Name: Proventil, Ventolin

Mechanism of Action:
β agonist (primarily β_2)—relaxes bronchial smooth muscle, resulting in bronchodilation
Also relaxes vascular and uterine smooth muscle

Indications and Field Use:
Treatment of bronchospasm from emphysema or asthma
Prevention of exercise-induced bronchospasm

Adult Dosage:
Give 2.5 mg; dilute 0.5 ml of the 0.5% solution for inhalation with 2.5 ml normal saline in nebulizer over 10-15 minutes
2 inhalations with metered-dose inhaler every 4-6 hours

Pediatric Dosage:
Not recommended in children younger than 12 years

Brand Name: Bretylol

Mechanism of Action:
Elevates ventricular fibrillation threshold
Biphasic autonomic (sympathetic) response—transient, slight adrenergic (sympathetic) response (increased heart rate, blood pressure, cardiac output, and possibly ventricular ectopy) due to norepinephrine release from nerve terminals, followed by a decrease in arterial pressure from vasodilation (due to norepinephrine depletion)

Indications and Field Use:
Intractable ventricular fibrillation and ventricular tachycardia as a second-line drug

Adult Dosage:
5 mg/kg (350-500 mg) initially, over 1 minute
10 mg/kg (700-1000 mg) second dose, if needed, 10 minutes later (second dose is twice the first dose); total dose generally 30 mg/kg followed by infusion of 2 mg/min

Pediatric Dosage:
Same as adult (rarely given)

Brand Name: Cyanide Antidote Package

Mechanism of Action:
Amyl nitrite - has affinity for cyanide ions; reacts with hemoglobin to form methemoglobin (low toxicity)
Sodium nitrite - same as amyl nitrite
Sodium thiosulfate - produces thiocyanate, which is then excreted

Indications and Field Use:
Cyanide or hydrocyanic acid poisoning

Adult Dosage:
Amyl nitrite—breathe 30 seconds out of every minute
Sodium thiosulfate and sodium nitrite—dose dependent on hemoglobin level

Pediatric Dosage:
Same as adult

Brand Name: Decadron, Hexadrol

Mechanism of Action:
Enters target cells and binds to cytoplasmic receptors, thereby initiating many complex reactions that are responsible for its anti-inflammatory and immunosuppressive effects

Indications and Field Use:
Elevated intracranial pressure (prevention and treatment)
Shock (as an adjunct to other treatment)
Anaphylaxis
Status asthmaticus
Croup

Adult Dosage:
1 mg/kg slow IV bolus

Pediatric Dosage:
40-60 mcg/kg slow IV bolus

atropine sulfate

adenosine

bretylium tosylate

albuterol

dexamethasone sodium phosphate

amyl nitrite,
sodium nitrite,
sodium thiosulfate

Brand Name: None

Mechanism of Action:
Rapidly increases serum glucose levels
Provides short-term osmotic diuresis

Indications and Field Use:
Coma of unknown origin
Hypoglycemia
Status epilepticus

Adult Dosage:
25-50 g IV bolus

Pediatric Dosage:
Give 25% dextrose 2-4 ml/kg IV bolus

Brand Name: Benadryl

Mechanism of Action:
Blocks cellular histamine receptors, but does not prevent histamine release; results in decreased capillary permeability and decreased vasodilation, as well as prevention of bronchospasm
Antiemetic - decreases motion sickness
Sedation

Indications and Field Use:
Anaphylaxis
Phenothiazine reactions
Blood administration reactions
Over-the-counter drug used for motion sickness, hay fever, and as a hypnotic
May also be used to treat side effects of some antipsychotic drugs

Adult Dosage:
25-100 mg IV push over 1-4 minutes
May also be given deep IM

Pediatric Dosage:
2-5 mg/kg IV push over 1-4 minutes
May also be given deep IM

Brand Name: Valium

Mechanism of Action:
Affects multiple levels of CNS to decrease seizures by increasing the seizure threshold
Transient analgesia
Amnesic
Sedative

Indications and Field Use:
Grand mal seizures, especially status epilepticus
Agitation secondary to head injury or hypoxia (treat the cause first)
Transient analgesia/amnesia for medical procedures (e.g., fracture reduction, cardioversion)
Delirium tremens

Adult Dosage:
5-10 mg slow IV push; can repeat at 10-15 minute intervals; administer no faster than 5 mg/minute

Pediatric Dosage:
0.2 - 0.3 mg/kg every 15-30 minutes (max. of 10 mg/kg); administer IV over at least 3 minutes or until seizure activity subsides

Brand Name: Intropin

Mechanism of Action:
Immediate metabolic precursor to norepinephrine
Effects are dose-dependent:
  1-2 mcg/kg/minute—acts on dopaminergic receptors to dilate vessels in kidneys and mesentery; no change in HR or BP; may increase urine output
  2-10 mcg/kg/minute—primarily β_1 stimulant action; increased chronotropy and inotropy
  10-20 mcg/kg/minute—primarily α stimulant; peripheral vasoconstriction
  20 mcg/kg/minute—reversal of renal effects by overriding α effects

Indications and Field Use:
Cardiogenic, septic, or spinal shock
Electromechanical dissociation

Adult Dosage:
2-20 mcg/kg/minute IV infusion

Pediatric Dosage:
Same as adult

Brand Name: Hyperstat

Mechanism of Action:
Non-diuretic antihypertensive—acts directly on arterioles resulting in dilation, probably by antagonizing calcium
Decreases afterload by causing arteriolar dilation

Indications and Field Use:
Hypertensive crisis, especially in pre-eclampsia

Adult Dosage:
5 mg/kg or 300 mg, undiluted; give rapid IV push over 10-30 seconds

Pediatric Dosage:
5 mg/kg

Brand Name: Adrenalin

Mechanism of Action:
α-bronchial, cutaneous, renal, and visceral arteriolar constriction
β_1-positive inotropic and chronotropic actions
β_2-bronchial smooth muscle relaxation and dilation of skeletal vasculature

Indications and Field Use:
Cardiac arrest
Severe bronchospasm, i.e., bronchiolitis, asthma
Anaphylaxis

Adult Dosage:
Cardiac dosage: use 1:10,000 solution; give 0.5-1.0 mg every 5 minutes, IV or ET
Anaphylaxis and asthma: use 1:1000 solution, give 0.1-0.5 mg SQ or IM; or use 1:10,000 solution; give 0.3-0.5 mg ET or IV if cardiovascular collapse occurs

Pediatric Dosage:
Cardiac: use 1:10,000 solution; give 0.01 mg/kg every 5 minutes, IV or ET.
Asthma/anaphylaxis/bronchiolitis: use 1:1000 solution; give 0.01 mg/kg SQ (maximum of 0.35 mg/dose)

diphenhydramine

dextrose 50%

dopamine

diazepam

epinephrine

diazoxide

Brand Name: Lasix

Mechanism of Action:
Potent diuretic—inhibits electrolyte reabsorption in the ascending Loop of Henle, and promotes excretion of sodium, potassium, chloride
Vasodilation, which increases venous capacitance and decreases afterload

Indications and Field Use:
Pulmonary edema; congestive heart failure

Adult Dosage:
0.5-1 mg/kg (usually 20-80 mg) IV, no faster than 20 mg/minute (if dose is > 40 mg, give at 4 mg/min)

Pediatric Dosage:
1 mg/kg IV

Brand Name: Bronkosol, Bronkometer

Mechanism of Action:
β_2 agonist: relaxes smooth muscle of bronchioles, vasculature, uterus

Indications and Field Use:
Acute bronchial asthma
Bronchospasm

Adult Dosage:
1-2 inhalations with metered-dose inhaler

Pediatric Dosage:
Not recommended in children less than 12 years

Brand Name: Apresoline

Mechanism of Action:
Vasodilator—decreases systemic vascular resistance; has a direct effect on vascular smooth muscle, more pronounced on arterioles than venules
Decreases diastolic blood pressure more than systolic
Increases heart rate, cardiac output, stroke volume
Increases blood flow to heart, brain, and kidneys

Indications and Field Use:
Moderate to severe hypertension (rarely used in the field)
Pre-eclampsia

Adult Dosage:
20-40 mg slow IV push over 1-2 minutes; titrate to effect; may repeat in 4-6 hrs; or 10-40 mg IM

Pediatric Dosage:
1.7-3.5 mg/kg daily; do not exceed 20 mg

Brand Name: Isuprel

Mechanism of Action:
β agonist, especially β_1 - positive inotropy and chronotropy
Bronchodilation
Relaxes GI, vascular, and uterine smooth muscle
Stimulates insulin secretion

Indications and Field Use:
Atropine-refractory bradycardia, including complete heart block
Refractory bronchospasm

Adult Dosage:
2-10 mcg/minute IV infusion and titrate for effect

Pediatric Dosage:
0.1 mcg/kg/minute

Brand Name: Solu-Cortef

Mechanism of Action:
Enters target cells and binds to cytoplasmic receptors, thereby initiating many complex reactions that are responsible for its anti-inflammatory and immunosuppressive and salt-retaining actions

Indications and Field Use:
Status asthmaticus
Shock due to acute adrenocortical insufficiency (abrupt cessation of cortisone therapy)

Adult Dosage:
4 mg/kg slow IV bolus
In anaphylaxis—500 mg bolus to prevent recurrence of symptoms (not a first-line drug)

Pediatric Dosage:
0.16-1.0 mg/kg slow IV bolus

Brand Name: Xylocaine

Mechanism of Action:
Decreases automaticity by slowing the rate of spontaneous phase 4 depolarization
Terminates re-entry by decreasing conduction in re-entrant pathways
Increases ventricular fibrillation threshold

Indications and Field Use:
Suppression of ventricular arrhythmias (ventricular tachycardia, ventricular fibrillation, PVC's)
Prophylaxis against ectopy in suspected acute myocardial infarction
Prophylaxis against recurrence after conversion from ventricular tachycardia or ventricular fibrillation
Frequent PVC's (more than 6 per minute, 2 or more PVC's in a row, multiform PVC's, or R-on-T phenomena)

Adult Dosage:
1 mg/kg IV bolus no faster than 50 mg/minute (may also be given IM, ET) followed by infusion of 1-4 mg/minute if bolus has been successful at terminating the arrhythmia

Pediatric Dosage:
Same as adult (rarely used)
Followed by infusion of 20-50 mcg/kg/min

isoetharine

furosemide

isoproterenol

hydralazine

lidocaine HCl (2%)

hydrocortisone sodium succinate

Brand Name: Nubain

Mechanism of Action:
Synthetic narcotic agonist/antagonist—analgesia occurs due to
activation of an opiate receptor in the limbic system of the CNS;
also acts as opiate antagonist due to competitive inhibition at
receptors

Indications and Field Use:
Moderate to severe pain—has less respiratory depressant effect
than opiate-derivatives

Adult Dosage:
10-20 mg slow IV push or IM

Pediatric Dosage:
Not recommended

Brand Name: Narcan

Mechanism of Action:
Competitive inhibition at narcotic receptor sites
Reverses respiratory depression secondary to depressant drugs

Indications and Field Use:
Antidote for:
  Narcotics
  Lomotil
  Talwin
  Darvon
Occasionally given for diazepam overdose
Differentiates drug-induced coma from other causes

Adult Dosage:
0.4 - 2.0 mg IV, IM, SQ, SL, ET
Titrate to respiratory effort and rate

Pediatric Dosage:
0.01 mg/kg

Brand Name: Procardia

Mechanism of Action:
Arterial and venous vasodilator; both actions reduce cardiac
work and oxygen demand (reduced afterload and preload)

Indications and Field Use:
Hypertensive crisis
Congestive heart failure
Angina

Adult Dosage:
10-20 mg sublingual

Pediatric Dosage:
Not used

Brand Name: Nitrostat, Tridil

Mechanism of Action:
Smooth muscle relaxant acting on vascular, uterine, bronchial,
and intestinal smooth muscle
Reduces workload on the heart by causing blood pooling
(decreased preload) and peripheral vasodilation (decreased
afterload).
Coronary artery vasodilation

Indications and Field Use:
Angina
Congestive heart failure

Adult Dosage:
IV (Tri-dil): 5 mcg/minute; increase in increments of 5 mcg,
monitoring pain and blood pressure
Sublingual (Nitro-stat): 1/150 gr (0.4 mg) tablet
Topical: 1 inch of paste
Aerosol: Spray preparation delivers 0.4 mg/metered dose. Spray
1-2 metered doses onto oral mucosa; no more than 3 doses/15
minutes should be used

Pediatric Dosage:
Not used

Brand Name: None

Mechanism of Action:
Exact mechanism unknown; affects phospholipids in CNS

Indications and Field Use:
Moderate to severe pain
Surgical or diagnostic procedures such as burn or abrasion
debridement, fracture reduction, dental procedures
Childbirth
Renal colic

Adult Dosage:
Less than 30 minutes/episode, mixed with oxygen (at least 50%
oxygen is required to prevent hypoxia)

Pediatric Dosage:
Same as adult

Brand Name: Levophed, Levarterenol

Mechanism of Action:
Potent α agonist (90% α, 10% β_1 effects), causing intense
vasoconstriction
Positive chronotropic action (can be overcome by vagal response
to increasing arterial pressure)
Increased inotropism (from β_1 effects) and increased cardiac
output, if bradycardia is not present

Indications and Field Use:
Second-line pressor for cardiogenic shock, other forms of shock
with low or normal peripheral vascular resistance (for example,
spinal shock)

Adult Dosage:
2-4 mcg/minute, up to 20 mcg/minute IV infusion and titrate to
desired blood pressure (usually 80-100 systolic)
Mix in D_5W, not 0.9% NaCl

Pediatric Dosage:
0.1 mcg/kg/min IV infusion

nitroglycerin

nalbuphine HCl

nitrous oxide

naloxone

norepinephrine

nifedipine

Brand Name: Osmitrol

Mechanism of Action:
Promotes rapid diuresis by increasing osmotic pressure in renal glomeruli - hinders water reabsorption in the renal tubules

Indications and Field Use:
Cerebral edema

Adult Dosage:
1.5-2 g/kg IV infusion

Pediatric Dosage:
2 g/kg IV infusion

Brand Name: Aramine

Mechanism of Action:
Direct effects: α and β stimulator, increases chronotropy, inotropy, peripheral vascular resistance
Indirect effects: causes release of norepinephrine from nerve endings
Results in severe vasoconstriction

Indications and Field Use:
Hypotension not due to hypovolemia
Not a drug of choice in the field

Adult Dosage:
0.5-5 mg IV push, then titrated to effect

Pediatric Dosage:
Same as adult

Brand Name: Demerol, Pethadol

Mechanism of Action:
Acts on opiate receptors in the sensory cortex of frontal lobes and diencephalon
Interferes with perception of pain

Indications and Field Use:
Moderate to severe pain

Adult Dosage:
50-150 mg IM every 3-4 hours when required
10-50 mg slow IV push

Pediatric Dosage:
1-1.8 mg/kg every 4 hours to maximum of 100 mg IM

Brand Name: Solu-Medrol

Mechanism of Action:
Enters target cells and binds to cytoplasmic receptors, thereby initiating many complex reactions that are responsible for its anti-inflammatory and immunosuppressive effects

Indications and Field Use:
Adjunct in treatment of:
  Hypovolemic shock
  Anaphylaxis
  Esophageal and airway burns
  Cerebral edema
  Septic shock

Adult Dosage:
15-30 mg/kg, up to 1 g slow IV bolus

Pediatric Dosage:
30-200 mcg/kg slow IV bolus

Brand Name: Alupent, Metaprel

Mechanism of Action:
β_2 agonist - acts directly on bronchial smooth muscle

Indications and Field Use:
Bronchospasm of COPD and asthma

Adult Dosage:
2.5 ml of an 0.4% or 0.6% unit dose (10 or 15 mg of drug, respectively) in nebulizer over 10-15 minutes

Pediatric Dosage:
Not recommended in children under 12 years

Brand Name: None

Mechanism of Action:
Alleviates pain by acting on the sensory cortex of frontal lobes and the diencephalon
Depresses fear and anxiety centers
Depresses brainstem respiratory centers—decreases responsiveness to changes in $PaCO_2$
Increases venous capacitance (venous pooling); and vasodilates arterioles, reducing afterload

Indications and Field Use:
Analgesia, especially in patients with burns, myocardial infarction, or renal colic
Pulmonary edema

Adult Dosage:
2-20 mg slow IV push; repeat as required; patient response is variable - use lowest effective dose

Pediatric Dosage:
100-200 mcg/kg slow IV push

metaraminol bitartrate

mannitol 20%

methylprednisolone
sodium succinate

meperidine

morphine sulfate

metaproterenol sulfate

Brand Name: Vaponefrin

Mechanism of Action:

α and β agonist: arteriole constriction; positive inotropic, positive chronotropic; bronchial smooth muscle relaxer (bronchodilator)

Also blocks histamine release, inhibits insulin secretion (can lead to hyperglycemia), relaxes GI smooth muscle

Indications and Field Use:

Croup

Post extubation edema

Laryngeal angioneurotic edema

Bronchospasm (as a second-line drug)

Adult Dosage:

0.5-0.8 ml in 4 ml normal saline by nebulizer over 10-15 minutes

Pediatric Dosage:

0.3-0.5 ml in 4 ml normal saline by updraft nebulizer over 10-15 minutes

---

Brand Name: Aminophylline

Mechanism of Action:

β_2 agonist: directly relaxes bronchial smooth muscle

Dilates pulmonary and coronary arterioles, decreasing pulmonary hypertension and increasing coronary blood flow

Indications and Field Use:

Asthma or bronchospasm

Bronchospasm secondary to asthma, COPD, or anaphylaxis

Pulmonary edema

Adult Dosage:

Loading dose of 6 mg/kg IV infusion diluted in 100 ml D_5W or normal saline over 20 minutes if patient has had no theophylline products in the last 36 hours

Loading dose of 1 mg/kg IV infusion diluted in 100 ml D_5W or normal saline over 20 minutes if patient has had theophylline products in the last 36 hours

Pediatric Dosage:

Over 1 year, same loading dose as adult; in $D_5 0.9\%NaCl$

Brand Name: None

Mechanism of Action:

Buffers H^+ in metabolic acidosis, lactic acid is the major source of H^+ in metabolic acidosis in cardiac arrest

Indications and Field Use:

Cardiac arrest

Overdose of aspirin, tricyclic antidepressants

With available blood gas results used in acidosis secondary to shock or other causes

Adult Dosage:

1 mEq/kg IV bolus

First dose usually 1 mEq/kg, with subsequent doses of 0.5 mEq/kg every 10 minutes in cardiac arrest; generally used in cardiac arrest after other standard treatment (defibrillation, intubation, epinephrine injection) has been used

Pediatric Dosage:

Same; used less liberally in children - can actually contribute to acidosis and cause fluid overload

---

Brand Name: Betalin

Mechanism of Action:

Required for carbohydrate metabolism

Deficiency leads to: anemia, polyneuritis, Wernicke's encephalopathy, cardiomyopathy

Administration may reverse symptoms of deficiency, but effects are dependent upon duration of illness and severity of disease

Indications and Field Use:

Alcoholism, delirium tremens

Other thiamine deficiency syndromes

Adult Dosage:

100 mg

Pediatric Dosage:

Rarely used

Brand Name: Bricanyl, Brethine

Mechanism of Action:

β_2 agonist - has an affinity for β_2 receptors of bronchial, vascular, and uterine smooth muscle

At increased doses, β_1 effects may occur

Indications and Field Use:

Bronchospasm (more prevalent in patients over the age of 40 or with coronary artery disease)

Used in-hospital to stop preterm labor

Adult Dosage:

0.25 mg SQ; repeat in 15-20 minutes

2 inhalations separated by a 60-second interval with a metered dose inhaler

Pediatric Dosage:

Not recommended for patients under the age of 12 years

Brand Name: Isoptin, Calan, Verelan

Mechanism of Action:

Blocks calcium influx into cardiac and smooth muscle cells, causing a depressant effect on the contractile mechanism and resulting in negative inotropy

Reduces contractile tone in vascular smooth muscle resulting in coronary and peripheral vasodilation

Slows conduction and prolongs refractory period in the AV node due to calcium channel blocking

Slows SA node discharge

Indications and Field Use:

Supraventricular tachycardia

Atrial fibrillation and atrial flutter with rapid ventricular response

Adult Dosage:

0.075-0.15 mg/kg (5-10 mg) IV over 2-3 minutes (maximum of 10-15 mg)

Pediatric Dosage:

0.1-0.3 mg/kg over 2-3 minutes, maximum 5 mg

theophylline
ethylenediamine

racemic epinephrine

thiamine (vitamin B)

sodium bicarbonate

verapamil HCl

terbutaline sulfate

Brand Name: Pitocin, Syntocin

Mechanism of Action:
Increases amplitude and frequency of uterine contractions
Dilation of vascular smooth muscle (increases renal, coronary, and cerebral blood flow)

Indications and Field Use:
Postpartum hemorrhage
Used in-hospital for induction of labor

Adult Dosage:
10-20 USP units/liter at rate of 1-4 ml/minute

Pediatric Dosage:
Not applicable

Brand Name: Luminal Sodium

Mechanism of Action:
Not well understood - cerebral depression by interference with transmission of impulses at the cerebral cortex
Also interferes with the reticular activating system

Indications and Field Use:
Seizures
Status epilepticus

Adult Dosage:
200-600 mg slow IV bolus at 25-50 mg/minute

Pediatric Dosage:
10-20 mg/kg slow IV push over 5-10 minutes

Brand Name: Dilantin

Mechanism of Action:
Inhibits cerebral seizure focus from spreading into adjacent areas
Depresses pacemaker automaticity
Improves AV conduction by decreasing AV node refractory period, especially in digitalis toxicity
Negative inotropy

Indications and Field Use:
Prophylaxis and treatment of recurrent seizures, in conjunction with more rapid-acting drugs such as diazepam
Not a first-line cardiac drug, except rarely in cases of digitalis toxicity
Ventricular arrhythmias

Adult Dosage:
16-18 mg/kg (700-1000 mg) slow IV push at 25-50 mg/minute or less; flush with saline

Pediatric Dosage:
Same as adult

Brand Name: Antilirium

Mechanism of Action:
Acetylcholinesterase inhibitor—increases concentration of acetylcholine at receptor sites by preventing its breakdown (parasympathetic stimulator)

Indications and Field Use:
Reverses atropine-like drugs (for example, street drugs, jimsonweed)
May inhibit CNS depressant effects of Valium, tricyclic antidepressants, antihistamines, phenothiazines

Adult Dosage:
1-4 mg slow IV push over 1-2 minutes (no faster than 1 mg/minute)
May repeat a 1-2 mg dose in 20 minutes if needed

Pediatric Dosage:
0.5 mg over 1 minute
May be repeated every 5-10 minutes to maximum of 2 mg

Brand Name: Pronestyl

Mechanism of Action:
Decreases automaticity by suppressing phase 4 depolarization, especially in the His-Purkinje system
Slows conduction velocity by depressing the rate of rise of phase 0
Prolongs effective refractory period and action potential duration in the His-Purkinje system
Shortens effective refractory period of AV node
Some anticholinergic properties which may affect SA and AV nodes to increase heart rate

Indications and Field Use:
Ventricular tachycardia
May also be used to treat PVC's, supraventricular tachycardia, atrial fibrillation with rapid ventricular response

Adult Dosage:
100 mg every 5 minutes (or 20 mg/minute) until ectopy is suppressed, to a maximum of 1 g
If successful, follow with infusion of 1-4 mg/minute

Pediatric Dosage:
Not given

Brand Name: Inderal

Mechanism of Action:
Blocks β receptor sites, causing the following:
  Decreased heart rate, cardiac output, contractility, and conduction
  Decreased myocardial oxygen consumption
Stabilizes myocardial cell membrane

Indications and Field Use:
Rarely used in the field
May be used for:
  Paroxysmal supraventricular tachycardia
  β agonist or digitalis-induced ventricular arrhythmias
  Hyperthyroid crisis

Adult Dosage:
0.5-3.0 mg slow IVP; may repeat in 2 minutes, give smallest effective dose
Patients may also be taking Inderal orally for hypertension, history of tachycardias, or as an adjunct to rehabilitation of post-myocardial infarction

Pediatric Dosage:
10-20 mcg/kg IV over 10 minutes

physostigmine salicylate

oxytocin

procainamide

phenobarbital sodium

propranolol

phenytoin sodium

Advanced cardiac life support treatment protocol for bradycardia. (© American Heart Association: Textbook of Advanced Cardiac Life Support, 2nd ed. p 242. Dallas. American Heart Association. 1987)

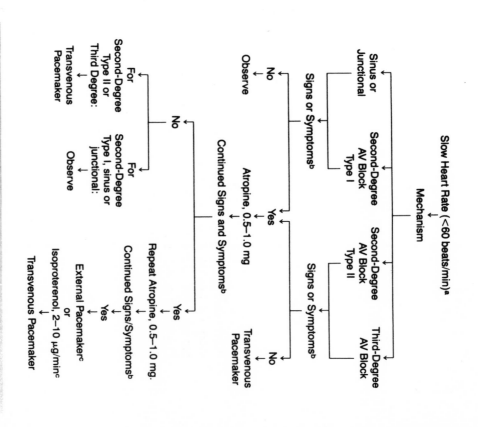

Bradycardia. This sequence was developed to assist in teaching how to treat a broad range of patients with bradycardia. Some patients may require care not specified herein. This algorithm should not be construed to prohibit such flexibility. AV = atrioventricular.

[a] A solitary chest (precordial) thump or cough may stimulate cardiac electrical activity and result in improved cardiac output. Either may be tried at this point.

[b] Hypotension (blood pressure <90 mmHg), premature ventricular contractions, altered mental status or physical symptoms (e.g., chest pain or dyspnea), ischemia, or infarction.

[c] Temporizing therapy.

Advanced cardiac life support treatment protocol for electromechanical dissociation. (© American Heart Association: Textbook of Advanced Cardiac Life Support, 2nd ed. p 240. Dallas. American Heart Association. 1987)

Advanced cardiac life support treatment protocol for paroxysmal supraventricular tachycardia. (© American Heart Association: Textbook of Advanced Cardiac Life Support, 2nd ed. p 244. Dallas. American Heart Association. 1987)

Continue CPR
↓
Establish IV access
↓
Epinephrine, 1:10,000, 0.5–1.0 mg IV push[a]
↓
Intubate when possible[b]
↓
(Consider bicarbonate)[c]
↓
Consider hypovolemia,
cardiac tamponade,
tension pneumothorax,
hypoxemia,
acidosis,
pulmonary embolism

Electromechanical dissociation. This sequence was developed to assist in teaching how to treat a broad range of patients with electromechanical dissociation. Some patients may require care not specified herein. This algorithm should not be construed to prohibit such flexibility. The flow of the algorithm presumes that electromechanical dissociation is continuing. CPR = cardiopulmonary resuscitation; IV = intravenous.

[a] Epinephrine should be repeated every 5 minutes.

[b] Intubation is preferable. If it can be accomplished simultaneously with other techniques, then the earlier the better. However, epinephrine is more important initially if the patient can be ventilated without intubation.

[c] The value of sodium bicarbonate is questionable during cardiac arrest, and it is not recommended for routine cardiac arrest sequences. Consideration of its use in a dose of 1 mEq/kg is appropriate at this point. Half of the original dose may be repeated every 10 minutes if it is used.

Unstable

Synchronous cardioversion
75–100 joules
↓
Synchronous cardioversion
200 joules
↓
Synchronous cardioversion
360 joules
↓
Correct underlying abnormalities
↓
Pharmacological therapy +
cardioversion

Stable

Vagal maneuvers
↓
Verapamil, 5 mg IV
↓
Verapamil, 10 mg IV
(in 15–20 min)
↓
Cardioversion, digoxin,
β-blockers, packing as indicated
(see textbook)

If conversion occurs but PSVT recurs, repeated electrical cardioversion is *not* indicated. Sedation should be used as time permits.

Paroxysmal supraventricular tachycardia (PSVT). This sequence was developed to assist in teaching how to treat a broad range of patients with sustained PSVT. Some patients may require care not specified herein. This algorithm should not be construed as prohibiting such flexibility. The flow of the algorithm presumes that PSVT is continuing. IV = intravenous.

Advanced cardiac life support treatment protocol for asystole. (© American Heart Association: Textbook of Advanced Cardiac Life Support, 2nd ed. p 243. Dallas. American Heart Association. 1987)

Advanced cardiac life support treatment protocol for ventricular ectopy (© American Heart Association: Textbook of Advanced Cardiac Life Support, 2nd ed. p 243. Dallas. American Heart Association. 1987)

If rhythm is unclear and possibly ventricular fibrillation, defibrillate as for VF.[a]

If asystole is present,[a]

↓

Continue CPR

↓

Establish IV access

↓

Epinephrine, 1:10,000, 0.5–1.0 mg IV push[b]

↓

Intubate when possible[c]

↓

Atropine, 1.0 mg IV push (repeated in 5 min)

↓

(Consider bicarbonate)[d]

↓

Consider pacing

Asystole (cardiac standstill). This sequence was developed to assist in teaching how to treat a broad range of patients with asystole. Some patients may require care not specified herein. This algorithm should not be construed to prohibit such flexibility. The flow of the algorithm presumes asystole is continuing. VF = ventricular fibrillation; IV = intravenous; CPR = cardiopulmonary resuscitation.

[a]Asystole should be confirmed in two leads.
[b]Epinephrine should be repeated every 5 minutes.
[c]intubation is preferable; if it can be accomplished simultaneously with other techniques, then the earlier the better. However, cardiopulmonary resuscitation (CPR) and the use of epinephrine are more important initially if the patient can be ventilated without intubation. (Endotracheal epinephrine may be used.)
[d]The value of sodium bicarbonate is questionable during cardiac arrest, and it is not recommended for routine cardiac arrest sequences. Consideration of its use in a dose of 1 mEq/kg is appropriate at this point. Half of the original dose may be repeated every 10 minutes if it is used.

Assess for need for
acute suppressive therapy

→ Rule out treatable cause
→ Consider serum potassium
→ Consider digitalis level
→ Consider bradycardia
→ Consider drugs

Lidocaine, 1 mg/kg

↓

If not suppressed,
repeat lidocaine, 0.5 mg/kg every 2–5 min,
until no ectopy, or up to 3 mg/kg given

↓

If not suppressed,
procainamide 20 mg/min
until no ectopy, or up to 1,000 mg given

↓

If not suppressed,
and not contraindicated,
bretylium, 5–10 mg/kg over 8–10 min

↓

If not suppressed,
consider overdrive pacing

Once ectopy is resolved, maintain as follows:
After lidocaine, 1 mg/kg .... Lidocaine drip, 2 mg/min
After lidocaine, 1–2 mg/kg ..... Lidocaine drip, 3 mg/min
After lidocaine, 2–3 mg/kg ..... Lidocaine drip, 4 mg/min
After procainamide .... Procainamide drip, 1–4 mg/min
(Check blood level.)
After bretylium .... Bretylium drip, 2 mg/min

Ventricular ectopy: acute suppressive therapy. This sequence was developed to assist in teaching how to treat a broad range of patients with ventricular ectopy. Some patients may require therapy not specified herein. This algorithm should not be construed as prohibiting such flexibility.

Advanced cardiac life support treatment protocol for ventricular tachycardia (© American Heart Association: Textbook of Advanced Cardiac Life Support, 2nd ed. p 241. Dallas. American Heart Association. 1987)

Advanced cardiac life support treatment protocol for ventricular fibrillation and pulseless ventricular tachycardia (© American Heart Association: Textbook of Advanced Cardiac Life Support, 2nd ed. p 238. Dallas. American Heart Association. 1987)

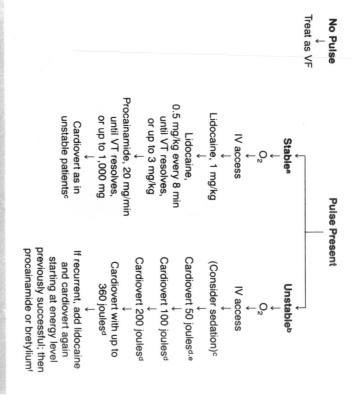

No Pulse
↓
Treat as VF

Pulse Present

Stable[a]
↓
IV access
↓
O₂
↓
Lidocaine, 1 mg/kg
↓
Lidocaine, 0.5 mg/kg every 8 min until VT resolves, or up to 3 mg/kg
↓
Procainamide, 20 mg/min until VT resolves, or up to 1,000 mg
↓
Cardiovert as in unstable patients[c]

Unstable[b]
↓
IV access
↓
O₂
↓
(Consider sedation)[c]
↓
Cardiovert 50 joules[d,e]
↓
Cardiovert 100 joules[d]
↓
Cardiovert 200 joules[d]
↓
Cardiovert with up to 360 joules[d]
↓
If recurrent, add lidocaine and cardiovert again starting at energy level previously successful; then procainamide or bretylium[f]

Sustained ventricular tachycardia (VT). This sequence was developed to assist in teaching how to treat a broad range of patients with sustained VT. Some patients may require care not specified herein. This algorithm should not be construed as prohibiting such flexibility. The flow of the algorithm presumes that VT is continuing. VF = ventricular fibrillation; IV = intravenous.
[a]If the patient becomes unstable (see footnote b for definition) at any time, move to "Unstable" arm of algorithm.
[b]Unstable indicates symptoms (e.g., chest pain or dyspnea), hypotension (systolic blood pressure <90 mmHg), congestive heart failure, ischemia, or infarction.
[c]Sedation should be considered for all patients, including those defined in footnote b as unstable, except those who are hemodynamically unstable (e.g., hypotensive, in pulmonary edema, or unconscious).
[d]If hypotension, pulmonary edema, or unconsciousness is present, unsynchronized cardioversion should be done to avoid the delay associated with synchronization.
[e]In the absence of hypotension, pulmonary edema, or unconsciousness, a precordial thump may be employed prior to cardioversion.
[f]Once VT has resolved, begin intravenous infusion of the antiarrhythmic agent that has aided resolution of VT. If hypotension, pulmonary edema, or unconsciousness is present, use lidocaine if cardioversion alone is unsuccessful, followed by bretylium. In all other patients, the recommended order of therapy is lidocaine, procainamide, and then bretylium.

Witnessed Arrest   **Unwitnessed Arrest**
Check pulse — If no pulse   Check pulse — If no pulse
↓
Precordial thump
↓
Check pulse — If no pulse
↓
CPR until a defibrillator is available
↓
Check monitor for rhythm — if VF or VT
↓
Defibrillate, 200 joules[b]
↓
Defibrillate, 200–300 joules[b]
↓
Defibrillate with up to 360 joules[b]
↓
CPR if no pulse
↓
Establish IV access
↓
Epinephrine, 1:10,000, 0.5–1.0 mg IV push[c]
↓
Intubate if possible[d]
↓
Defibrillate with up to 360 joules[b]
↓
Lidocaine, 1 mg/kg IV push[e]
↓
Defibrillate with up to 360 joules[b]
↓
Bretylium, 5 mg/kg IV push[e]
(Consider bicarbonate)[f]
↓
Defibrillate with up to 360 joules[b]
↓
Bretylium, 10 mg/kg IV push[e]
↓
Defibrillate with up to 360 joules[b]
↓
Repeat lidocaine or bretylium
↓
Defibrillate with up to 360 joules[b]

Ventricular fibrillation (and pulseless ventricular tachycardia).[a] This sequence was developed to assist in teaching how to treat a broad range of patients with ventricular fibrillation (VF) or pulseless ventricular tachycardia (VT). Some patients may require care not specified herein. This algorithm should not be construed as prohibiting such flexibility. The flow of the algorithm presumes that VF is continuing. CPR = cardiopulmonary resuscitation.
[a]Pulseless VT should be treated identically to VF.
[b]Check pulse and rhythm after each shock. If VF recurs after transiently converting (rather than persists without ever converting), use whatever energy level has previously been successful for defibrillation.
[c]Epinephrine should be repeated every 5 minutes.
[d]Intubation is preferable. If it can be accomplished simultaneously with other techniques, then the earlier the better. However, defibrillation and epinephrine are more important initially if the patient can be ventilated without intubation.
[e]Some may prefer repeated doses of lidocaine, which may be given in 0.5-mg/kg boluses every 8 minutes to a total dose of 3 mg/kg.
[f]The value of sodium bicarbonate is questionable during cardiac arrest, and it is not recommended for routine cardiac arrest sequences. Consideration of its use in a dose of 1 mEq/kg is appropriate at this point. Half of the original dose may be repeated every 10 minutes if it is used.